Cochlear Implant Rehabilitation in Children and Adults

Cochlear Implant Rehabilitation in Children and Adults

Edited by
Dianne J. Allum, PhD
University Hospital of Basel

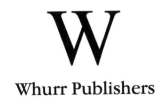

Whurr Publishers

© 1996 Whurr Publishers Ltd
First published 1996 by
Whurr Publishers Ltd
19b Compton Terrace, London N1 2UN, England

Reprinted 1998

British Library Cataloguing-in-Publication Data
A catalogue record for this book is available from the British Library.

ISBN 1-897635-54-0

Photoset by Stephen Cary
Printed and bound in the UK by Athenaeum Press Ltd, Gateshead, Tyne & Wear

Contents

List of Contributing Clinics

AUSTRIA
Vienna
Brigitte Eisenwort and Ulrike
Willinger
Allgemeines Krankenhaus der
Stadt Wien
Währinger Gürtel Straße 18-20
A-1090 Wien
Austria

Wolfgang Baumgartner and
Wolfgang Gstöttner
HNO-Universitätsklinik
Klinische Abteilung für
Phoniatrie-Logopädie
Alser Straße 4
1090 Wien
Austria

AUSTRALIA
Melbourne
Shani Dettman, Elizabeth Barker,
Gary Rance, Richard Dowell,
Karyn Galvin, Julia Sarant, Robert
Cowan, Marisa Skok, Rod Hollow,
Merran Larratt and Graeme Clark
Cochlear Implant Clinic
The Royal Victorian Eye and Ear
Hospital
32 Gisborne Street
Melbourne, Victoria 3002
Australia

FRANCE
Montpellier
Martine Sillon, Adrienne Vieu, Jean-
Pierre Piron, Reine Rougier,
Michel Broche, Françoise Artieres-
Reuillard, Michel Mondain and
Alain Uziel
Montpellier Cochlear Implant Center
Centre Hôpitalier Régional
Service ORL
Hôpital St.-Charles
300, rue A. Broussonet
34059 Montpellier
France

Paris
Claude Fugain, Michel Ouayoun,
Lucile Monneron and Claude-
Henri Chouard
Service d'ORL et de Chirurgie
Cervico-Faciale
Hôpital Saint-Antoine
184, rue du Faubourg Saint-Antoine
75012 Paris
France

GERMANY
Aachen
Helmut L. Neumann and Renate
Meixner
Audiologisches Zentrum Aachen
Vetschauer Straße 16-18
52072 Aachen
Germany

Hannover
Bodo Bertram
"Wilhelm Hirte" Cochlear Implant
Center (CIC)
Gehägestraße 28-30
30655 Hannover
Germany

Angelika Strauß-Schier and Ute Rost
Medizinische Hochschule Hannover
Zentrum HNO
Postfach 1 80
Konstanty-Gutschow-Straße 8
30625 Hannover
Germany

ITALY
Rome
Ersilia Bosco, Deborah Ballantyne
and Maria Teresa Argirò
IIIrd Clinico ORL
Università "La Sapienza"
Policlinico Umberto 1
Viale del Policlinico 155
00161 Rome
Italy

JAPAN
Tokyo
Masae Shiroma, Sotaro Funasaka,
Kumiko Yukawa and Shukuko
Kawanami
Department of Otorhinolaryngology
Tokyo Medical College
Office 6-7-1, Nishishinjuku
Shinjuku-ku, Tokyo, 160
Japan

RUSSIA
Moscow
George A. Tavartkiladze, Elsa V.
Mironova, Raisa A. Borovleva,
Inna A Belyantseva and Gregory I.
Frolenkov
Research Center for Audiology &
Hearing Rehabilitation
Bakuleva Street 18
Moscow 117513
Russia

SPAIN
Barcelona
Carmen Pujol and Teresa Amat
Clinica Claros
Los Vergos 31
08017 Barcelona
Spain

Pamplona
Alicia Huarte Irujo, Maite Molina and
Manuel Manrique
Clínica Universitaria Navarra
Facultad de Medicina
Universidad de Navarra
Apartado 4209
31080 Pamplona
Spain

SWEDEN
Stockholm
Göran Bredberg and Ewa Martony
Karolinska Institutet
Hörselkliniken
Södersjukhuset
118 83 Stockholm
Sweden

SWITZERLAND
Basel
Dianne J. Allum
Gehörlosen- und Sprachheilschule
Riehen
University Hospital of Basel
4031 Basel
Switzerland

John H. J. Allum
Abteilung für exp. Audiologie und
Neurootologie
HNO-Klinik
Kantonsspital Basel
4031 Basel
Switzerland

Riehen
Rene Müller
Gehörlosen- und Sprachheilschule
Riehen
Inzlingerstrasse 51
4125 Riehen
Switzerland

UNITED KINGDOM

Nottingham

Sue Archbold, Kevin P Gibbin,
  Barry McCormick and
  Gerard M O'Donoghue
Nottingham Paediatric Cochlear
  Implant Group
1st Floor Ropewalk House
113 The Ropewalk
Nottingham NG1 6HA
England

Southampton

Mark E Lutman
Human Science Group
The Institute of Sound and Vibration
  Research
University of Southampton
Highfields
Southampton SO17 1B5
England

UNITED STATES OF AMERICA

Baltimore

J. Robert Wyatt and John K. Niparko
The Johns Hopkins University
Department of Otolaryngology, Head
  & Neck Surgery
P.O. Box 41402
Baltimore, MD 21203-6402
USA

Iowa City

Linda Spencer and Shelley Witt
University of Iowa Hospitals & Clinics
Department of Otolaryngology
  Speech and Hearing
200 Hawkins Drive
Iowa City, Iowa 52242-1078
USA

New Jersey

Mary Ellen Nevins
Program for Hearing Impaired
Keen College
1000 Morris Avenue
Union, New Jersey
USA

New York

Patricia M. Chute and Simon C.
  Parisier
Cochlear Implant Center
Manhattan Eye, Ear and Throat
  Hospital
210 East 64th Street
New York, 10021
USA

St. Louis

Jean S. Moog, Ann E. Geers, Nancy
  Tye-Murray and Elizabeth Gilbert
  Bedia
Central Institute for the Deaf
909 South Taylor
St. Louis, Missouri 63110
USA

Preface

The idea behind producing a volume about international rehabilitation methods originated because of a respect I gained for the skills and insights of many clinicians I personally visited around the world. The challenge was to provide a forum in which their ideas could be represented in a common language so that they could reach beyond their own countries. It was a difficult task to select the representative clinics because there are so many highly qualified individuals concerned with the rehabilitative care of cochlear implant recipients. Included here are chapters from 17 different clinics representing four continents, 12 different countries and eight different languages. The aggregate number of patients seen by these teams totals more than 3800, or about one-fifth of the current implant users worldwide. Most of the major cochlear implant devices have been used for the rehabilitation of deafness by one or more of the authors.

A second purpose was to bring together rehabilitation concepts that described wide-based service programmes as well as specific training methods. Authors were asked to provide information that could be adapted, to some extent, for international use. This meant that some of the excellent, language-specific materials could not be preserved in their original form. The final outcome, however, has produced a text that can be used as a basis for developing cochlear implant programmes throughout the world. The careful reader will find details in each of the chapters that can be pieced together to create entirely new applications.

The final purpose of this book was to provide a means for dealing competently with cochlear implant patients in terms of training them to utilise their device in the most effective manner. It has only been during the last decade that clinicians have begun to address the issues associated with the rehabilitation of cochlear implant users, in particular children. This, then, is the first book concerned with rehabilitation after cochlear implantation that deals both with adults and children in a non-device-specific manner. The primary readers of this book will be those involved in the immediate training of cochlear implant users. It is of interest, however, to all professionals interested in the treatment of deafness and to families and support persons associated with the deaf individual. The ideas expressed in this book are timeless. Concepts included are those that can be generalised to the rehabilitation of all hearing-impaired individuals, not just those who have cochlear implants.

I would like to express my appreciation to the many colleagues who have contributed to this book. The effort to produce manuscripts in the English language was Herculean for some. The constraint to keep information only to that which could be adapted for international application was limiting and challenging for others. The collaborative effort has resulted in a book that will serve as a reference point for the rehabilitation of individuals with cochlear implants, no matter how the technology advances.

I want to thank András Szigeti and Wanda Brunetti for their excellent help in compiling and correcting all the manuscripts. I am grateful to Colin Whurr for his sympathetic support throughout the process of editing and producing this volume. Finally, I wish to thank my husband, John Allum, for his understanding during the many hours consumed by this project.

Dianne J. Allum-Mecklenburg
June, 1996
Basel, Switzerland

Introduction

The word 'habilitate' originates from the Latin *habilitare* meaning to enable. An original meaning of this word was 'to impart an ability or a capacity'. The goal of the cochlear implant (re)habilitationist, then, is to impart to the recipients of these devices the ability to use their electrically activated auditory sensations of hearing as an effective means through which communication can take place. The reader will notice, however, the omission of the word habilitation. We collapse the terms habilitation and rehabilitation. Habilitation usually refers to training of congenitally deaf children or prelingually deafened adults and children and the word rehabilitation is reserved for adults and shorter-term deafened children. In this text, however, the decision to use (re)habilitation, omitting the parentheses, was chosen to describe a method for re-establishing a communication mode whether it be from a gestural or signed language to a newly acquired spoken language communication mode or a retraining in the use of audition. It describes the rehabilitation of auditory-oral communication. One other feature in the writing style of this book is that major efforts have been made to avoid gender-specific references. We hope that the reader will accept the use of *he* when a general reference to a patient is meant.

Most rehabilitation programmes developed as an outgrowth of a medical model of care for patients who undergo a major surgery. The programmes required methods for careful selection, preoperative evaluations and postoperative management, as well as the surgical skills. Little was known about the amount of postoperative training needed to support the learning of novel listening skills. The challenge, at the time, was not about the type of rehabilitation but about how much rehabilitation training was needed. As would be expected in a medical model, the aim was to release the patient from hospital care as soon as possible. This was not possible with cochlear implant users because of the long-term, fine tuning needed to fit the speech processor. The hospitals and clinics had both the programming systems needed to adjust the processors and the skilled professionals involved in fitting and maintaining the external equipment. This meant that once a patient was in the hospital system, he would always return for rechecks and refitting. In the world of treatment for hearing impairment, this ongoing responsibility belonged to hearing aid dealers and audiologists. Thus, in terms of cochlear implant patient care, the need for a change in patient service was realised. Further, the clinical facility became involved with the social integration of its patients. The challenge was, and is, that an individual receiving an implant will have an active medical device that needs monitoring, care and possible upgrade for the rest of that person's life. Thus, a union between all health care professionals concerned with cochlear implant users has evolved through the years. The individuals who are in direct contact with cochlear implant users represent a truly multidisciplinary group with basic scientists, engineers, surgeons, teachers of the deaf, audiologists, speech therapists, psychologists and a variety of paediatric specialists working together. A recent enquiry found that only two courses on cochlear implants are offered at the postgraduate level in the United States, none in Europe, two in Australia and none in Asia. It took several years for cochlear implantation to become an accepted medical treatment for deafness, and many more for the field of cochlear implant rehabilitation to evolve. Fully active programmes have been around for less than 15 years, as of this writing.

All clinics concern themselves with preoperative selection procedures and evaluation of performance, as well as intraoperative monitoring, device programming, and postoperative testing and results. This is because cochlear implantation demands a holistic treatment plan for patients. The following chapters, however, focus attention on the practical orientation of providing aftercare training and support. Topics include counselling, expectations, preparatory response training techniques, educational integration and programmes, language training, psychological support, parent education and other methods that generally focus on adults, teenagers or young children. The programmes represented here describe themselves as providing rehabilitation within their clinic or both within and externally through outreach programmes. Programmes such as those described by teams in Nottingham, Iowa City, Manhattan, Basel, Paris and Hannover have a greater emphasis on acting as resource centres rather than as centres for auditory training. Other facilities with either localised populations (Moscow, Vienna, Tokyo, Rome, Barcelona) or direct cooperation with a school or rehabilitation centre (Montpellier, Melbourne) provide long-term training for auditory perception and spoken language. It should be pointed out that this division is artificial because there is no such thing as a rehabilitation programme that does not extend its services into the community or an outreach programme that does not include clinical therapy.

Some special issues are also discussed. Economic concerns regarding the provision of any health care service, especially long-term care, beg the question of whether or not cochlear implantation is a rational treatment in terms of its cost and its potential use. Cochlear implants require a surgical procedure and the accompanying expenses of hospital care and postoperative care are relatively high for the first few years after implantation. The subject has been investigated by Wyatt and Niparko who have calculated the cost and potential benefit to the American economy.

Another issue is how best to provide rehabilitation training in an environment that is hostile to a cultural emphasis on hearing. This topic is discussed in the chapter by the Swedish team who have needed to adapt their programme to meet the demands of a bilingual society: one that uses oral speech and another that does not. Monitoring changes that occur during implant use supports therapeutic methods, encourages families and helps to rationalise the effectiveness of cochlear implants. Teams from Nottingham, Montpellier, St Louis and Moscow describe a number of assessment tools, many of which can be adapted for international use, and indications that are helpful for setting goals and expectations.

The emphasis throughout the book is on the rehabilitation strategies and services that have evolved as a result of the large number of individuals requiring ongoing aftercare. The most significant feature that is revealed after a thorough reading is that there really are no therapies that are specific to cochlear implant users or directly related to a particular device. The training itself is an extension of many of the techniques that have been applied to hearing aid wearers. The major difference seems to be the inclusion of more materials that contain high-frequency information. Other differences exist in the expectations of the rehabilitationists.

The message of this book is that rehabilitation of cochlear implant users is a process rather than a series of training tasks. The amount and type of rehabilitation differ for children and adults and between those who have had auditory experience during their lives or not. A careful reading of each chapter will reveal at least one unique aspect about the rehabilitation process. The clinician looking for a variety of exercises will find them dispersed throughout the texts. Most of these are adaptable for different language. Thus, exercises described for a German patient are applicable to French-, Spanish-, English-speaking (and so forth) patients. All the chapters are self-contained so that readers can select from the many approaches described.

Communication is one of the major characteristics that separates man from other living entities on the planet. Cochlear implants directly influence communication style. There is no single technique that is superior to another and it is not possible to provide a clearly structured approach that will apply to all cochlear implant users. What we learn in the end is that rehabilitation is an art as well as a method that requires the skills of a motivated, informed and competent team of health care professionals.

Chapter 1
Basics of Cochlear Implant Systems

DIANNE J. ALLUM

Introduction

A cochlear implant device provides a unique opportunity for the rehabilitation of deaf individuals who are unable to utilise other assistive devices such as hearing aids or tactile devices for the purpose of understanding speech. Current implant systems offer useful auditory information about acoustic signals that occur naturally in the environment. This is accomplished by sending electrical impulses to different locations along the auditory nerve. Two basic principles are inherent in the idea of cochlear implants: first, foreign, biocompatible materials can be placed within the human body without being rejected (Shepherd, Franz & Clark, 1990); and, second, auditory nerve fibres respond to electrical stimulation (Luxford & Brackman, 1985).

Commercially obtainable cochlear implant systems became available in the 1980s. Until that time, they were investigational devices that had been developed by pioneers in the field of otology and engineering. In France, the first wearable unit was worn by a patient of Dr Charles Eyries in 1957. It was a simple, single-wire stimulating system that provided a sensation of sound to the user. The patient reported that it was even possible to understand some words through electrical stimulation. William House and Jack Urban received news of the possibility of providing auditory sensations to totally deaf individuals and began investigation into developing a multichannel electrode system in 1962 (House & Berliner, 1991). Their first efforts yielded interesting results, but the technology for multichannel implementation was not available in the 1960s.

They focused their attention on a single-channel, single-ball electrode device that transmitted information without significant need to analyse and transform the signal. Eventually, this system became the 3M/House device implanted in more than 200 patients. In the meantime, research

1

continued in Austria, France, Belgium and Australia (Parkins & Anderson, 1983) on the application of multichannel implants. The development of single- and multichannel systems moved hand in hand into the 1990s, each finding its use. The single-channel implants experienced successful use in terms of providing basic access to acoustic information with some patients able to make exceedingly successful use of the simple stimuli (Hochmair-Desoyer & Hochmair, 1996).

Multi-electrode, multichannel systems are highly dependent on the ability to apply sophisticated speech coding strategies and safety features. Thus, their development required advanced technologies of chip design, miniaturisation, battery consumption and other engineered capabilities. The favourable results obtained from multichannel implementations led to a broader acceptance of cochlear implants. At the time of this writing, more than 17 000 individuals, throughout the world, have received some type of cochlear implant device. As an implantable medical device, intra- and postsurgical complications are low (Hoffman & Cohen, 1995) and the postoperative outcomes for the perception of meaningful speech information are more than satisfactory (Clark & Cowan, 1995).

Normal cochlea

A brief overview of the important features of a normal cochlea is worthwhile. Sound waves enter the outer ear canal and travel to the tympanic membrane. Movement of the tympanic membrane sets the ossicles (malleus, incus, stapes) into motion. The stapes rests on the oval window leading to the fluid-filled cochlea. The pumping action of the stapes sets off a wave of motion within the fluid-filled cochlea. The cochlear hair cells, sitting relatively at rest, bend as the sound wave passes along the scala vestibuli. The hair cells have synaptic contacts to fibres of the auditory nerve. When a hair cell bends, it causes a chemical reaction in its cell body that is transformed into an electrical impulse that synapses with awaiting nerve fibres. The impulse activates the neural elements (spiral ganglion cells) within Rosenthal's canal, travels onward along the auditory nerve, up the brain stem and to the cortex.

The purpose of a cochlear implant is to provide a non-functioning peripheral auditory system (pathology at the level of the hair cells) with the possibility to perceive information about environmental sounds, speech and music in a way which is as physiologically natural as possible. This means that cochlear implant users, ideally, should be able to perceive sound through their remaining functional auditory pathway. Given that there is a pathological cochlea that no longer functions effectively, the logical procedure would be to bypass the cochlea and stimulate the auditory nerve directly. Indeed, this is how cochlear implants operate; they activate neurons that are located after the cochlear hair cells and their dendrites. Auditory signals then pass through the body's natural auditory system to the brain, where comprehension can take place.

Pathological cochlea

The primary criterion for cochlear implantation is a majority of missing or non-functioning cochlear hair cells. It means that information from the acoustic environment transmitted through a normal or near-normal middle ear and into the cochlea cannot be transduced into effective electrical signals that then travel along the auditory nerve. A breakdown of auditory information transmission can also occur at the level of the brain stem or the cortex. However, a cochlear implant is applicable only to *cochlear pathology*. If there is a non-functioning VIIIth nerve (acoustic nerve) or if there is other retrocochlear pathology (brain stem or cortical), a cochlear implant will not be of assistance in ameliorating the deafness. For a non-functioning cochlear nerve, new implants called 'brain stem implants' have been developed (Laszig et al., 1995). If the problem lies at the level of the cortex, little can be done in today's technology. Thus, we will discuss only the implications of cochlear pathology.

The types of deafness that have been associated with individuals receiving cochlear implants range from unknown, genetic or inherited pathology to unpredictable, accidental deafness due to trauma or infection. The severity of the pathology affects cochlear hair cell activity and/or cochlear nerve fibres and how they transmit information through the cochlea. Figure 1 schematically illustrates this point. The normal, cochlea is shown in Figure 1.1a. There is a full complement of spiral ganglion cells and neural fibres. A sound wave entering the cochlea will excite the neural fibres in a pattern similar to the incoming signal. Figure 1.1b shows the partially unrolled cochlea and open cochlea where pathology has reduced the number of hair cells, spiral ganglion cells and/or neural fibres. In such a case, the acoustic signal cannot pass to the awaiting fibres and little or no response pattern can be observed. If few or no hair cells are present, the mechanism for setting into action the necessary chemico-electrical changes cannot be produced. The link between the middle ear and the auditory nerve is broken. Sound is transmitted to the cochlea and a functioning auditory nerve awaits excitation, but no signal can pass between the two. Finally, Figure 1c shows the implanted cochlea. The electrodes electrically activate spiral ganglion cells and their nerve fibres to stimulate a pattern which represents the original acoustic signal. Note that the schematically represented, electrically elicited pattern is not as complete as that produced in a normal cochlea.

The reason that it is possible to transmit along the auditory pathway without placing electrodes directly on the auditory nerve is because of

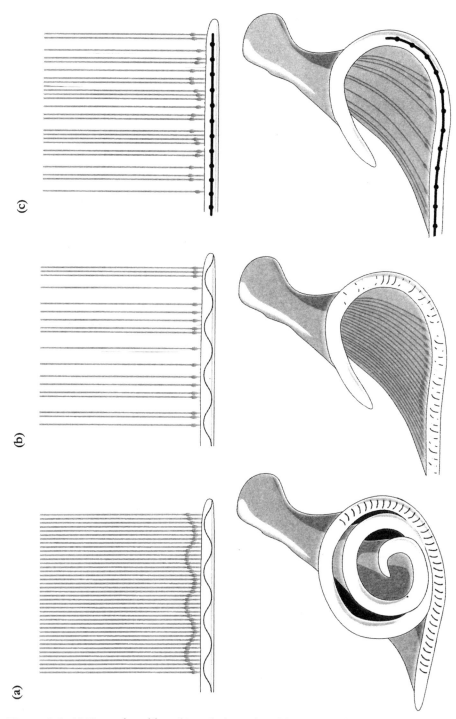

Figure 1.1: (a) Normal cochlea; (b) Pathological cochlea; (c) Implanted cochlea

electrolytic conduction within the cochlear scalae; that is, the fluid there is a good conductor of electricity. The scala tympani is a fluid-filled space close to the acoustic nerve. When electrical current is passed to an electrode which is sitting in the perilymph of the scala, the current spreads outward, activating spiral ganglion cells of frequency-specific regions of the acoustic nerve. There have been efforts to place stimulating electrodes directly in the auditory nerve (Simmons, 1966) but this proved more complicated and less reliable than placing electrode(s) within the scala tympani of the cochlea. Electrolytic conduction is also possible even in ossified or dry cochlea because there is always some interstitial fluid in the bony regions. The efficiency of the transmission, however, may be reduced and higher stimulating currents may be required to provide an auditory sensation to the cochlear implant user.

Fibres from the auditory nerve extend to the cochlea in a very orderly fashion. This is known as tonotopic order. The nerve fibres that transmit high-frequency information are located at the basal end of the cochlea nearest to the middle ear cavity. The fibres that transmit low-frequency information are located at the apical end of the cochlea. This predictable arrangement makes it possible to offer frequency-specific details of speech, or other acoustic signals, to the auditory nerve when placing transmitting electrodes within the scala tympani. The location of the electrodes along the scala helps to define the frequency information and the amount of current (microamperes) defines the amplitude. In psychoacoustic terminology, the pitch and loudness of a signal are thus provided to the acoustic nerve. Tonotopic organisation of the cochlea is very important for speech information. It can be likened to a series of frequency band filters lying along the cochlea. The spectral information associated with speech passes through these filters reuniting in the brain to form meaningful units of spoken language. The word tonotopic literally means place–pitch: tono = pitch and topic = place.

When there are remaining functional hair cells (known as residual hearing), a hearing aid can amplify the incoming sound and recruit (activate) a large number of neural fibres so that an auditory sensation can be perceived by the listener (see Figure 1.2). However, if too few hair cells remain within widespread regions of the cochlea, no amount of amplification will create a sensation of pitch in the regions of missing hair cells. Deaf individuals who depend on hearing aids possibly lack a wide tonotopic representation of pitch because they do not have enough hair cells located in different regions of the cochlea to represent different pitch percepts. Such hearing aid users may obtain some acoustic information but not enough to understand speech. They may be candidates for cochlear implants. The electrical signals transmitted through the implanted electrodes activate nerve fibres that begin the process of signal propagation along the VIIIth nerve leading to the brain stem and cortex.

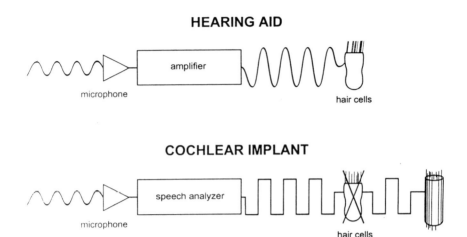

Figure 1.2: Schematic representation of the difference between a hearing aid and cochlear implant system. The hearing aid requires an adequate supply of hair cells to transfer signals to the auditory nerve. A cochlear implant bypasses the hair cells and stimulates the auditory nerve directly

Components of a cochlear implant system

The peripheral elements of the auditory system can be supplemented for deaf individuals by cochlear implants. There are common features of all implant systems (Mecklenburg, 1990a). There must be a pick-up microphone to receive acoustic signals from the external environment (Figure 1.3a). There must be a method for amplifying, analysing, coding and transmitting the signals (Figures 1.3b–c). Finally, there must be a means to receive the electrical signals produced by the speech processor, to decode them and to transmit them to the auditory nerve (Figures 1.3d–h).

External Components

A cochlear implant system derives its name from the actual implant. In fact, there are many components that are worn externally; these include a receiving microphone, connecting cables, a speech processor and a transmitting antenna. These external parts collect, analyse, code and transmit auditory information to the internally implanted parts which receive, decode and transmit the auditory information to the acoustic nerve. Some devices are capable of housing the speech processor in a

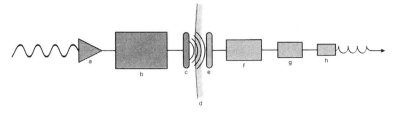

a mic b speech processor c transmitter coil d skin e receiver f stimulator g electrodes h hearing nerve

Figure 1.3: Schematic of a cochlear implant system

hearing aid-like processor that can be worn behind the ear. The auditory signals which have been gathered by the microphone (instead of the external ear) need to be amplified and partially filtered (middle ear function) and then analysed and coded in an appropriate manner for the auditory nerve to respond (inner ear function).

The speech processor is a sophisticated device that analyses sound in near real time. Sounds are filtered, amplitude is adjusted and signals are coded within the processor. Next, the coded signals are passed to a transmitting antenna. This is usually held in place by magnetic attraction to another magnet that is located under the skin so that signals pass across the skin via transcutaneous transmission. Up to this point, all of the equipment is external. A user of an implant device puts the microphone and antenna (usually known as a headset or headpiece) and the speech processor on and off each day. When this equipment is not being worn, the person is again unable to hear.

Internal Components

The implant itself holds the receiving antenna, electronics package, the electrode array and, perhaps, a lead with a ground electrode. The internal equipment is permanently placed under the skin in the mastoid bone behind the external ear with the electrodes usually passing into the scala tympani of the cochlea. Depending on the sophistication of the device, this small ceramic (Schindler & Kessler, 1989) or titanium package (Crosby et al., 1984) contains electronics that allow it to transmit the coded information received from the speech processor, either near-simultaneously (Schindler & Kessler, 1989) or very rapidly (Peeters et al., 1993; Hochmair-Desoyer & Hochmair, 1996) to one or more electrodes. The electrodes are often referred to as an electrode carrier or electrode array. Tiny wires from the electronics package are embedded in a biocompatible material to protect against body fluids. The electrodes are exposed balls, plates or rings at the end of the wires (Mecklenburg, 1990b).

Characteristics of multichannel cochlear implant systems

Factors that influence the effectiveness of cochlear implant systems are the number and location of activated electrodes, the method of current transmission, the stimulation rate and the speech coding strategy. Some characteristics of the five major cochlear implant systems are summarised in Table 1.1. It is worthwhile to understand differences between implant devices. A description of commonly used terminology is useful for this purpose.

Number of Implanted Electrodes

An electrode is merely a tiny piece of exposed metallic material, usually platinum in the case of intracochlear electrodes. An electrode can also be a metallic substance located outside the cochlea. Such electrodes are usually referred to as ground electrodes. The number of implanted electrodes in current multichannel systems varies between 15 and 24 (see Table 1.1). These electrodes may be referred to as electrode contacts.

Table 1.1: Overview of the five major companies providing cochlear implant systems in Europe. Note that Clarion and LAURA devices are also capable of implementing simultaneous compressed analogue strategies

CIS	MED-EL	CLARION	LAURA	MXM	NUCLEUS
Information	Full Spectrum	Full Spectrum	Full Spectrum	FFT	Maximal Peaks
RATE per ave.channel	Max 18,180 1,500	Max 6,667 833	Max 12,500 1,500	4,500 145–400, FO	Max 1,500 250
Actual Channels per stimulation cycle	12 monopolar	8 mono-/ bipolar	8 mono-/ bipolar	15 com. ground	3–10: ave 6 bipolar, com. ground
Electrode contacts	24+ground	16+ground	16+ground	15+ground	22
Electrode spacing	2.6 mm	2.0 mm	2.05 mm	0.70 mm	0.75 mm
Telemetry	Yes	Yes	Yes	No	No
CIS strategy	Yes	Adapted	Adapted	No	No
Stored programs	3	3	1	2	1

Update information. It was reported that the Nucleus C124M is capable of providing a CIS strategy which is specified to stimulate at a maximum overall rate of ca. 15,000 pps on 12 channels. The implant has telemetry capability and adds a monopolar configuration. The associated speech processor has a capacity for 4 stored programs.

Electrode Spacing

The distance between two adjacent electrodes is the electrode spacing. Some electrodes may be located very near each other while others may be widely spaced. Spacing can vary from as close as 0.5 mm apart (Clarion) to 2.8 mm (Med-El: eight-channel).

Electrode Array

The carrier for the electrodes may be described as the electrode array. It consists of the wires that extend from the electronics package to the exposed electrodes plus the biocompatible material covering the wires. The proximal part of the electrode array is the portion that extends between the end of the inserted array and the body of the electronics package. Fixation of the electrode array is applied to the proximal electrode array with cement or suture during a cochlear implant operation. It is also referred to as the redundant electrode array.

Electrode Array Extent

The distance between the first electrode and the last electrode is the array extent. In most cases, however, insertion depth is described by the total length of the inserted electrode array into the cochlea which is *ca* 32–35 mm long (Denes & Pinson, 1993). This includes the portion on the array where no active electrodes are located. For instance, the Nucleus system has 22 electrodes, each 0.75 mm apart. This results in an electrode extent of 16.5 mm, a distance of 17 mm for total insertion of the 22 electrodes and a total insertion depth of 25 mm when its 10, non-active stiffening rings are included. The length of the cochlea that can be electrically stimulated, then, is approximately 16.5 mm. The Clarion has pairs of electrodes located 2 mm apart, where each member of the pair is separated by 0.5mm. Thus, eight pairs of electrodes have an extent of 14 mm (7 [separations] x 2 mm). The total insertion depth may be as great as 25 mm for the Clarion. To date, the longest insertion depth (30 mm) and electrode extent (26 mm) are associated with the Med-El 12-channel array.

Active/Inactive Electrodes

An electrode is active when it has an assigned threshold and comfortable level (MCL) and is programmed to transmit current. It is possible for an electrode to have a defined threshold and comfort level without being active; that is, the electrode selected to transmit current. It is called an inactive electrode. There are several reasons why a clinician might choose to deactivate an electrode.

Channels (Active)

Channels describe the number of electrodes that transmit current within a set frame of reference, which is usually time (i.e. 1 millisecond) or a full pass of all electrodes, as in CIS. Depending on the characteristics of the signal, active channels within a stimulation cycle range from an average of six for Nucleus up to 15 for MXM. This means that anywhere from three electrodes to 15 electrodes will transmit an electrical impulse within a given stimulation cycle (see Table 1.1).

Stimulation Cycle

A series of electrodes is stimulated within a particular cycle. The devices that implement CIS usually have a cycle which is dependent upon the pulse width (pulse duration) of the signals transmitted through the implant, if there is not an adjustable time gap between the pulses. For these systems, when the pulse width is increased the stimulation rate per channel decreases. A cycle may also be limited by a maximum time.

Sampling Rate

Generally, this can be described as the number of points (or amplitudes) measured digitally at a particular frequency for any input signal received through the microphone. The higher the sampling rate, the better the digital output of the speech processor. An excellent reference to explain this principle is provided by Rosen and Howell (1989). Essentially, the faster the sampling rate, the more representative the reconstructed (or decoded) signal. One could imagine this as a connect-the-dots game. The more dots (sampled points), the easier it is to recognise the picture. The fewer the dots, the more possibility exists to misinterpret, or poorly indicate, the picture represented by the dots.

Stimulation Rate (per Channel and Overall)

The number of times electrodes transmit a pulse during one second is referred to as stimulation rate and is written as pps (pulses per second). Pulses are usually biphasic. This means that a particular polarity of pulse (positive or negative) is immediately followed by a pulse of the opposite polarity. Biphasic pulses are implemented in most cochlear implant systems in order to avoid excess DC (direct current) charge, which can be harmful to neural tissue. Therefore, most implant systems describe the use of biphasic, charge-balanced pulses. The method used by MXM differs. It stimulates with a monophasic pulse which is passed through a capacitor. Capacitive coupling protects against unwanted DC charge effects.

The overall stimulation rate is the aggregate number of pulses occurring for all the electrodes within a second. Most CIS systems use an overall stimulation rate which is constant. This suggests that if only one electrode were chosen, the overall stimulation rate and the rate per channel could be the same: that is, it is the maximum number of pulses that can be delivered through the implant system in a second. When the overall stimulation rate and the number of active channels per cycle are known, it is usually possible to determine the stimulation rate per channel. This is calculated by dividing the overall rate by the number of channels. An eight-channel system with an overall biphasic rate of 12 000 would yield a rate per channel of 1500 (12 000 divided by 8). However, if there were only seven channels activated, the rate would be 1714 per channel: for six channels the rate would be 2000, and so forth. This differs for SPEAK (Seligman and McDermott, 1995), which has an average stimulation of 250 pps and the standard coded strategy implementation by MXM (Beliaeff et al., 1993), which has a stimulation rate that varies with the fundamental frequency of the input signal.

Table 1.2 Summary of external and internal components of a cochlear implant system

External	
receiving microphone	directional, omnidirectional, mono/binaural (Nucleus) input, sensitivity control (Med-El)
cables	microphone-to-speech processor microphone-to-coil
transmitting antenna	with/without magnet (usually adjustable) variable magnet strengths available (Note: the Clarion headpiece has an integrated microphone and antenna)
speech processor	on/off switch, volume control, sensitivity control, program switch (memory slots), indicator LEDs, external-input jack, alarm signal, battery compartment
Internal	
receiving antenna	outside or inside the electronics package single or multiple-wound coil
electronics package	titanium or ceramic
multichannel electrode array	straight or preformed, short or long
ground electrodes	separate lead or located on electronics package

Frequency Boundaries

The frequency band width related to any particular electrode is described as the upper and lower frequency boundary. Implant systems using CIS describe overall frequency ranges between 300 and 5500 Hz. The MXM system has a range from 100 to 7800 and the Nucleus system reports a range from 180 to 10 000 Hz. A wide overall frequency range may be a factor influencing effective access to speech information (Lawson et al., 1995). In the most simplistic view, the frequency range for a particular electrode can be estimated for a linear assignment by dividing the frequency range (5500 minus 300 = 5200) by the number of channels, i.e. eight (5200 divided by 8 = 650). A six-channel system would have a band width per channel of approximately 867 Hz. Regardless of the number of channels, the full frequency range is always analysed in the speech processor. Note that band widths are usually assigned logarithmically, although it is also possible to combine linear and logarithmic assignments.

Stimulation Mode

The mode of stimulation usually refers to the way in which electrodes are referenced to each other, or coupled, for the purpose of directing the flow of current. Three modes of stimulation exist in present implant systems: bipolar, monopolar and common ground. Electrodes which are linked to each other as bipolar pairs mean that one electrode acts as the active electrode and the other serves as the return, or ground. In cochlear implant terminology, bipolar electrodes are always located within the cochlea. Bipolar pairs can be composed of electrodes that are immediately next to each other or can be more widely spaced. Monopolar describes stimulation between an active electrode located within the cochlea and a remote electrode located somewhere outside the cochlea. It can either be a free electrode or a strip of metal located on or near the electronics package. Common ground is a term specifically applied to the Nucleus and MXM systems and describes a technique used to activate one electrode against all other implanted electrodes, which are momentarily connected together to serve as a single (common) ground. This has also been labelled pseudo-monopolar (Parkins & Houde, 1982).

Speech coding strategies

A brief overview is provided here for analogue and pulsatile (Feature Extraction, SPEAK, CIS and HR-SB) strategies. The interested reader is referred to more detailed descriptions for most of the strategies (Eddingdon, 1983; Crosby et al., 1984; Schindler & Kessler, 1989; Patrick et al., 1990; McKay et al., 1991; Tyler & Tye-Murray, 1991; Beliaeff et al., 1993; Peeters et al., 1993; Wilson, 1993; Seligman & McDermott, 1995; Hochmair-Desoyer & Hochmair, 1996).

Analogue Strategies

The principle underlying analogue strategies is to transmit acoustic information without selective filtering of the incoming signal. A significant criterion is the capability of the implant system to activate a number of electrodes simultaneously (Eddington, 1983; Schindler & Kessler, 1989; Patrick et al., 1990; Peeters et al., 1993). A series of bandpass filters covers the full spectrum of speech and details from each of the filters are always transmitted, i.e. not selected as in feature extraction strategies. A segment of speech passes through each filter band which is associated with a particular electrode. Depending on frequencies present in a particular speech segment, the associated electrodes will be activated at a particular amplitude. In a digital implementation of an analogue strategy, as in the Clarion, the amplitudes within each band are updated rapidly and simultaneously for all active electrodes. This type of coding requires significant power demands from the implant because of the simultaneity. The maximum number of channels stimulated for an analogue strategy is eight (Clarion).

Feature Extraction Strategies

The principle is to provide selected information with emphasis on elements of a signal that relate specifically to speech. An essential feature of speech is the fundamental frequency (F0), which provides significant suprasegmental details. Other features revolve around formant information for vowels such as the first formant (F1) and the second formant (F2), and higher frequency elements that support the perception of consonants. Each of these features is associated with specific frequencies (Peterson & Barney, 1952); for instance, the fundamental frequency is the lowest frequency (mean of 135 Hz for male speakers, 235 Hz for female speakers and 375 Hz for children). The first formant will range between 270 and 1000 Hz and the second formant from *ca*. 1000 Hz to as high as *ca*. 3200 Hz. This means that it is possible to emphasise these features simply through filtering. Bandpass filters sort (analyse) the incoming signals for the defined frequencies and then transmit them to related electrodes. The maximum number of channels stimulated per cycle in the Nucleus versions of feature extraction is four, and electrodes stimulate non-simultaneously.

SPEAK Coding

Electrodes are activated depending on which filters receive information that is greater than a certain defined amplitude (McKay et al., 1991; Tyler & Tye-Murray, 1993; Wilson, 1993). This means that a signal within a certain bandwidth must have an intensity great enough to be recognised. Three to 10 highest amplitudes are selected and corresponding electrodes are instructed to stimulate. The principle is called maximal spectral peak detection. The particular implementation is also dependent on the threshold and comfort levels of a specific patient because as stimulus units increase the pulse width (duration) is increased. Generally, for the Nucleus system, the number of channels to be selected will be influenced by the intensity of the incoming signal and the defined output at the electrodes. If an input signal is soft, fewer frequencies will be detected in the filter bands (fewer peaks that reach a maximal level) and, thus, fewer channels/electrodes will be selected for stimulation. Another factor is the influence of intensity. The louder a signal must be for the implant user to hear a soft sound and to listen at a comfortable level (the programmed values), the fewer number of channels will stimulate. This occurs for high levels of stimulation because they require wide pulse widths for the Nucleus device, where a stimulation cycle is defined by time. Fewer active electrodes will be chosen for stimulation when pulse durations are longer. A final characteristic of SPEAK is that several channels will usually be activated where electrodes are located immediately next to each other. This is because maximum energy usually occurs across closely related frequencies. Channels of stimulation vary for the SPEAK strategy between three and ten with an average of six, and electrodes stimulate non-simultaneously at an average stimulation rate of 250 Hz.

CIS (Continuous Interleaved Sampler)

The main principle of CIS is always to stimulate all active electrodes for each cycle but non-simultaneously (Wilson, 1993). It differs from feature extraction and SPEAK in this respect because these two strategies select electrodes for stimulation (channels) from a number of active electrodes. It differs from analogue strategies because it is non-simultaneous. A second principle is related to speed. The CIS strategies stimulate electrodes at very rapid rates, as fast as 2500 pps in laboratory implementations (Wilson et al., 1991). The maximum number of channels stimulated for a commercial CIS strategy is 12 per cycle with an overall rate of 18180 pps (Med-E1). Simultaneous and overlapping CIS strategies are alternative coding methods investigated for the Clarion device (Loeb, 1995).

High-Rate/Selective Band (HR-SB)

This new strategy may be referred to by different names, but for the purpose of this chapter it describes using the selective channels employed by analogue and SPEAK strategies combined with the underlying principle of high-rate stimulation of CIS strategies (Lawson et al., 1995). The two major requirements for this strategy's implementation are, first, there should be a larger number of electrodes available for activation than the number that will be stimulated in a particular cycle and, second, that stimulation rate be rapid. Channel selection is similar to that used for pitch-extracted sampler (Dillier, Boegli & Spillman, 1993) and is similar to analysing the maximum spectral energy within a particular bandwidth. Stimulation rate can be *ca*. 800 pps per channel or faster. Another characteristic may be that each channel stimulates at a different, optimised rate. This strategy chooses a selective set of channels to be activated non-simultaneously and stimulates at a fast rate during each stimulation cycle (Wilson, 1996).

Psychophysical characteristics associated with cochlear implants

The psychophysical results obtained from a cochlear implant user supply the information that defines the individualised speech processor programs regardless of strategy. They are usually obtained and/or described behaviourally by the patient during the fitting procedures (Roberts, 1991). In some cases, it is possible to define some of the parameters objectively (Abbas & Brown, 1991; Spivak & Chute, 1994; Battmer, Gnadeberg & Allum-Mecklenburg, 1995). The parameters may directly affect rehabilitation outcomes and should be well understood by cochlear implant specialists.

Threshold

The definition of threshold in audiometric terms is the softest point at which an individual can identify a signal 50% (Delk, 1973). This varies slightly for cochlear implants. Some devices require that the patient be able to identify the softest signal 100% of the time (Feature Extraction and SPEAK) but CIS strategies are similar to audiometric threshold, or even softer. Depending on the strategy, threshold may be defined as current output (microamperes or dB), charge (microcoulombs) or stimulus levels (a function of pulse duration and amplitude).

Comfortable Listening Level

The description of a comfortable listening level usually refers to a maximum comfortable listening (MCL) level which means that the signal is as loud as an individual would want to listen to over a long period of time. Depending on the strategy, comfortable listening level may be defined as current output (microamperes or dB), charge (microcoulombs) or stimulus levels (a function of pulse duration and amplitude).

Dynamic Range

The difference between the maximum comfortable listening level and the threshold is the dynamic range. These ranges may vary slightly from electrode to adjacent electrode. Acoustically, dynamic range is between the uncomfortable listening level (UCL) and the threshold: however, UCL is not a usable level for cochlear implant programs. Dynamic range, then, refers to the usable range of hearing available through the implant.

Pitch Perception

The ability to distinguish different pitch at different electrode sites or for different rates of stimulation is pitch perception. The former is called place-pitch perception and the latter is referred to as rate-pitch discrimination. The major effect is obtained by changing place of stimulation to take advantage of tonotopic representations of frequency (Wilson, 1996).

Loudness Perception

The ability to detect differences in charge per phase (pulse duration x amplitude) is loudness perception. Low charge is perceived as a soft sound and greater charge is perceived as a louder sound. An increase in pulse width (duration) and/or current usually results in the cochlear implant user detecting a louder sound.

Loudness Growth

This is the rate/slope at which differences in loudness occur. A rapid/steep loudness growth indicates a small dynamic range. For instance, if the loudness between comfortable and uncomfortable is very small, it is described as having a very steep loudness growth. Conversely, a slow loudness growth relates to a wide dynamic range. It is possible for a cochlear implant user to have a slow loudness growth for soft-to-medium sounds and a rapid loudness growth for more intense sounds. It is also possible to observe a slow, or lack of, loudness growth at high levels of stimulation. This is usually a function of the output of a particular electrode (compliance voltage) rather than a function of the cochlear implant user's auditory system. Slow loudness growth at threshold levels is also possible (Allum & Mortlock, 1993).

Implications of speech processor parameters on rehabilitation

Thresholds

Inappropriately set thresholds for CIS strategies can result in a continuous low buzzing sound or low-level background noise that is always present when the speech processor is turned on. Thresholds that are set too low or high alter the effective dynamic range for speech if there is a true comfortable level. It is possible that thresholds can be set incorrectly for some electrodes and not for others. This may affect the loudness growth function on each electrode because the dynamic ranges differ. In such a case, depending on the amount of variance between the channels, speech may sound distorted. Invalid thresholds may also result in poor postoperative, sound-field audiometric levels so that it appears that speech is received at very high levels during sound-field testing. The clinician should take care with such interpretations, however, because sound-field results will vary for different implant systems depending on whether they stimulate simultaneously or not and how rapid the stimulation rate is per channel. Settings for threshold are relatively easy to obtain because they are a simple estimation of the presence of 'something versus nothing'.

Comfortable Levels

Most pulsatile cochlear implant systems attempt to stimulate at levels near the comfortable level because that should provide the most useful levels for receiving easily audible sounds. If the comfortable levels vary significantly from channel to channel, then speech is reported to sound uneven or choppy. Unfortunately, comfort levels are the most difficult setting to determine both for adults and children. The problem exists because loudness judgements are subjective and the person listening must voluntarily decide whether or not a particular sound is 'comfortable'. For some deaf listeners, the desire to hear overrides the decision to choose a comfortable listening level because they inherently believe that 'more is better'. They allow settings to be inappropriately high. For other deaf listeners, the increase in loudness is stressful because they do not understand what it feels like to hear a signal that is too loud. Adults with this worry may choose settings that are too low. In very young children, the ability to indicate a comfortably loud level simply does not exist because any listener must first learn how to make comparisons before the possibility to choose between different alternatives exists. These children may only have the possibility to react to sound. The result can be rather distressing because the child does not realise, or indicate, that a sound is loud until it is very apparent. That is, the sound suddenly is too loud and the child may respond with an aversion response (removing the headset, crying, becoming angry or aggressive, refusing to cooperate for further testing, etc.). The same circumstance exists for hearing aid fittings, as well. It is possible for clinicians to devise methods for children that allow even very young listeners to express relative loudness through play. Intraoperative (Battmer, Gnadeberg & Allum-Mecklenburg, 1995) and postoperative (Spivak & Chute, 1994) objective stapedius thresholds are an aid to estimating comfort levels.

Dynamic Ranges

Dynamic ranges should be relatively similar across any series of channels. This suggests that thresholds and comfortable levels are also similar across all channels. It is not necessarily the case because the dynamic ranges, although relatively constant across channels, may be at different intensity ranges. An example is a threshold of 8 dB and comfortable level of 20 dB for one electrode and a threshold of 20 dB and comfortable level of 32 dB for another. The dynamic ranges for the two electrodes are equal, but the threshold and comfortable levels are not. The dynamic range, depending on the way in which the speech coding strategy maps loudness, will relate to the loudness growth and thus how sounds are perceived for different input levels. If the loudness growth function varies too greatly across channels, the listener may have an inability to distinguish loudness changes for soft sounds or for loud sounds. The loudness imbalance may be reported as rough or uneven quality of speech; sometimes even as a popping sound, if the dynamic ranges vary greatly from electrode to electrode. A challenge to clinicians and therapists is to find ways to balance (equalise) loudness percepts on neighbouring electrodes and across the array, because pitch influences loudness perception. Usually, the higher the pitch, the louder the percept. Testing electrodes that elicit different pitch sensations may confuse the listener about relative loudness.

Pitch Perception

Discriminating pitch differences is one of the more important abilities needed for deaf individuals to learn speech understanding. Spoken language is composed of sound images of different frequencies and intensities. If we use an analogy of the ability to distinguish between two neighbouring piano keys and two piano notes played in differnt octaves, it may be easier to imagine the brain's ability to distinguish between closely spaced electrodes and those slightly further apart. More widely spaced active electrodes provide a basis for better distinguishable channels (Blamey, Parisi & Clark, 1995; Wilson, 1996). The further apart the electrodes (or channels) are spread out on the electrode array, the easier it is for the listener to identify them as being different. The enhancement of pitch differentiation is also available in some systems with adjustable bandpass filters (Aronson & Arauz, 1995).

Other Programmable Parameters

Variables that can be adjusted during fitting differ between systems and some devices offer more than others. With the exception of the above-mentioned parameters, the following can be changed: the order of electrode stimulation (sequential or staggered), smoothing cut-off filter, automatic channel selection, noise suppression, input dynamic range, compression, rectification, mode, pulse width, active electrode status, pulse polarity, pulse rate per channel, time between biphasic pulses and more. Many of these have been discussed in this chapter but others are beyond the scope of this discussion because they are either rarely altered from a default setting, require a thorough understanding of the effects of discrete changes or are used mainly for the purposes of research. The future flexibility and applicability of these parameters may yield even more natural quality for cochlear implant users as well as more effective implementation of speech coding strategies.

Summary

The accuracy of threshold and comfort listening levels, equivalency of dynamic ranges across electrodes and optimum channel selection are the most significant behaviourally influenced measurements that specifically relate to performance.

Conclusion

Cochlear implants represent a relatively new technology that is useful in providing auditory signals to individuals who do not have access to speech information because of auditory deficits. Their use requires an understanding of the characteristics and programmable features that make individualised and optimal fittings possible. The rehabilitationist who is well aware of these characteristics will be able to work more closely with the specialist who fits the speech processor. It will also be possible to generalise from the performance of cochlear implant users about the parameters that might need adjusting for more successful implant use. The most effective application of cochlear implants results from strong cooperation between all professionals working together with the implant user to offer the best opportunity for achieving speech understanding and improved auditory/oral communication.

References

Abbas PJ, Brown CJ (1991) Electrically-elicited auditory brain stem responses: growth of responses with current level. Hearing Research 51: 123–38.

Allum DJ, Mortlock A (1993) Interactive software for setting cochlear implants in children. Advances in Otology, Rhinology and Laryngology 48: 191–98.

Aronson L, Arauz SL (1995) Fitting the Nucleus-22 cochlear implant for Spanish speakers. Annals of Otology, Rhinology and Laryngology 104 (Suppl. 166): 75–76.

Battmer R-D, Gnadeberg D, Allum-Mecklenburg D (1995) Algorithmic representation of common ground programming in children with the Nucleus device. Advances in Otology, Rhinology and Laryngology 50: 83–90.

Beliaeff M, Dubus P, Leveau J-M, Repetto J-C, Vincent P (1993) Sound signal processing and stimulation coding of the Digisonic DX10 15-channel cochlear implant. In Hochmair-Desoyer IJ, Hochmair ES (Eds) Advances in Cochlear Implants. Innsbruck: Manz, pp 198–203.

Blamey PJ, Parisi ES, Clark GM (1995) Pitch matching of electric and acoustic stimuli. Annals of Otology, Rhinology and Laryngology 104 (Suppl. 166): 220–22.

Clark GM, Cowan RSC (1995) International Cochlear Implant Speech and Hearing Symposium – Melbourne 1994. Annals of Otology, Rhinology & Laryngology 104 (Suppl. 166).

Crosby PA, Seligman PM, Patrick JF, Kuzma JA, Money DK, Ridler J, Dowell RC (1984) The Nucleus multi-channel hearing prosthesis. Acta Otolarygologica (Stockh) (Suppl.) 411: 111–14.

Delk JH (1973) A comprehensive dictionary of audiology. Hearing Aid Journal 1: 151.

Denes PE, Pinson EN (1993) The Speech Chain: The Physics and Biology of Spoken Language. New York: WH Freeman, p 85.

Dillier N, Boegli, Spillmann T (1993) Speech encoding strategies for multielectrode cochlear implants: a digital signal processor approach. Progress in Brain Research 97: 301–11.

Eddington DK (1983) Speech recognition in deaf subjects with multichannel intracochlear electrodes. Annals of the New York Academy of Science 405: 241–58.

Hochmair-Desoyer I, Hochmair E (1996) Implementation of coding strategies in cochlear implant systems and comparative results. Central East European Journal of Otology, Rhinology, Laryngology, Head & Neck Surgery 1(1): 33–41.

Hoffman RA, Cohen NL (1995) Complications of cochlear implant surgery. Annals of Otology, Rhinology & Laryngology 104 (Suppl. 166): 420–22.

House W, Berliner K (1991) Cochlear implants: from idea to clinical practice. In Cooper H (Ed) Cochlear Implants: A Practical Guide. London: Whurr.

Laszig R, Sollmann WP, Marangos N, Charachon R, Ramsden R (1995) Nucleus 20-channel and 21-channel auditory brain stem implants: first European experiences. Annals of Otology, Rhinology and Laryngology 104 (Suppl. 166): 28–33.

Lawson DT, Wilson BS, Zerbi M, Finley CC (1995) Speech processors for auditory prostheses. First Quarterly Progress Report, NIH Contract N01-DC-5-2103.

Loeb GE (1995) Flexible continuous interleaved sampling (FCIS): A new era for MultiStrategy Clarion Research. Paper presented at the Third International Congress on Cochlear Implant, Paris, 27–29 April, Abstract No. 157.

Luxford WM, Brackman DE (1985) The history of cochlear implants. In Gray R (Ed) Cochlear Implants. San Diego, CA: College Hill Press, pp 1–26.

McKay C, McDermott H, Vandali A, Clark G (1991) Preliminary results with a six spectral maxima sound processor for the University of Melbourne/Nucleus multiple-electrode cochlear implant. Journal of the Otolaryngology Society of Australia 6: 354–59.

Mecklenburg DJ (1990a) Cochlear implants and rehabilitative practices. In Sandlin R (Ed) Handbook of Hearing Aid Amplification, Vol II. Boston: College Hill Press, pp 179-88.

Mecklenburg DJ (1990b) In Sandlin RE (Ed) Handbook of Hearing Aid Amplification, Vol I. Theoretical and Technical Considerations. Boston: College Hill Press, pp 180–83.

Parkins CW, Anderson SW (1983) Cochlear Prostheses: An International Symposium. Annals of the New York Academy of Science 405.

Parkins CW, Houde RA (1982) The cochlear (implant) prosthesis: theoretical and practical considerations. In Sims DG, Walter GG, Whitehead RL (Eds) Deafness

practical considerations. In Sims DG, Walter GG, Whitehead RL (Eds) Deafness and Communication. Baltimore: Williams & Wilkins, pp 332–56.

Patrick JF, Seligman PM, Money DK, Kuzma JA (1990) Engineering. In Clark GM, Tong YT, Patrick JF (Eds) Cochlear Prosthesis. Melbourne: Churchill Livingstone, pp 102–08.

Peeters S, Offeciers E, Kinsbergen J, van Durme M, van Enis P, Dijkmans P, Bouchataoui I (1993) A digital speech processor and various speech encoding strategies for cochlear implants. Progress in Brain Research 97:283–89.

Peterson GE, Barney HL (1952) Control methods for a study of the vowels. JASA 24: 175–84.

Roberts S (1991) Speech-processor fitting for cochlear implants. In Cooper H (Ed) Cochlear Implants. London: Whurr, pp 201–18.

Rosen S, Howell P (1989) Signals and Systems for Speech and Hearing. New York: Academic Press.

Schindler RA, Kessler DK (1989) State of the art of cochlear implants: the UCSF experience. American Journal of Otology 8: 79–83.

Seligman P, McDermott H (1995) Architecture of the Spectra 22 speech processor. Annals of Otology, Rhinology and Laryngology 104 (Suppl. 166): 139–41.

Shepherd RK, Franz B, Clark GM (1990) The biocompatibility and safety of cochlear prostheses. In Clark GM, Tong YT, Patrick JF (Eds) Cochlear Prosthesis. Melbourne: Churchill Livingstone, pp 69–98.

Simmons FB (1966) Stimulation of the acoustic nerve as a treatment for profound sensorineural deafness in man. Archives of Otolaryngology 84: 2–54.

Spivak LG, Chute PM (1994) The relationship between electrical acoustic reflex threshold and behavioral comfort levels in children and adult cochlear implant patients. Ear and Hearing 15(2): 184–92.

Tyler R and Tye-Murray N (1991) Cochlear implant signal-processing strategies and patient perception of speech and environmental sounds. In Cooper H (Ed) Cochlear Implants. London: Whurr, pp 58–67.

Wilson BS (1993) Signal processing. In Tyler RS (Ed) Cochlear Implants. London: Whurr, pp 35–85.

Wilson B (1996) Strategies for representing speech information with implants. Paper presented at the Sixth Symposium on Cochlear Implants in Miami, FL, 2–3 February.

Wilson BS, Lawson DT, Finley CC, Wolford RD (1991) Coding strategies for multi-channel cochlear prosthesis. Annals of Otology, Rhinology and Laryngology 12 (Suppl.): 56–61.

Chapter 2
Evaluation of the Benefit of the Multichannel Cochlear Implant in Children in Relation to its Cost

J. ROBERT WYATT AND JOHN K. NIPARKO

Introduction

The cochlear implant is a medical intervention applied to both adults and children diagnosed with severe-to-profound deafness. Candidates for the implant do not gain practical benefit from alternative listening devices such as tactile devices (Phonator, Tactaid) or high-powered hearing aids. Benefit is defined as providing useful information for the understanding of speech. Although understanding speech is the most critical outcome, a full assessment of benefit is likely to require an evaluation of other life attributes in addition to sensory function.

Recent trends in clinical research (Gafni & Birch, 1993) have increasingly emphasised the importance of assessing the impact of a medical intervention (treatment) on an individual's day-to-day life. Termed 'outcomes research', these studies survey an intervention's performance in real life, when implemented by many professionals on broad populations of individuals (Feeny & Torrance, 1989). There are several facets of an outcome that might be considered and then compared with a baseline. For example, pre-implant status may be compared with post-implant status. Comparisons can also be made with other conventionally used alternative treatments, or even comparable treatments that may have similar costs (Drummond & Maynard, 1993). The most practical method is to assess the outcome with respect to the costs associated with the care, rehabilitation and maintenance for a particular treatment.

Outcomes research as applied to cost-effectiveness

The effectiveness of an intervention may be evaluated in the context of its cost in several ways. The methods differ in the manner in which outcomes are valued. In cost-benefit analysis, outcomes are valued in financial terms. Specifically, this means that the benefit usually relates to the amount of money that will be saved for health care in the future. In cost-effectiveness analysis, outcomes are valued in terms of a specific or general health care outcome. Cost-utility analysis is a form of cost-effectiveness analysis that rates outcome in terms of generic changes in life expectancy *and* quality of life. Although treatments for hearing rehabilitation have little impact on longevity, they do result in improved sensory function and enhanced communication (Cohen, Waltzman & Fisher, 1993; Miyamoto et al., 1992; Osberger, Maso & Sam, 1993). These two factors alone can presumably produce a change in quality of life. For this reason, cost utility provides the most appropriate measure of hearing rehabilitation.

A standard unit of measure of cost-effectiveness in performing a cost-utility assessment is the quality adjusted life year (QALY). A QALY yields a measure of benefit provided by an intervention. This measure relates to gains in overall health. The cost per QALY represents the value of a particular intervention in terms of its economic impact on society, as well as on the individual. The duration of quality-of-life effects is also incorporated in the QALY measure. Substantial improvement in the quality of life resulting from an intervention dramatically decreases the assumed cost per QALY. A further use of the QALY is for comparisons between different interventions (treatments). This is because each QALY, regardless of treatment, incorporates the generic changes in life expectancy and quality of life that result from an intervention. Thus, one treatment's cost per QALY is comparable to another's cost per QALY because they consider similar factors. The lower the cost per QALY, or the greater the number of QALYs obtained at a given cost, the greater the cost-effectiveness of an intervention.

Cost utility of the cochlear implant in adults

Studies of the cost utility of the cochlear implant in postlingual adults are now available. Several studies have used a multi-attribute utility index to model the quality-of-life impact of the multichannel cochlear implant (Summerfield & Marshall, 1995a; Wyatt, Niparko, Rothman & DeLissovoy, 1995; Wyatt, Rothman, DeLissovoy & Niparko, 1995). The cost per QALY for the cochlear implant was initially determined by using clinical cost data. The cost included all phases of treatment and the cost for potential complications. It also used a health-utility outcome based on the communication gains obtained with the device. The gains were established in large clinical trials (Cohen, Waltzman & Fisher, 1993). In the United States, cochlear implantation costs were estimated to be US$15 600 per QALY. Sensitivity analysis, a technique that systematically varies the assumptions of costs, risks and benefit that underlie the calculations, indicated a range from as little as US$12 000 to as much as US$30 000 per QALY. These modelled results placed the multichannel cochlear implant well within the 'cost-effectiveness range' occupied by a vast array of common medical and surgical procedures available in the United States.

We recently performed a cost-utility analysis on survey data from profoundly deaf implant users ($n = 226$) and compared it with 32 candidates awaiting cochlear implantation (Wyatt, Rothman, DeLissovoy & Niparko, 1995). Health status was assessed using the Ontario Health Utilities Index, Mark III (Feeny et al., 1992). Table 2.1 illustrates the differences in hearing, speech and cognitive function. It also reveals differences in the emotional status between the implanted and non-implanted groups. The analysis demonstrated a substantial impact by the cochlear implant on quality-of-life measures. Relating this to overall health status, the results of the Mark III index yielded a substantial utility index improvement of 0.204 ($P < 0.001$). Cost-utility calculations based on this utility value indicated a cost per QALY of US$15 928. Use of a 'feeling thermometer' method (Hurst, Jobanputra & Hunter, 1994) in this patient population yielded an even more favourable result. The cost-utility result using these data was US$9325.

Other investigators have also performed cost-utility analyses for use of cochlear implants in adults. Summerfield and Marshall (1995b) and Summerfield (1995) have performed two separate analyses, one of

Table 2.1: Health status by attribute measured by the Ontario Health Utilities Index in implant candidates (pre-implant group; $n = 32$) and implant users ($n = 226$)

Attribute	Pre-implant group	Implant user group	Prob> |T|
Hearing	*2.97*	*5.07*	*0.000*
Speech	*4.73*	*5.51*	*0.000*
Vision*	4.87	4.52	0.026
Emotion	*3.10*	*3.58*	*0.003*
Pain	3.10	3.10	0.968
Ambulation	5.72	5.71	0.953
Dexterity	5.86	5.90	0.635
Cognition	6.30	6.65	0.017
Self-care	2.93	2.97	0.32

Note: See Wyatt, Rothman, DeLissovoy and Niparko (1995). Significant difference ($p < 0.01$) in raw scores by attribute in italics. Note that in contrast with all other significant findings, the visual score was greater for the pre-implant than the implanted group (*).

which uses a visual-analogue 'feeling thermometer' scale. In a study of 208 adult implant users, they found a health utility improvement of 32% and a cost utility (based on United Kingdom cost data) of US$13 200. Harris, Anderson & Novak (1995) carried out a prospective analysis using the Quality of Well-Being Scale (Kaplan, Bush & Berry, 1976) to assess health status in seven adult cochlear implant recipients. They were able to demonstrate a health-utility improvement of 11% and a cost utility of US$31 711.These studies are summarised in Table 2.2. At the most recent NIH consensus conference on Cochlear Implants (Consensus Statement, 1995), these results were discussed, and the panel concluded that implantation of adults compares very favourably with commonly utilised medical procedures ranging from those with extremely high cost utility (e.g. neonatal intensive care) to those with relatively low cost utility (e.g. dialysis); see Wyatt, Niparko, Rothman and DeLissovoy (1995) for review.

Cost utility of cochlear implantation in children

Assessments of quality-of-life effects and the cost-effectiveness of cochlear implants in children are likely to be increasingly important. Controversy surrounds the use of the cochlear implant in children because they receive it through parental consent rather than with independent informed consent. Communication enhancement with the cochlear implant requires a strong family and professional commitment, particularly in the first two years of use.

Pressure on federal, state and local budgets has forced scrutiny of programmes of special education. In the United States, the current era of health care reform has placed increased pressure on the medical profession to provide cost-effective and efficient care. This is particularly important because, within the USA, much of the recent increase in health care expenditure can be traced to advances in medical technology. In using such technologies, care providers are now required to justify medical and surgical interventions based not only on safety and efficacy, but also on cost-effectiveness.

Determining the cost utility of cochlear implantation in children also presents a particular challenge. Significant audiologic and speech and language benefits have been demonstrated for children who use a cochlear implant (Cohen, Waltzmn & Fisher, 1993; Miyamoto et al., 1992), but there exist a vast array of developmental and maturational outcomes to be assessed in determining the quality-of-life changes in children (Hutton, Politi & Seeger, 1995). Methods for assessing quality of life are not as well established for children as for the adult population. Most assessments rely on parental opinion or reporting. For example, an early study by Cunningham (1990) examined the impressions of parents of children who had a single-channel device. They found that, in addition

Table 2.2: Summary of cost-utility assessments of the multichannel cochlear implant

Gain in quality of life due to multichannel cochlear implant	Quality of life measurement instrument	Method	Cost-utility result (US$)	Country	Authors
10%	EuroQol	Theoretical mapping	12 500	UK	Summerfield & Marshall (1995b)
11%	Quality of Well-Being Scale	Prospective by patients (*n* = 7)	31 711	USA	Harris, Anderson & Novak (1995)
18%	Health Utilities Index	Theoretical mapping	15 593	USA	Wyatt, Rothman, DeLissovoy & Niparko (1995)
20.4%	Health Utilities Index	Comparison of implanted and non-implanted patients (*n* = 258)	15 928	USA	Wyatt, Rothman, DeLissovoy & Niparko (1995)
30%	Visual-Analogue Scale	Retrospective by patients (*n* = 229)	9000	USA	Wyatt, Rothman, DeLissovoy & Niparko (1995)
32%	Visual-Analogue Scale	Retrospective by patients (*n* = 208)	13 200	UK	Summerfield & Marshall (1995)

to noting subjective improvements in speech, language and attention, 98% would recommend the device to other parents. Cost-effectiveness considerations in children depend heavily on several factors:

- the utilisation of special educational and rehabilitation services;
- the degree to which the expected speech and language benefits lead to improved reading comprehension, speech reception/production and other functional capabilities that would result in improved employability and lifetime earning potential;
- the impact of the device on general measurements of quality of life.

Research on speech-and-language-impaired populations indicates that the development of an aural concept of language is critical to the development of visual language comprehension (reading) and expression (writing). For example, mathematic computation ability among 15-year-old, hearing-impaired individuals lies below the seventh grade level, when the average ability of 15-year-old, hearing students is at the tenth grade level (Allen, 1986). Even more striking is the disparity in reading comprehension. In the same study, mean reading comprehension ability among the hearing-impaired students was at the third grade level; the mean ability among 15-year-old, hearing students, again, was at the tenth grade level.

Auditory perception appears to be critical in a number of other areas as well. Tests of selective visual attention revealed that hearing-impaired children have deficits in their selective visual attention, suggesting that auditory input affects the development of attention skills (Quittner, Katz & Mitchell, 1992). Profoundly hearing-impaired children who receive a cochlear implant demonstrate improved visual attention skills that eventually reach those of age-matched peers with less severe hearing impairments than those who use hearing aids.

Low employment rates of congenitally deaf adults, even among those who are gifted (those with unusually high intelligence) have been reported (Vernon & LaFalce-Landers, 1993). There is also a documented gap in earning potential for hearing-impaired individuals, in general, relative to the hearing population. The most recent study to address this issue found significantly higher unemployment among the profoundly hearing impaired. Those who were employed had a personal income which was 70.3% of the national median (Schein, 1977). If the cochlear implant were able to restore auditory perception leading to an increased income of 22% because of employment opportunity, this group would have a personal income comparable to 92.3% of the national median. A simple cost-benefit analysis based on personal income that ignores all other quality-of-life benefits, then, would more than offset all costs of the implant and its associated rehabilitation.

Against this background, a theoretical analysis of cost-effectiveness of cochlear implantation of children may be performed. The validity of such an assessment depends heavily on assumptions about the impact of the implant on educational needs. Costs associated with manual strategies of deaf education are highly variable, depending on programme size, residential facilities and transportation. Student-to-staff ratios for most early education schools for the deaf average less than 4:1 (Education Programs and Services, 1990). The overall cost of educating students in schools for the deaf, despite wide variation, are uniformly recognised to be substantially higher than those associated with the mainstream educational setting. For our analysis, we have chosen to use US$35 000: a figure consistent with previously published cost data (Northern & Downs, 1991), and recently budgeted campus costs per deaf student in the state of Maryland, USA (Maryland State Board of Education, 1995).

With the above information, a cost-benefit ratio for childhood implantation can be estimated. These estimations use cost projections that are adjusted for inflation and time value of money using a discount rate of 5% per year. This equalises present and future expenditures so that the final result is expressed into today's dollars. Let us assume that a child is implanted at the age of four years at a cost of US$53 058 for the surgical procedure and associated rehabilitation. At a rate of 50% mainstreaming three years post-implant, and a 90% rate of partial mainstreaming six years post-implant (as has been the early experience in the Johns Hopkins and in the Hannover, Germany implant programmes), cost savings in middle and upper levels of education can be determined. Under these assumptions, the cochlear implant saves approximately US$152 000 in educational costs and yields a *net* present-value-of-implant placement of US$99 501 (cost savings minus cost). An alternative interpretation suggests that if 41% of early childhood implant recipients are partially mainstreamed within six years after implantation, educational savings will completely offset the total cost of implantation.

Note that this analysis is purely economic in nature and does not consider non-economic benefits and limitations. Detailed cost-utility studies in children are now under way. These studies will undoubtedly give a fuller view of quality-of-life effects of implanting young children.

Systematic study of the cost utility of hearing rehabilitation with the multichannel cochlear implant will require several avenues of study:

- analysis of the impact of sensorineural hearing impairment on quality of life for children and their families, stratified by severity, pattern, time of onset of hearing impairment and communication/educational strategy;
- appraisal of existing scales of quality of life and general health perception for sensitivity to hearing-related changes in children;

- determination of effects of auditory rehabilitation interventions on the above measures.

Conclusions

Severely and profoundly deaf individuals face limitations in their social and vocational opportunities. This places these individuals at a noticeable economic disadvantage. Based on traditional measures of quality of life, recent interventions appear to provide benefit that dramatically, and favourably, impacts on these limitations. Such studies are important in analysing the needed components of programmes of rehabilitation and future directions for clinical intervention. Furthermore, third-party payers, consumers and health care providers now need to make decisions based on economic and health outcomes data. While cochlear implants are covered by many insurance plans in the United States, there is a growing trend for exclusion or low reimbursement by managed care programmes and self-insured employers. These policies will potentially limit access to auditory rehabilitative interventions and threaten to constrain the development of newer technologies.

References

Allen T (1986) Patterns of academic achievement among hearing-impaired students: 1974 and 1983. In Schridroth A, Karchman M (Eds) Deaf Children in America. San Diego, CA: College Hill Press.

Cohen NL, Waltzman SB, Fisher SG (1993) A prospective, randomized study of cochlear implants. The Department of Veterans Affairs cochlear implant study group. New England Journal of Medicine 328(4): 233–7.

Consensus Statement (1995) NIH Consensus Development Conference: Cochlear Implants in Adults and Children. Bethesda, MD: Office of Medical Applied Research, NIH, Federal Bldg, No. 618, Bethesda, MD 20892.

Cunningham JK (1990) Parents' evaluations of the effects of the 3M/House cochlear implant on children. Ear and Hearing 11(5): 375–81.

Drummond MF, Maynard J (1993) Purchasing and Providing Cost-effective Health care. Edinburgh: Churchill Livingstone.

Education Programs and Services (1990) US schools and classes. American Annals of the Deaf 135: 88–134.

Feeny D, Furlong W, Barr R, Torrance G, Rosenbaum P, Weitzman S (1992) A comprehensive multiattribute system for classifying the health status of survivors of childhood cancer. Journal of Clinical Oncology 10: 923–8.

Feeny DH, Torrance GW (1989) Incorporating utility-based quality-of-life assessment measures in clinical trials: two examples. Medical Care 27(Suppl):190–204.

Gafni A, Birch S (1993) Guidelines for the adoption of new technologies: a prescription for uncontrolled growth in expenditures and how to avoid the problem. Canadian Medical Association Journal 148(6): 913–17.

Harris JP, Anderson JP, Novak N (1995) An outcomes study of cochlear implants in deaf patients: audiologic, economic and quality of life changes. Archives of Otolaryngology, Head and Neck Surgery 121: 398–404.

Hurst N, Jobanputra P, Hunter M (1994) Validity of EuroQol – a generic health status instrument. British Journal of Rheumatology 33: 655–62.

Hutton J, Politi C, Seeger T (1995) Cost-effectiveness of cochlear implantation of children. In Uziel A, Mondarin M (Eds) Cochlear Implants in Children. Advances in Otorhinolaryngology. Basel: Karger 50: 201–6.

Kaplan R, Bush J, Berry C (1976) Health status: types of validity and the index of well-being. Health Services Research 11: 478–507.

Maryland State Board of Education (1995) State Budget for Maryland Schools. Baltimore, MD: Maryland State Board of Education.

Miyamoto RT, Osberger MJ, Robbins AM, Nyres WA, Kessler DK, Pope ML (1992) Longitudinal evaluation of communication skills of children with single- or multi-channel cochlear implants. American Journal of Otology 13(3): 215–22.

Northern J, Downs M (1991) Hearing in Children. 4th edn. Baltimore: Williams & Wilkins, pp 28–9.

Osberger MJ, Maso M, Sam LK (1993) Speech intelligibility of children with cochlear implants, tactile aids, or hearing aids. Journal of Speech and Hearing Research 36(1): 186–203.

Quittner SL, Katz D, Mitchell T (1992) The development of attention in hearing-impaired children. In Proceedings of the First European Symposium on Pediatric Cochlear Implants 1: 86.

Schein JD (1977) Economic Status of Deaf Adults. New York: New York University School of Education Thesis.

Summerfield AQ (1995) Cost-effectiveness considerations in cochlear implantation. Abstracts of the NIH Consensus Conferences: Cochlear Implants in Adults and Children, 75–9.

Summerfield AQ, Marshall D (1995a) Costs and cost-utility of cochlear implantation. In Cochlear Implantation in the UK 1990–1994. MRC–INR, London: HMSO.

Summerfield AQ, Marshall D (1995b) Cochlear implantation: demand, costs, and utility. Annals of Otology, Rhinology and Laryngology 104 (9, Part 2, Suppl 166): 245–8.

Vernon M, LaFalce-Landers E (1993) A longitudinal study of intellectually gifted deaf and hard of hearing people. Educational, psychological and career outcomes. American Annals of the Deaf 138: 427–34.

Wyatt J, Niparko J, Rothman M, DeLissovoy G (1995) Cost-effectiveness of the multi-channel cochlear implant. American Journal of Otology 16(1): 52–62.

Wyatt J, Rothman M, DeLissovoy G, Niparko J (1995) Cost-effectiveness of the multi-channel cochlear implant in 258 profoundly deaf adults. Laryngoscope, in press.

Chapter 3
Monitoring Progress in Young Children with Cochlear Implants

MARK E. LUTMAN, SUE ARCHBOLD, KEVIN P. GIBBIN,
BARRY McCORMICK AND GERARD M. O'DONOGHUE

Introduction

The Nottingham Paediatric Cochlear Implant Programme was formed in 1989 and remains unusual in many respects because it:

- focuses on young children mainly below the age of five years;
- covers a large geographical area and conducts rehabilitation primarily via an outreach programme, sharing skills with families and a range of support professionals;
- places only limited emphasis on directed individual training of auditory and speech skills, preferring to enable the implanted child to acquire and develop spoken language in natural everyday contexts;
- engages in research, including the development of a computer database devised specifically to monitor the functioning of the device and the progress of communication skills in these young children.

This chapter outlines the rationale behind the Nottingham approach and describes some of the methods used to monitor the rehabilitation phase following implantation. Outcome measures are described as essential benchmarks of progress.

Historical background

The decision to start a child-only implant programme was influenced by several factors (McCormick, 1991). In the first place, and most importantly, there was a pressing demand from parents of deafened children and results from work outside the United Kingdom, especially in the USA and Australia, were demonstrating clearly the effectiveness of multichannel cochlear implants in children. The findings, however, were mainly based on school-aged children who were older than we had in mind and who were able to undertake the performance tests required to demonstrate progress objectively. We also had a strong basis of expertise, stemming from an advanced paediatric audiology service in Nottingham with specialisation in the audiological assessment and rehabilitation of very young children, and an active research background. Experimental studies had already been conducted by one of the authors (GMO) on the electrical stimulation of the cochlea. Further, there were educational and other facilities in place to deal with profoundly deaf children from which a developing cochlear implant programme could tap resources. These facilities included local, well-developed itinerant services for children with special needs.

The public health care perspective added other influencing factors because it was perceived that young children offer the greatest potential for cumulative health gain, when compared with older children and adults. This idea of increased potential for benefit arose from anecdotal accounts that better performance is achieved when children are implanted at a young age and that early implantation offers the added benefit of enabling a child to develop spoken language during linguistically formative years and the potential for improved educational attainment. Additionally, there is the greater number of years over which these benefits can be expected to accrue. Finally, there is the potential to achieve some savings in the cost of long-term special education, further enhancing the cost utility of cochlear implantation. This last factor is consistent with the trend in the UK towards increased parental choice in education and a leaning toward less restrictive educational environments for children with special needs.

Rationale for the Nottingham approach

There are three major beliefs that have influenced our rehabilitation approach. First, because of the impact that implantation has on development of spoken language in young implanted children, special skills and interests are needed in the team that will work to facilitate the development of auditory skills. There are only minor differences between the rehabilitation of children who can make successful use of hearing aids and those who obtain access to audition through cochlear implants. This means that the necessary skills are already familiar to many paediatric audiologists, educators and speech and language therapists. Hence, building a cochlear implant team is achieved most easily by harnessing the existing skills of individuals and adapting their use to implant technology. This is more efficient than developing rehabilitation skills in personnel who are primarily specialists in implants.

The second belief is that high quality of service is best achieved by focusing on a limited range of objectives; in our case this entailed focusing primarily on children under the age of five years at implantation, and meeting their needs over the next few years. Today, with the benefit of hindsight, we can see that the decision to implant children without prior experience in adults has had major advantages. The implant team was able to focus skills on a specific client group, and this has allowed us to achieve levels of expertise that would have been difficult without such concentration.

The third belief is that the development of spoken language is driven by a natural desire to communicate efficiently with others. In very young children, this communication will be primarily with parents and other family members. As the child grows older, communication needs will expand to include friends, teachers, school peers and many others. For this and other reasons, a naturalistic approach is preferable to highly intensive clinic-based training methods, which are neither necessary nor desirable for most children. Our emphasis, therefore, has been to share skills and strategies with families and key-worker professionals who directly influence the child. This includes an emphasis on the use of audition in everyday life. It is our expectation that skills learned under such everyday circumstances will generalise more readily than those learned under highly structured clinical conditions. This expectation is supported by outcomes and parental perspectives reported by Lloyd (1994).

Process of rehabilitation

Although cochlear implantation is a complex major surgical procedure, surgery is only a brief part of the overall process, which may take several years to complete. This is especially true for children, and even more so for very young children. The surgical phase is preceded by an extended period of pre-assessment to ensure that the child is suitable from primarily an audiological and medical point of view. The pre-assessment includes developmental, communication and educational considerations, as outlined in Figure 3.1. We have found that an adapted form of the ChiP profile devised by Hellman et al. (1991) provides invaluable multidisciplinary insights during the pre-assessment phase. Such insights will become even more important as we reconsider our selection criteria to include children with marginal hearing aid benefit and children with additional needs.

Electrophysiological and behavioural measures obtained during the pre-assessment period provide important baseline information for monitoring progress during the rehabilitation phase. The device may be fine-tuned on many occasions after the initial fitting and the process of obtaining suitable dynamic range settings runs in parallel with rehabilitation (Figure 3.1). Although the fine-tuning and rehabilitation are conceptually distinct, they cannot be separated completely in practice. Performance characteristics reported during rehabilitation sessions

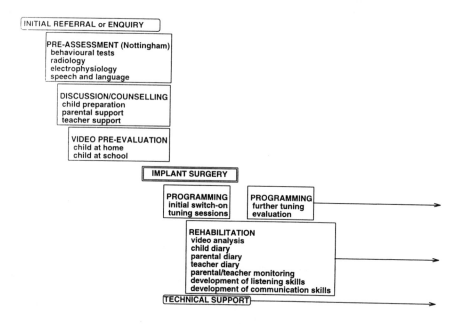

Figure 3.1: The process of cochlear implantation with time running from left to right

often influence fine-tuning decisions, and adjustment to device settings may lead to altered practices and expectations during rehabilitation.

Implant team

Examination of the rehabilitation box shown in Figure 3.1 indicates that the rehabilitation team consists of a large group of individuals. Not only are members of the implant team involved, but also many others who work closely with the child at a local level. Parents are a very important component of the rehabilitation process, as are other family members, teachers and local professionals. Hence, the team of rehabilitators consists of two parts: those from the implant centre and those local to the child. The need for local input is emphasised in our programme which serves the whole of the UK because our implanted children may live at a considerable distance from the implant centre. An essential element of any successful programme is the partnership between the implant centre and the local teams.

The implant centre team consists of more than a dozen individuals contributing in varying amounts. They include surgeons, audiological scientists, teachers of the deaf, speech and language therapists and medical physicists. Table 3.1 shows the breakdown of human resources currently employed in our programme, expressed in whole-time equiva-

Table 3.1: Human resources for a programme implanting 36 young children per year

Staff category	Whole-time equivalents
Coordinator	0.5
Surgeon	0.5
Audiological scientist	4.1
Teacher of the deaf	4.0
Speech & language therapist	3.5
Medical physicist	0.2
Secretary/administrator	2.6

lents. The numbers are based on a programme that is implanting children at the rate of 36 new cases per year, and which includes an intensive follow-up of all children for three years after implantation. After this three-year period, follow-up continues at a reduced frequency that may be as little as one home visit and one clinic visit per year. In many cases, however, a need remains for further visits and the numbers in the table account for such extra time. However, because the rate of implantation has increased progressively and is only just approaching 36 per year, the workload has not yet reached a steady state in our clinic, and somewhat greater staff numbers will be required in future even without an increase in the rate of implantation.

Figure 3.2 illustrates the change in the pattern of human resource input from the implant centre over the four years following implantation. Rehabilitation, assessment and counselling represent the major commitment for the first three years. There is also a large component of

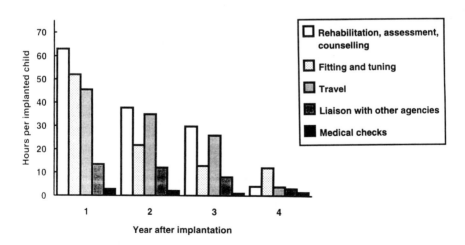

Figure 3.2: Pattern of human resource input as a function of time since implantation. The columns represent the mean hours per child in each year. Note that pre-assessment is classified within year one

travel deriving from the outreach element of the programme. After year three, the resource input drops radically as the rehabilitation changes from intensive to occasional support; however, the fitting and fine-tuning components continue unaltered. These changes from year three to year four reflect the fact that responsibility for rehabilitation can be transferred almost entirely to the local team after year three whereas the fine-tuning and device troubleshooting remain the responsibility of the implant centre at present. Note, however, that the period covered by the figure was one where relative stability of technology existed. If the data had been collected over a more recent period, they would have reflected a greater concentration on refitting. This is because an updated sound processor became available in 1994. The policy of our programme is to move to improved technology wherever appropriate, and the contracts we have negotiated with purchasing health authorities anticipate this need.

The roles of the team members over the four years generally divide on professional lines. The audiological scientists perform the assessment and tuning, while the rehabilitation work is performed by speech and language therapists and by teachers of the deaf. In accordance with the outreach philosophy, the rehabilitation role is primarily one of an itinerant (peripatetic) adviser. The aim is to encourage the provision of suitable listening and learning conditions for implanted children. This recognises that the amount of time that can be spent by implant centre team members with the children is limited, both by resource constraints and geographical separation. Therefore, the greatest benefit to the children is achieved indirectly by providing support to local team members. The implant team members also play an important role in monitoring progress by ensuring standardisation in testing across the diverse situations in which the children are placed. They enable the use of specialised techniques that may not be available locally owing to limitations of equipment or required assessment skills. Supervision by the implant team members also ensures that the outcomes database is as complete as possible. An associated benefit of the programme is that specialist outreach support promotes innovative good practice, thereby potentially enhancing the assessment and rehabilitation of other profoundly deaf children.

Educational and communication considerations

Children with cochlear implants are found in a variety of educational settings available for deaf children, including residential and day schools, units attached to mainstream schools, mainstream schools themselves with various levels of support and at pre-school and nursery facilities. Within these settings, there may be differing communication styles: auditory/aural, Total Communication (Lynas, 1994) and those with an emphasis on manual systems of communication. Three-quarters of our implanted children are in Total Communication settings with the remainder in auditory/oral settings. This reflects the educational policy in the UK for deaf children rather than specific judgements made on the needs of each child. Wherever the children are placed, responsibility for post-operative management of the child will fall largely on the local teacher (Archbold, 1994; Geers & Moog, 1991; Goin & Parisier, 1991; Somers, 1991). In the year following implantation, children spend only 1% of their waking hours on average at the implant centre; the rest of the time is predominantly at home and at school. Thus, to ensure the optimal use of the implant system throughout the child's waking hours, our rehabilitation staff focus on working with the local teachers of the deaf, classroom teachers, speech and language therapists and the child's family. This is preferable to working exclusively with the child, as effort spent with the local professionals and the family can benefit the child during the 99% of waking hours when the child is away from the implant centre.

The philosophy adopted by our team is to 'make the normal happen' (Tait & Wood, 1987). That is, we provide situations that are known to promote the development of spoken language in both hearing and deaf children. Highly structured, adult-controlled methods of rehabilitation are not encouraged; instead, the parent or teacher structures the learning situations experienced by the child, bearing in mind the child's stage in the development of auditory skills. Before implantation, the emphasis on audition may well have been inappropriate; after implantation, the emphasis changes so that parents and local teachers must adapt their approach and expectations to provide the necessary conditions for obtaining the maximum benefit from the implant. The role of the implant centre staff is to support the parents and local professionals and to help them make the necessary transitions. This is achieved via the educational outreach programme which maintains direct contact with home and school, and with other local professionals not based at the school. The programme of in-service training is adapted to the educational needs of each child and has been described elsewhere (Archbold, 1994).

Contact with the local professionals begins at the start of the assessment period, before the child receives the cochlear implant. At least two visits by a member of the implant centre staff to the child's locality occur before surgery. These increase to monthly visits in the year immediately after implantation, then reduce to every two months in the second and third post-implant years. These rates are the minimum levels of support provided, and may be increased in specific cases as the need arises. During these visits, assessment of emerging listening skills of the child takes place using the methods outlined above. The rehabilitation being provided for the child and its effectiveness are monitored and appropriate activities and developments are discussed with parents and local staff. Some time may be spent working with the child on activities other than those concerned with assessment, such as educational activities, but the main focus is on supporting the local team of parents and professionals.

In the UK, responsibility for educational placement and communication setting rests with the local authorities with additional advice received from local professionals. The ability of the implant centre to influence these factors is limited and varies between authorities in different regions. Experience of implanted children has made it increasingly clear that emphasis on a strong auditory/aural component is essential to optimise the use of, and benefit from, the implant (Cooper, 1991; Somers, 1991; Tye-Murray, 1993). Hence, there may be a need for negotiation by the implant team with local education providers before and after implantation, to ensure that appropriate circumstances prevail. Educational approaches considered appropriate before implantation may no longer be appropriate when the child has access to useful audition. This requires flexibility; however, sudden changes in educational setting close to the time of implantation may be unsettling for the child and therefore counter-productive. Careful assessment of each child, the current placement of the child and the availability of facilities locally are required to provide useful advice to those making decisions on behalf of the child. This advice needs to be updated from time to time as the child's communication skills develop and the ability to function in a more challenging environment increases.

Increasing numbers of implant centres in the UK are providing such a programme of support. With more implant centre teachers of the deaf and speech therapists working in this way, there is a need for consistency of support and expectations across centres. Several school classes contain more than one implanted child, each under the care of a different implant centre. This means that it is important to ensure that the local professionals are not subjected to inconsistent information or advice. To avoid such inconsistency, the implant centre teachers of the deaf have developed guidelines for their practice, supported by the British Association of Teachers of the Deaf, the British Cochlear Implant Group, the National Deaf Children's Society and the Department for Education. It is hoped that universal adoption of the guidelines within the UK will maximise the teamwork within and between implant centres to provide the greatest benefit for children.

Monitoring performance

Monitoring progress forms an important part of the rehabilitation process. The outcome measures used vary throughout the rehabilitation period, unlike the situation for programmes involving older children or adults, because young children undergo rapid development during the period after implantation. This includes both the natural cognitive development that accompanies the particular age span, and also the development of spoken language skills and concepts that are accelerated from a low starting point as a result of receiving acoustical information through the implant. Therefore, the ability of these young children to undertake specific performance tests may be severely limited by cognitive and linguistic development. Consequently, it can be very difficult to demonstrate and monitor progress in this young population. These considerations have necessitated the development of observational and proxy techniques that do not place a heavy linguistic load on the child. Measures that rely on stricter performance testing are not applicable, in general, until after at least 18 months of post-implant experience. Hence, the nature of the monitoring procedures changes over the rehabilitation period with greater emphasis on performance-based outcomes in the later years. This is true for measures of spoken language and, to a lesser extent, for measures of speech perception.

Outcome measures

The measures used to monitor the performance of the cochlear implant device itself, and the performance of the child with the device, provide important information for the rehabilitation programme. This includes departures from the expected pattern (based on current experience in our programme), which would entail either adjustments to the device or changes to rehabilitation methods. Moreover, further accumulation of these measures across children, over time and as a function of age, provides the background against which future children can be compared. Further, changes in functioning of the device picked up by monitoring lead to further appropriate behavioural fine-tuning sessions (see McCormick, Archbold & Sheppard, 1994 for further details).

Monitoring the device

Although the implanted parts of current devices are reliable, failures do occur. Sudden, total failures are relatively simple to detect, even in young children. However, some failures may be partial or intermittent and can, therefore, be extremely difficult to detect, especially in children functioning at the pre-verbal level. The exact incidence of intermittent problems is unknown but there is a strong possibility that in any sizeable paediatric implant programme one or more children will be underfunctioning because of such problems. It is generally believed that consistency of input from any auditory prosthesis is important to allow the user to acclimatise to its characteristics. This is likely to be the case with cochlear implants, especially for young children who are developing percepts and the fundamental precursors of spoken language. Hence, monitoring of device performance *per se* is an important aspect of the rehabilitation programme. Physiological changes that affect the signals passing from the cochlea to the brain, such as further loss of cochlear nerve ganglion cells, may also occur, and these changes may require changes in strategy.

Evaluation of device performance is checked by using behavioural responses. When behavioural checks suggest a problem, there is a need to conduct further tests to establish device performance objectively. For this purpose, we rely on electrophysiological measures obtained routinely from all children at the time of surgery. These measures can be repeated, whenever necessary, to establish if there is a decrement (or change) in functioning. This practice provides a baseline for each child against which later results can be compared. Such longitudinal comparisons are more sensitive to small changes than comparisons across children. Two measures are used, both obtained using conventional auditory brainstem response (ABR) apparatus. The baseline measurements are obtained in the operating theatre once the device has been positioned in the ear: an electrical signal is sent to stimulate the ear electrically in the same way as when fitting the device post-operatively. The electrical auditory brainstem response (EABR) to single biphasic pulses resembles the ABR for acoustical stimuli, although with a shorter latency. The threshold for recording the Wave-V component is measured for a selection of electrodes, usually numbering four, and distributed evenly along the electrode array (Mason, 1994). The second measure uses the same equipment and stimuli, but focuses on the electrical artefact produced by the implanted device. This is much larger than the EABR and is obtained quickly with only limited averaging. All electrodes are measured to check that the artefact magnitudes are appropriate. This second measure is equivalent to the 'integrity test' that is performed in most centres by the manufacturer's representative using the Nucleus device.

These tests are readministered post-implant if there is reason to suspect a device malfunction. The device is stimulated in a manner similar to that used for fitting, but with the repetitive transients required for time-domain averaging replacing the stimulus bursts used for behavioural testing. As the child must keep still for an extended period to obtain clear responses, younger children are usually either anaesthetised or sedated for testing while asleep. It is axiomatic that rehabilitation with a cochlear implant can only reach its full potential if the device is functioning properly.

Checks of conventional hearing aids should occur daily, and the same is true for cochlear implant systems. A parent or teacher of the deaf is unable to listen to the output of a cochlear implant, unlike a conventional hearing aid, so a practical means of monitoring the quality of system performance must be established for all children. Some children will lack the functional language to describe what they hear, but the system performance can be assessed, nonetheless, using a suitable game format. One way in which this can be achieved is to use Ling's Five Sounds (oo, ah, ee, sh, ss) to assess the ability of the child to respond to and discriminate between the phonemes (Ling, 1988). The child's responses can be linked to a game; for example, the child moves a snake on hearing (ss) or a monkey on hearing (oo). In this way, even children functioning at the preverbal level quickly become able to provide the necessary responses. Although this is not a comprehensive assessment, the fact that the five sounds cover the speech spectrum of Western languages makes the check functionally adequate for the purpose. Using this simple technique, it is possible to perform the essential daily check on the system's performance, and we request children's teachers to carry out this check every day.

Monitoring language development

One of the primary goals of cochlear implantation in young children is to promote the development of spoken language. A broad description of language development is given by the Classification of Linguistic Performance (Dyar, 1995). It examines the linguistic competence of the child at five, interrelated levels: communication, receptive language, expressive language, voice and speech. Ratings at these five levels are combined to give an overall classification into one of three categories: preverbal, transitional and functional. Preverbal is where the deaf child has not yet reached the level of recognisable words. Transitional language describes a child using recognisable word or phrase patterns as reported by the deaf child's family and adults who know the child well. Language is also classified as transitional if it is possible to elicit some word or phrase patterns in a familiar or closed-set context on a minimum of two occasions. Functional language describes a deaf child who demonstrates the ability to use language(s) spontaneously and in a systematic way; for example, consistent use of emerging speech patterns in more than one context where the child demonstrates an apparent knowledge of meaning and syntactic rules. Equivalent features of language are noted in the case of deaf children who use sign language as the primary means of everyday communication. An important feature of this scheme is that multiple classifications can be accommodated when a child uses more than one language; for example English, Welsh or British Sign Language.

The resulting profile has several purposes. It substantiates the findings from conventional speech and language assessments and recorded samples. It illustrates the differing skills of prelingual and sign-language dominant children from a bilingual perspective. It identifies potential non-sensory complications and it indicates specific deterioration in spoken language skills that may result from profound deafness of acquired origin. In the context of the overall rehabilitation programme, we expect to see progress towards functional spoken language in implanted children.

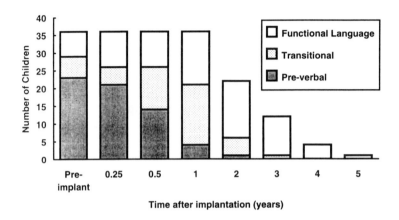

Figure 3.3: Classification of linguistic status of children before implantation and at subsequent intervals. Note that the classification may have been achieved in spoken language or sign language

Figure 3.3 illustrates the pre-implant status of the first 36 children in the Nottingham implant programme. Approximately 80% of the children were classified as either preverbal (64%) or transitional (17%) at the time of implantation. By the 12-month interval, almost 60% were still at the preverbal and transitional stages. Results from 22 children at the 24-month interval indicated 73% had attained the functional language stage and only one child remained at the preverbal stage. These findings emphasise the long timescale of progress and the need for realistic expectations in the early years after implantation.

Monitoring sound detection

The most basic measure of sound perception with a cochlear implant, or for any hearing aid for that matter, is sound-field threshold for warble tones. All children who can perform the threshold detection task should be able to perform sound threshold audiometry. This is because it is the same task required to set the lower limit of the dynamic range for electrical stimulation. For cochlear implants, this testing has a slightly different role than for hearing aids. In one respect, the test is redundant: electrical threshold has already been determined and set to correspond to the lower end of the acoustical (input) dynamic range of the sound proces-sor. The sound-field threshold is merely a reflection of the sensitivity of the microphone and input circuitry of the processor. However, the test has two other roles that are important. First, it provides a clear demon-stration to parents and any local professionals in attendance about the lowest sound detectable levels voluntarily given by the child. It is impor-tant that the results are shown as a function of frequency. A common experience, especially among teachers familiar with profoundly hearing-impaired children wearing hearing aids, is surprise when the child responds well to high-frequency sounds at low and moderate levels. This experience is useful in setting expectations in teachers and parents, and illustrates how effective cochlear implants are in transmitting the high-frequency cues that are often absent with hearing aids. The second role of the test is to provide the baseline for a quick and easy check that the device is functioning under circumstances that reflect its everyday use. This is in contrast with the synthetic stimulation and selection of individual channels used for tuning of the processor.

Monitoring word detection

Many young children are unable to perform rigorous tests of word discrimination until they have achieved substantial competence in spoken language. This may not occur until they have experience with their implant for two or three years. However, speech discrimination is one of the main goals of cochlear implantation, and is an underlying basis of spoken language development. Hence, there is a need for word discrimination tests that can be undertaken by young children as early as possible in the rehabilitation programme. One such test is the Auto-mated McCormick Toy Discrimination Test (Ousey et al., 1989), an auto-mated computer-based form of the live-voice test (McCormick, 1977). This test presents digitally stored word tokens at precisely calibrated levels to obtain the threshold level for correct identification with a stan-dard adaptive algorithm. The child simply points to the toy correspond-ing to the word token; no spoken response is necessary. The test is validated in young, English-speaking children with normal hearing and with hearing-impaired children (Summerfield et al., 1994). (It is possi-ble, in principle, to use this type of test in languages other than English. However, selection of suitably contrasting word pairs, production of test materials and validation of the new test would be needed before it was used.) In the present context, the test is used to measure an aided sound-field threshold for word identification. In this way, it is an indica-tor of speech perceptual ability. The threshold gives a composite measure that combines auditory sensitivity with the ability of the child to organise the incoming acoustical information into a meaningful word. The proportion of young children who can successfully complete the test ranges from 20% one year after implantation to 83% three years after implantation. Furthermore, the thresholds achieved improve over that time from approximately 60 to 55 dB(A) on average, indicating increasing ability to utilise speech cues. The test can be performed earlier, and thresholds decrease further and faster, in children who have an established spoken language base before implantation.

Monitoring sound perception through observation

Only a few children are able to perform the above tasks for sound and word detection before they have experienced about 18 months of implant use. The following observational methods were developed in our centre to fill this gap.

Listening Progress (LiP) is a profile of early listening skills, including listening to environmental and speech sounds. It assesses changes in listening skills as the child demonstrates the ability to respond to and identify sounds in play situations. An example is responding to a musical instrument or discriminating between long and short speech sounds. Details of the profile and its record sheet are given by Archbold (1994). It is particularly useful in children with little or no language who are unable to report verbally what they hear. The profile quantifies responses to environmental, instrumental and speech sounds at the lower end of the scale, through discriminating one sound from another, to identification of sounds in isolation. It includes responses to, and discrimination between, Ling's Five Sounds (Ling, 1988). LiP has also proved useful for picking up malfunctions of the implant system, monitoring limitations of the speech coding strategy and evaluating the appropriateness of the learning environment. Figure 3.4 illustrates the changes that can be expected by summarising the mean progress of a group of 28 children over the 12 months following implantation. The results are expressed simply as a score out of the maximum of 42. There are wide variations in the rates of progress across children. Nonetheless, each child showed a positive change at each successive assessment interval. Older children, and those deafened after the age of five, tend to demonstrate these basic skills earlier, as might be expected (although in the longer term, children implanted younger tend to achieve higher levels of spoken language skills).

Early communicative behaviour measured by video analysis is another observational technique adapted for use in our centre. Communicative behavioural patterns, such as turn-taking and eye contact with the speaker, are precursors of normal language development (Bruner, 1983). These patterns can be observed in young children before they are able to speak or understand spoken language. Video recordings and their analysis provide a useful method for verifying and quantifying observations. Children who make good use of conventional hearing aids

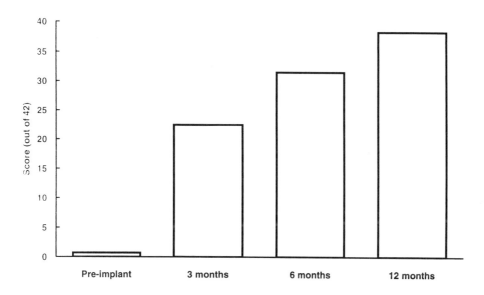

Figure 3.4: Mean scores on Listening Progress (LiP) profile before implantation and at subsequent intervals (*n* = 28 children)

have been shown by this technique to become more proficient at vocal turn-taking over time. They also take fewer turns which are silent because of the use of sign or gesture. Conversely, very deaf children who are not able to make good use of hearing aids develop silent turn-taking skills by using gesture (Tait, 1987). We have adapted this technique for use in the implant rehabilitation programme to monitor progress in the first year after implantation (Tait, 1993). Video recordings of each child in conversation with someone they know well are made at regular intervals. Analysis of the results for preverbal children implanted in the first five years of the programme showed that our implanted children all took turns silently before implantation, or did not take any turns at all. Our aim is that the implant should allow them to follow the pattern of good hearing aid users and take turns using vocalisation, and ultimately words. This has turned out to be true.

Figure 3.5 illustrates progress in early communicative skills for vocal turn-taking, over a 12-month period, for nine children under five years of age implanted in the programme (Tait & Lutman, 1994). They are compared in the figure with two other matched groups of nine children tested by the same method in the mid-1980s: good hearing aid users and poor hearing aid users. The poor hearing aid users would all be candidates for cochlear implantation today. The findings illustrate clear differences between the good hearing aid users and implantees. In fact, the implantees seem to be showing more rapid progress than the good hearing aid users. If such measures are predictive of ultimate speech percep-

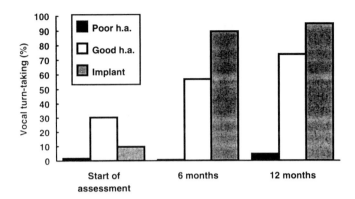

Figure 3.5: Comparison of mean vocal turn-taking scores obtained from video analysis amongst age-matched groups of (1) poor hearing-aid performers, (2) good hearing-aid performers, and (3) cochlear implantees, taken before implantation and at subsequent intervals. Each group consisted of nine children with a mean age of three years at the start of assessment

tion and production performance, these data suggest that the implantees may even out-perform children with severe hearing impairments currently considered to be doing well with hearing aids. Out of the various measures we employ, this video analysis provides the earliest formal indication of benefit from the implant.

Observational measures of speech production and vocalisation

Because of the difficulty in conducting formal evaluations on newly implanted young children, there is a strong reliance on observational measures. We have found several techniques useful.

Profile of Actual Speech Skills

We have adapted the Profile of Actual Speech Skills (PASS) from a video analysis procedure devised by the Indianapolis Cochlear Implant Programme (Osberger et al., 1991). It is a sensitive method for documenting the quantity and quality (or variety) of speech production of the child after implantation. The PASS profile categorises the utterances of young or low-verbal deaf children as actual phonemes or speech sounds, speech-like sounds, non-speech vocalisations or noises and silent speech postures. The types of utterances are characteristic of the speech of many profoundly deaf children. Any of three additional procedures can be used to examine consonant and vowel systems, place of articulation, and to summarise place, voice and manner features once the initial profile is made.

PASS analysis has provided extremely useful information on the changing status of speech and voice skills following implantation in children who do not have established speech. We have been able to perform the analysis on approximately 80% of children with low-level speech within the first year after implantation. This technique allows us to analyse representative samples of a child's spoken language in a relaxed and stress-free setting at specified assessment intervals. Results from our children show a marked increase in the quantity of vocalisations produced. Further, there is a change in quality of vocalisations shown by the children. Our study reveals that the emergence of recognisable speech sounds or phonemes of English takes at least 12 months in many cases. This can be frustrating for families and professionals alike. However, the rate of speech acquisition appears to become more rapid once the early precursors and linguistic rules of spoken language have been established.

Speech Intelligibility Rating

The purpose of the Speech Intelligibility Rating (SIR) is to document the intelligibility of emerging speech and voice skills. The speech and language therapists at our centre apply a rating scale based on recorded and live assessments. The scale has a set of six ordered categories. At the time of this writing, the scale is under development and the categories are arbitrary. We plan to evaluate the categories against appropriate objective measurements and formal speech tests. This will only be possible when more implanted children have reached the three-year assessment interval. It is also planned to evaluate the categories against judgements of independent listeners presented with recorded audio samples of the children's speech.

The preliminary findings with this new tool revealed the following. Before implantation, only one child was classified as intelligible to a listener who concentrates and lipreads. In other words, their everyday speech was generally unintelligible to inexperienced listeners. Some 91% were predominantly unintelligible in everyday situations where speech is not accompanied by gesture or contextual cues. By the 12-month interval, 25% were at least intelligible to a listener who concentrates and lipreads. By the 24-month interval, approximately 60% had reached that level; that is, they were using speech effectively as the primary means of everyday communication. This percentage had reached 91% by the 36-month interval. Based on these results, it is predicted that up to 90% of children implanted at the pre-school stage will produce intelligible speech within five years of implantation. These data are useful for setting appropriate expectations for those involved in rehabilitation both at the implant centre and local to the child.

Monitoring progress through questionnaires

In parallel with the behavioural measures described above, proxy measures of the child's performance and benefit from the implant are obtained through formal questionnaires. The questionnaires outlined below are completed by parents and teachers.

The Meaningful Auditory Integration Scale (MAIS)

This questionnaire was developed in Indianapolis by Robbins (1990). All parents receive the questionnaire with the aim of monitoring the child's use and reliance on the implant. It also focuses on reliance on audition and increasing ability to attach meaning to sound. Parents and teachers are asked to score the child regularly, responding to questions about the child's wearing of the device, awareness of environmental sounds and ability to deduce more subtle meaning from sound; for example, to distinguish one speaker from another. Aside from revealing increasing acceptance and use of the implant, our findings on 36 children showed a difference between parents' and teachers' scores. Lower scores were given by the teachers, which probably illustrates the greater length of time taken to attach meaning to sound in the noisier environment of the classroom than at home.

Environmental Sound Awareness and Identification

For the safety of their child, awareness of environmental sounds is a major aim of implantation for many parents. We ask parents to comment on their child's responses to a range of 50 common environmental sounds and the increasing ability to identify these sounds. Immediately following the initial fitting of the device, many children show an awareness of environmental sounds. The ability to identify sounds and to monitor the environment through audition develops more slowly. Completing the questionnaire enables parents to document listening progress when their child may be unable to cooperate with more formal tests. Our findings show that although there is a wide variation amongst children, the vast majority of children learn to monitor their non-linguistic environment via audition over the first year following implantation.

Monitoring progress through parental reports

Parents provide more general information through structured interviews. These allow parents more freedom to explain their observations than is possible within the questionnaire format. Interviews take place prior to implantation and then annually asking about their expectations of the device. Parents are asked about the changes seen in the year after implantation. The probing investigates communication skills, spoken language, listening skills (for speech and environmental sounds) and behaviour.

Summary and conclusions

Cochlear implantation is a well-established means to manage children with profound hearing impairments who are unable to benefit from conventional hearing aids. It is a complex process requiring long-term commitment to rehabilitation, and harnessing the skills of many professionals. However, these skills have much in common with those required to manage profoundly deaf children who are able to benefit from hearing aids. The Nottingham programme is founded on the concept that management of cochlear implant children is an expansion of that provided for profoundly deaf hearing-aid users. It also supports the need to provide circumstances in which normal, everyday situations can be utilised to facilitate the learning of communication skills through the new sensation of hearing.

An important element of the rehabilitation programme is the monitoring of progress over a period of at least five years after implantation. This ensures adequate device performance, identifies problems and sets suitable expectations for parents and professionals local to the child. A wide range of tests is needed because the ages of children implanted in Nottingham are often low, and their linguistic status varies from preverbal through transitional to having functional language. The tests include measures of sound perception, word discrimination and speech production and vocalisation. Many of these tests were specifically developed by our team for this purpose.

Appropriate expectations are important for rehabilitation. Results from children implanted below the age of five years, whether congenitally deaf or deafened after a period of normal hearing, indicate that most children will develop spoken language to communicate effectively with normal-hearing people. In general, this status is reached after approximately five years. Based on our experience, outcomes appear to be less promising for children implanted at older than five years, but further data are required to confirm this observation. Our hope is that earlier implantation will be the rule in future. As more children are implanted at a younger age, and as children with additional handicaps are included in implant programmes rehabilitation programmes will need to adapt both their methods and expectations.

Acknowledgements

The authors wish to acknowledge the substantial input to the work described in this chapter from all members of the Nottingham Paediatric

Cochlear Implant Team. Special thanks are due to Dee Dyar, Margaret Tait and Tracey Twomey for their helpful comments on an earlier draft of this text. Invaluable advice and assistance were provided by David Marshall of the Institute of Hearing Research, who also analysed the resource utilisation of the programme. Parts of the research outlined in this chapter were supported by the Hearing Research Trust, 330/332 Gray's Inn Road, London WC1X 8EE.

References

Archbold S (1994) Monitoring progress in children at the pre-verbal stage. In McCormick B, Archbold S, Sheppard S (Eds) Cochlear Implants for Young Children. London: Whurr, pp 197–213.

Bruner JS (1983) Child's Talk: Learning to Use Language. Oxford: Oxford University Press.

Cooper H (1991) Training and rehabilitation for cochlear implant users. In Cooper H (Ed) Cochlear Implants: A Practical Guide. London: Whurr, pp 219–39.

Dyar D (1995) Assessing auditory and linguistic performances in low verbal implanted children. Advances in Otolaryngology, in press.

Geers AE, Moog JS (1991) Evaluating the benefits of cochlear implants in an educational setting. American Journal of Otology 12: 116–25.

Goin DW, Parisier SC (1991) Implementing a cochlear implant team in private practice or academic setting. American Journal of Otology 12: 213–17.

Hellman SA, Chute PM, Kretschmer RE, Nevins ME, Parisier SC, Thurston LC (1991) The development of a children's implant profile. American Annals of the Deaf 136(2): 77–81.

Ling D (1988) Foundations of Spoken Language for Hearing Impaired Children. Washington DC: Alexander Graham Bell Association for the Deaf.

Lloyd H. (1994). Family perspectives. In McCormick B, Archbold S, Sheppard S (Eds) Cochlear Implants for Young Children. London: Whurr, pp 269–84.

McCormick B (1977) The Toy Discrimination Test: an aid for screening the hearing of children above a mental age of two years. London: Public Health 91: 67–9.

McCormick B (1991) Paediatric cochlear implantation in the United Kingdom – a delayed journey on a well marked route. British Journal of Audiology 25: 145–9.

McCormick B, Archbold S, Sheppard S (1994) Cochlear Implants for Young Children. London: Whurr.

Osberger MJ, Robbins AM, Berry SW, Todd L, Hesketh LJ, Sedey A (1991) Analysis of spontaneous speech samples of children with a cochlear implant or tactile aid. American Journal of Otology 12 (Suppl): 151–64.

Ousey J, Sheppard S, Twomey T, Palmer AR (1989) The IHR-McCormick Automated Toy Discrimination Test – description and initial evaluation. British Journal of Audiology 23: 245–9.

Robbins A (1990) Developing meaningful auditory integration in children with cochlear implants. Volta Review 92: 361–70.

Somers MN (1991) Effects of cochlear implants in children: implications for rehabilitation. In Cooper H (Ed) Cochlear Implants: A Practical Guide. London: Whurr, pp 322-45.

Summerfield Q, Palmer AR, Foster JR, Marshall DH, Twomey T (1994) Clinical evaluation and test–retest reliability of the IHR-McCormick Automated Toy Discrimination Test. British Journal of Audiology 28: 165–79.

Tait DM (1987) Making and monitoring progress in the pre-school years. Journal of the British Association for Teaching of the Deaf 11: 143–53.

Tait DM (1993) Video analysis: a method of assessing changes in pre-verbal and early linguistic communication following cochlear implantation. Ear and Hearing 14: 378–89.

Tait DM, Lutman ME (1994) Comparison of early communicative behavior in young children with cochlear implants and with hearing aids. Ear and Hearing 15: 352–61.

Tait DM, Wood DJ (1987) From communication to speech in deaf children. Children Language Teaching and Therapy 3(1): 1–16.

Tye-Murray N (1993) Aural rehabilitation and patient management. In Tyler RS (Ed) Cochlear Implants: Audiological Foundations. San Diego, CA: Singular, pp 87–143.

Chapter 4
An Integrated Rehabilitation Concept for Cochlear Implant Children

BODO BERTRAM

Introduction

A profound hearing impairment in early childhood has lasting and serious effects on the development of the personality of affected children. This is because important stimuli needed for normal development are not accessible (Alich, 1987). To limit the consequences of hearing handicap as much as possible, it is essential to obtain an early diagnosis. This will help to define the type and aetiology of the loss and to quantify the degree of hearing impairment so that critical phases of development can be exploited effectively. This also means that these diagnosed children should be provided immediately, upon detection, with technically high-quality, well-fitted hearing aids. Also, at that time, extensive and intensive auditory training with educational support must be introduced. Although the emphasis is on the treatment for the child, the interaction with the parents and their cooperation are major prerequisites for successful education of these children (Heinemann, 1984).

The whole child: need for treatment

As early as the 1950s and 1960s, there was evidence suggesting the need for comprehensive psychosocial support of all children, whether they had normal hearing or not. Jussen (1991) says, 'The psychosocial development of a human being is obviously carried out in a relatively uncontrolled sequence of definable stages of development'. Further, he writes, '[development] can be impaired considerably if; for example, there is an unrecognised hearing impairment. The maturational processes that are fixed in the biologic system continue to develop, but without the accompanying, age-appropriate learning processes being carried out' (1991, p 258). Thus, it is essential that diagnosis and treatment of deafness take place as early as possible.

The cochlear implant is, at present, the only option for symptomatic treatment of sensory inner ear deafness for children who, in spite of intensive efforts by parents, doctors and educators and early and adequate hearing aid application, have not obtained enough benefit from hearing aids. It serves to bypass the middle ear and as a functional replacement for the defective cochlea. It accomplishes this with the help of stimulation to the hearing nerve by means of specially configured electric biopotentials (Lehnhardt, 1993). In other words, it should provide (at least) a sensation of hearing to the children who receive it.

Receiving a cochlear implant, however, may not reduce the actual hearing deficit with regard to speech perception because there are many other consequences of hearing loss. Equally important is the fact that acoustic information will continue to be perceived in an incomplete manner because 'Listening is an active process, in which emotion, motivation, concentration and communication are of crucial importance' (Kiphardt, 1989). Consequently, the mere medical treatment of children with cochlear implants is not a responsibly implemented procedure. Rather, an intensive and long-term, special education is necessary which takes into account the educational needs of the hearing-impaired child.

The postoperative rehabilitation of deaf-born or deafened children with a cochlear implant must not be confined only to hearing and speech therapy. In such a case, treatment is deficit orientated and does not consider the needs of the whole child. Our viewpoint is that all facets of personality must receive integrated support.

Results of psycholinguistic research support this idea when reporting that 'structures of perception and behavior are developed in a complex interrelationship between sensorimotor, emotional and social experiences. The inter-linked inventory of experiences operates on the fundamental premise that the interactions of linguistic structures can be constructed' (Jussen, 1991, p 260).

Organisational aspects of postoperative cochlear implant care

Cochlear implantation for congenitally deaf and deafened children is justified only if the following criteria are met. (1) An interdisciplinary approach involving physicians, audiologists, teachers for deaf children, psychologists, movement therapists and parents is guaranteed. (2) Comprehensive educational rehabilitation takes place after the surgery and it involves the parents, who participate actively in the rehabilitation process. (3) Local educators are involved in the rehabilitation after having been instructed by a cochlear implant centre, specifically relating to the auditory-verbal education of the implanted children. (4) The integration of cochlear implant children takes place on an individual basis along with educational and social integration in a speech-intensive environment. (5) Continuous counselling and cooperation with the parents, as well as the psychological well-being of the children, are the main focus of the educational work, and if the availability of professional and competent long-term support is guaranteed. One additional comment: the rehabilitation must not only focus on auditory-verbal aspects but also take the personal development of the child into consideration.

Preoperative evaluations

The selection of children requires consideration of the otological, medical, psychological and educational aspects of hearing impairment. Therefore, the cochlear implantation programme for children in Hannover involves close collaboration between the cochlear implant team at the ENT clinic of the Medical School of Hannover (Medizinische Hochschule Hannover – MHH), the Rehabilitation Center 'Wilhelm Hirte' (Cochlear Implant Center – CIC) Hannover and specialists in other clinics or children centres, as well as teachers or local therapists from the children's home communities. Weeks or even months before conversations take place with the parents at our centre, we contact the local preschool educators, teachers for the deaf or therapists of the children in order to obtain educational, paediatric-neurological and paediatric-psychological reports.

Preoperative visit: baseline studies and counselling

Several examinations and counselling sessions take place at the MHH (see Table 4.1) and at the CIC. The baseline performance is measured by the Hannover Hearing Test (Bertram, 1995) presented in aided and unaided conditions; an assessment of linguistic and motor development specially designed at our centre, a diagnostic questionnaire and a motor development test (Bertram et al., 1994).

The initial counselling is solely for the purpose of supplying information to the parents. For this counselling to take place, it is not necessary for the parents already to have agreed to implantation and it binds them in no way. It serves as a forum for answering questions the parents may have about a cochlear implant and, more specifically, about the potential for their child.

The exchange aims to show parents the possibilities and the limitations of a cochlear implant in an objective and non-threatening way. We discuss their hopes, their doubts, their fears, as well as their motivation and expectations. Discussions also encompass the critical views of deaf organisations. The opinions of these groups are reflected openly. The psychological stress of the parents concerning the eventual support needed for the cochlear implant is also considered. These conversations

Table 4.1: Medical and therapeutic support for children with a cochlear implant at the Cochlear Implant Center (CIC), Hannover

Medical and therapeutic assistance	
• wound healing	• pre-training
• healing of the mastoid area	• first fitting of the speech processor (SP)
• periodic otoscopic examinations of the eardrum	• fine-tuning the speech processor
	• audiometry
	• technical inspection of the speech processor
	• speech therapy measures
	• tests of auditory abilities and oral speech development
	• motor control therapy*
	• occupational training*

Note: *in future

are detailed and always maintained on a confidential basis.

Most of the parents who come to us usually have already taken their children through many otologic and audiologic examinations. They have exhausted, with little success, all the present-day technical possibilities for providing hearing improvement to their children. Thus, we believe it is essential that the parents feel that they have been advised with serious consideration by our specialists.

We provide them with the possibility to form an impression of the rehabilitation work that will take place at the CIC with the help of videos that describe the hospitalisation and show conversations with parents of children who have already been operated on. The addresses and telephone numbers of parents' self-help groups, as well as extensive information materials, are also made available to them at this early visit. The parents are given the opportunity for further consultations before making a decision for or against receiving a cochlear implant for their child. Table 4.2 summarises the contents of the pre-implant discussions.

The multidisciplinary team

In order to guarantee qualified, interdisciplinary, postoperative care, our team consists of 13 specialists, including: two teachers of the deaf, four speech therapists, one speech pathologist, one specialist in education,

Table 4.2: Elements of early counselling at the CIC

Discussion topics:
- history of the hearing impairment
- psychosocial situation of the family
- how the family deals with the hearing impairment of the child
- social environment of the parents
- psychological effects of the child's deafness on the parents
- experiences relating to deafness issues: own and others
- communication styles between parents and child
- motivation of the parents
- expectations of the parents
- willingness to support the postoperative measures
- effectiveness of previous hearing aids, as well as hearing and speech training from the parents' point of view
- prospects for success
- possibilities for integrating into different types of schools

General information:
- educational and medical criteria
- details about the operation (possible risks)
- function and demonstration of the speech processor
- methods for detecting faults in the device
- aims and contents of pre-training for the first fitting of the speech processor
- rehabilitation after the operation
- organisational (logistic) issues
- cooperation between the rehabilitationists, kindergartens, schools and therapists

Other:
- videos
- written material (booklets, instruction leaflets)
- residential possibilities for the parents, as well as the children
- conversation by parents with children already operated on
- parents' self-help group
- open opportunity for further conversations
- no obligation on the part of the parents to make a decision

one movement therapist, one specialist in voice and breath control and three engineers. The CIC, Hannover is a part of the Stiftung Hannoversche Kinderheilanstalt and is supported by the Deutsche Cochlear Implant Gesellschaft e.V. Hannover.

Pre-training after surgery and initial fitting of the processor

The family visits the CIC only a few days after the surgery. This is a precursor to the extended visit they will make during the initial fitting phase which usually takes place six weeks after surgery. In this way, the child is already prepared for the early rehabilitation and has established confidence in coming to the CIC.

Pre-training occurs both at this early visit and at a second training session shortly before we start the initial fitting. The pre-training phase is characterised by several steps. The mother, father or both parents and child stay at the centre for one day where they have the opportunity to participate in the morning activities with other children, parents and therapists. They observe the rehabilitation of several children who already have their implant and see the fitting process with experienced children.

The parents have the opportunity to have discussions with other parents about their own experiences with rehabilitation and school integration of their children (see Table 4.3). Finally, practical training for the fitting takes places with the child.

Six weeks later, the postoperative rehabilitation programme starts with the first fitting of the speech processor. This is a very important moment for the child and parent. During this procedure one must consider, particularly with young children, that a number of factors influence the fitting: the child's fear of being touched in the area of the scar, the fear of the computer and, in particular, the actual headset; the limited ability for concentration and perseverance by the child; the limited ability of the child to cooperate depending on the age of the child; the inability to provide exact estimations of hearing levels (threshold and comfort); and usually the intense attachment to the mother or the father.

Moreover, it is important to consider the emotional strain on the child and parent simply because of the special situation. These considerations point to the need for good cooperation between engineer-audiologist, therapist and parents.

Table 4.3: Techniques applied to encourage parental cooperation

- Individual conversations
- Group discussions
- Role playing
- Consultation
- Instruction
- Family therapy*
- Release from guilt

Note: * in future

Overview of the rehabilitation programme

The CIC cares for 18 children per week, with the mother or father staying in one of three single-family houses. There is a separate building for rehabilitation. Every child participates in 25 lessons of 30 minutes each during the week. The children also have free time to play or do craft activities. This is important for social development. Although we initially plan a 12-week programme for each child, the time frame for the programme to be completed may be as long as two years (see Figure 4.1). This depends mainly on scheduling.

The rehabilitation programme of the centre involves special hearing training, and the development of spoken language and communication skills. The child's cognitive, emotional and social development are also part of the programme; additionally, the children receive rhythm and movement training.

The local specialists who care for the children are invited to be present during the hospitalisation at the Hannover School of Medicine and during discussions and therapy sessions at the CIC. The fact that the teachers come to the CIC on a regular basis shows their intention and desire to actively take responsibility for the ongoing auditory rehabilitation of the children. In this way, the CIC serves a multi-faceted function of linking the hospital, the parents and the institutes for hearing-impaired children.

Special features of the hearing and speech education of children with a cochlear implant

Testimonial reports about children receiving cochlear implants may leave parents with an impression that nearly all problems associated with hearing impairment are gone after implantation. That, of course, is not correct. In the first place, deafness does not disappear simply with the transmission of auditory information because 'cortical recognition, or comprehension of linguistic information, occurs beyond the peripheral analyses which belongs to the neocortical area' (Sendlmeier, 1992 p.9). Even with the help of the implant, auditory input is reduced both quantitatively and qualitatively. Only if the rehabilitation technique matches the technology will there be positive effects from implantation.

It is true that the children 'hear' directly after the first fitting of the speech processor. However, the parents must realise that this does not mean that they understand. This difference is sometimes overlooked. Before children can take advantage of their new ability to perceive auditory speech information through the cochlear implant, they will need a suitable period of listening experience and appropriately long and

PREPARATORY TRAINING FOR THE INITIAL FITTING

INITIAL FITTING OF THE SPEECH PROCESSOR:
DETERMINING AN INDIVIDUALIZED PROGRAM

OBSERVATIONS OF CHILD'S FIRST REACTIONS TO HEARING
DURING WALKING HOURS: ACCEPTANCE OF THE SP

EARLY AUDITORY PERCEPTION
FIRST REACTION OF ACOUSTIC SIGNALS, DEVELOPMENT OF A
SIGNAL-ORIENTATION-WARNING FUNCTION

AUDITORY DISCRIMINATION TRAINING
AID TO STRUCTURED LISTENING EVERYDAY SOUNDS, ANIMAL
SOUNDS, VEHICLE SOUNDS,
ACTION WORDS (WALK, WAKE-UP, SIT DOWN)

DEVELOPMENT OF BASIC SPEECH PERCEPTION
AUDITORY FEEDBACK SELF-MONITORING AND PERCEPTION OF
OTHER SPEAKER'S VOICES: ENCOURAGE BABBLE AND WORD PLAY
USE PHONEME SEQUENCES, INTERJECTIONS, ETC.

OPEN-SET SPEECH TRAINING WITHOUT LIPREADING

DEVELOPMENT OF SPEECH UNDERSTANDING
SUPRASEGMENTALS: NUMBER OF SYLLABLES AND WORDS,
INTONATION, SENTENCES LENGTH SEGMENTALS: PHONEMES,
WORDS, SENTENCES

LONG-TERM GOAL: DEVELOPMENT OF ARTICULATION SKILLS AND
COMPETENCE IN ORAL SPEECH

DEVELOPMENT OF INTEGRATED SPEECH PERCEPTION
ACTIVE COMMUNICATION AT PLAY
PRACTICE OF SPOKEN LANGUAGE AND ITS COGNITION IN DAILY
COMMUNICATION

OTHER ASPECTS INFLUENCING THE CHILD'S PERSONALITY AND
REHABILITATION

- SOCIAL ENVIRONMENT (FAMILY, SCHOOL, ETC.)
- MUSICAL-RHYTHMIC EDUCATION
- MOTOR DEVELOPMENT
- DEGREE OF SUPPORT FOR COGNITIVE, SENSORIMOTOR,
  SOCIAL AND EMOTIONAL DEVELOPMENT
- MEMORY TRAINING–DISCOVERY OF EXTENT AND
  STIMULABILITY OF NEW CAPABILITIES
- "THE ACTION ALWAYS DETERMINES THE CREATION OF
  SPEECH"
- MOTIVATION FOR COMMUNICATION BY MAKING USE OF
  THE VARIOUS SITUATIONS THAT OCCUR IN THE COURSE OF
  THE DAY

Figure 4.1: The Integrated Rehabilitation Concept of the Cochlear Implant Center in Hannover (CIC). Initial hearing/speech education as a developing, integral process with parent participation

intensive hearing and speech training. Admittedly, not all children will be able to develop the abilities needed for open-set speech recognition. This is because every child has very different circumstances.

The hearing and speech education of these children starts under very different conditions compared with those of normal-hearing children. One of the most important considerations for developing the ability to recognise speech is the delayed activation of the auditory pathways. This means that the development of hearing strategies for the auditory sensory system, which uses electrically evoked hearing patterns, will take time.

The change from using other sensory modalities to using the auditory sense is also difficult. Children first have access only to visual, vibro-tactile, kinesthetic and, depending on the severity of their hearing impairment, some acoustic features of speech. Consequently, in contrast with children who have normal-hearing abilities, congenitally deaf or early deafened children are not equipped with a basic set of auditory capabilities during the period when speech acquisition takes place. They lack the fundamental ability needed for localising sound sources, listening in noise, identifying different speakers, identifying events that are directly associated with acoustic events and auditory closure (Lindner, 1991).

With a cochlear implant, the possibility arises for these children to use the genetic potential of the brain and to initiate its function with adequate stimuli from the environment, i.e. sounds and speech (Radigk, 1987).

Auditory perception will gradually develop, starting from the development of elementary capabilities for the perception of acoustic characteristics, and continue with the development of high-level strategies of hearing for speech understanding. This includes the step-by-step development of the phonemic-phonologic and semantic-lexical levels of speech as well as its syntactic-morphologic and pragmatic levels.

The alert rehabilitation team realises that there are many factors involved in the training process. This makes it difficult to design a single rehabilitation programme that is applicable to all children. Other considerations are voice production and whether the child even uses the basic function of vocalisation. Characteristics of speech such as voicing onset and breath control enter into the strategy for rehabilitation. General body tension is also a factor and may require movement therapy (see Figure 4.2).

Articulation, the ability to produce different phonemes and the type of phoneme errors will guide therapeutic choices. Language development, linguistic understanding and the appropriate use of linguistic structures which are demonstrated through spontaneous speech will lead to different needs for each child. The child's attention span directly affects rehabilitation. Seemingly, nothing can be overlooked. Lipreading ability, reading ability, gross and fine motor skills, and oral speech skills all interact to support specific training paradigms. Table 4.4 lists some of the activities applied to children in our centre. All of these factors are influenced by the emotional and cognitive development of the child, his/her social behaviour and environment and how he/she interacts in the classroom, i.e. how the child deals with changing environments. Also the rehabilitation approach should consider the circumstances in which these children live their daily lives with their families and the children's general learning abilities and willingness to cooperate in the education setting (auditory/verbal, manual/signing).

The role of parents in the process of rehabilitation

Close collaboration with parents is an important requirement for a high level of postoperative success. Therefore, they need sufficient information about both the possibilities and the limitations of the cochlear implant. They, ultimately, will be responsible for the effective development of high verbal skills that are associated with good speech and spoken language.

The parents should realise that only after an adequate period of rehabilitation can they expect improvement in voice quality, more exactness

Table 4.4: Support given to cochlear implant children at the CIC

Special educational support

Auditory-verbal education:
- hearing education
- hearing training
- development of perception: self and others
- initiation of speech
- development of speech understanding
- correction of speech production
- training of memory
- cognitive education

Movement training: perceptual motor activities:
- rhythmic and musical education
- training of movement

Education of behaviour:
- social behaviour
- emotional education
- group play

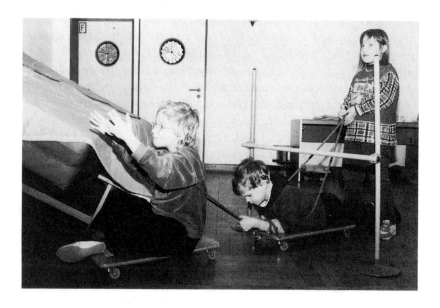

Figure 4.2: Movement therapy

of articulation, an increase in the repertoire of phonetic abilities and better language abilities (Mecklenburg, 1988).

The role of the teacher

Teachers and therapists need to support the parents' efforts in finding an acceptable means of promoting communication skills in their young child. This takes place step by step and is based on a model of auditory-verbal, interactive communication. It may be difficult to implement because the majority of the parents have used sign language to communicate with their children. It requires significant change by the parents in their communication strategy and also the time needed to make the change. One of the primary responsibilities of the teacher is to provide good guidance to the parents during this transitional phase. The teachers and therapists must have confidence that parents are able to learn the new communication strategy and they must trust in the child's abilities. Experts can guide the parents in the best way to achieve these goals.

Conclusion

The task of providing paediatric rehabilitation is constantly in a state of reassessment regarding the training of auditory speech perception and the use of auditory/oral methods of communication. We, as rehabilitationists, would like to believe that our methods provide children with the opportunity to make the best use of their implant. However, the development for each child is dependent on many factors, which include onset of deafness (pre-, peri- or postlingually deafened), duration of deafness, age when the implant was surgically placed, the degree of functionality left in the auditory system and the intellectual abilities of the child. These organic factors are influenced by the development of the child's personality, the circumstances surrounding education and the family's background. Further, the intensity of the special educational intervention and the conditions at school and its social environment will have an effect on the maturational process of the child.

The philosophy at the CIC is to provide holistic treatment and real-world experience for each individual child. The programme provides special support for children, parents, teachers and other involved individuals. Receiving the implant and the speech processor are only the first steps towards the new world of hearing. The CIC has an ongoing programme that continues to provide information and service to cochlear implant users and their families throughout their lives.

To understand the individual child as a unique personality who has integrity, to give him/her a feeling of high regard, of love and security and to meet that child with respect for his/her feelings and emotions, without considering him/her simply as an object that has deficits requiring educational intervention and theoretical considerations, should be the rehabilitationist's maxim. That is, in spite of all the rehabilitation measures and intentions, the growing child must, as a first priority, be what it is meant to become: a personality, who wins the world through inquisitiveness and creativity, with confidence and pleasure.

A final remark. It should naturally follow that those concerned with the child's rehabilitation accept the parents of these children as competent partners who have great personal experiences concerning their child's hearing impairment and the associated difficulties gathered through daily contact with their child. This means that there must exist an open, serious dialogue for understanding their hopes and their worries. In the end, there must be the establishment of a high priority for supporting and maintaining a safe and broad parent–child relationship.

References

Alich G (1987) Zur Problematik der Terminologie bei Höegeschaedigten. In Gegner U (Ed) Orientierungen der Höergeschaädigtenpaedagogik. Journal Hörgeschädigtenpädagogik (Suppl), 21: 11–22.

Bertram B (1995) Hannover Hörtest. Medizinische Hochschule Hannover, unpublished dissertation.

Bertram B, Irion A, Maneke J, Sefke S (1994) Diagnostikbogen zur Sprachentwicklung. Hannover, Germany: Cochlear Implant Center.

Heinemann M (1984) Hörgeräteversorgung bei Kindern. Tagungsbericht: Erziehung zur Sprache im Wandel. In Proceedings from the Berufsverband Deutscher Hoergeschaedigtenpaedagogen, 12–14 May, Leipzig, p 111.

Jussen H (1991) Hörgeschädigtenpädagogik im Wandel. Hörgeschädigtenpädagogik 45: 258–66.

Kiphardt E (1989)Vorwort des Herausgebers. In Olbrich I, Auditive Wahrnehmung und Sprache. Dortmund:Verlag Modernes Lernen.

Lehnhardt E (1993) Cochlear Implantate bei Kindern. HNO-aktuell 1(1): 19.

Lindner G.(1991). Frühkindlich erworbene Fähigkeiten zur Invarientenbildung als Basis für die Lautsprach-perzeption Stuttgart/New York: Georg Thieme Verlag, pp 152–6.

Mecklenburg DJ (1988) Cochlear implants in children: nonmedical considerations. American Journal of Otology 9(2):163–8.

Radigk W (1987) Kognitive Entwicklung und zerebrale Disfunktion. Dortmund: Verlag modernes lernen, p 17.

Sendlmeier F (1992) Sprachverarbeitung bei pathologischem Gehör . Stuttgart/New York: Georg Thieme Verlag.

Chapter 5
Parent- and Patient-Centred Aural Rehabilitation

NANCY TYE-MURRAY, LINDA SPENCER, SHELLEY WITT, ELIZABETH GILBERT BEDIA

Introduction

The mission of the cochlear implant programme at the University of Iowa Hospitals is twofold: to provide clinical services to profoundly deafened individuals and to conduct research related to cochlear implant efficacy. Table 5.1 presents an overview of the cochlear implant programme, indicating the stages of the cochlear implant process and the professionals involved at each stage (Tye-Murray, 1993). In this chapter, we will focus only on the sixth stage, aural rehabilitation. We provide rehabilitation services to children's families, young cochlear-implant users and adult cochlear-implant users.

Description of patient population

Both adults and children are implanted at the University of Iowa Hospitals. Most of the recipients do not live in Iowa City or the surrounding communities, so they must travel a fair distance to receive services. As a result, many of the aural rehabilitation services that we provide were designed for use in the patient's home, community setting or during a short training period at the Center (anywhere from two hours to several days). For children, staff at the cochlear implant centre primarily serve as consultants for educators and parents.

With a few exceptions, most of the children in our programme use simultaneous communication (speech and manually coded English) and are prelingually deafened. This means that they had a profound, bilateral hearing loss before the age of 24 months. They live in their home community and attend a public school. They range from age 2 to 13 years at the time of implantation.

Table 5.1: Six stages of the Iowa Cochlear Implant Program and the personnel involved with each stage (see Tye-Murray, 1993, for more details)

Stage/Personnel	Description
Initial contact: Clinical coordinator	Provide general information about cochlear implants and candidacy to those who contact the cochlear implant centre
Pre-implant: Audiologist	Provide specific information about counselling candidacy, benefits, commitments and cochlear implant hardware/software to potential candidates
Formal evaluation: Audiologist, surgeon, psychologist, speech-language pathologist	Perform medical, hearing, speech, language and psychological evaluation to determine candidacy
Surgery: Surgeon	Implant the internal hardware
Fitting: Audiologist	Fit the device and provide instruction about use and maintenance
Aural rehabilitation: Cochlear implant speech-language pathologist, school speech-language pathologist, audiologist, classroom teacher	Provide auditory training, speechreading training, speech and language therapy, counselling and communication strategies training

Parent-centred intervention

Our parent-centred aural rehabilitation efforts are based on two premises. The first is that parents or primary caretakers must be intimately involved in a child's post-implantation programme. We have learned that although an involved family does not necessarily guarantee a successful cochlear implant user, a child will probably not be a successful user without one. Here, we define success as gains made on speech, language and audiological measures. Involved parents demonstrate all or many of the following behaviours. They ensure that the child wears the cochlear implant regularly and that it is in good working order. They provide consistent auditory speech stimulation and a good language model, and stimulate the child's language production (see Table 5.2). They engage their child frequently in conversation and maintain regular contact with school personnel. Finally, involved parents participate in the development and implementation of the child's educational programme. A primary goal of our parent-centred intervention is to nurture parental involvement.

The second premise of our parent-centred aural rehabilitation is that conversation during everyday activities is one of the most effective means to develop a child's listening, speaking and language skills following implantation (see Tye-Murray, 1994, for a representative conversation training programme). Parents are encouraged to become effective conversational partners, in part by adhering to the guidelines presented

Table 5.2: Techniques that parents can use to stimulate their child's language development*

Signaling expectation	Wait for the child's response. Indicate a response is expected, by tilting the head and raising eyebrows
Describing: self-talk	Use an event or idea the child is interested in and describe aspects. Illustrate that language to organise, analyse and direct actions by talking through the process aloud. The child has access to the thoughts
Parallel-talk: modelling and expansion	An adult provides language to an activity a child is performing. An adult copies the meaning of a child's utterances but modifies/expands the grammar of the message
Question stimulation	An adult uses questions to provide the child with models of how to ask and answer questions
Time talk	Linking time words to events or routines that are significant to a child to help the child develop the concept and language of time
Violation of a routine	Changing an established routine to draw out a comment and promote longer and more complex messages on the child's part
Withholding or hiding an object	Keeping an important object or item to stimulate the language used for requests
Natural reinforcement	Monitor the child's language and give reinforcement for attempts to use language appropriately
Reading	Use reading to build vocabulary, make predictions and illustrate different language and grammatical forms

*A complete description is available in Spencer (1994), pp 51–84.

in Table 5.3. They also are encouraged to create many listening experiences, in the context of everyday conversations with their child (Tye-Murray, 1992a). For instance, waking up in the morning might be transformed into a sound detection activity. In this case, the young child listens beneath the covers for the mother to say, 'peek-a-boo' (Tye-Murray & Fryauf-Bertschy, 1992).

Assessment

The parent-intervention programme has two components, assessment and training. In the assessment component, the primary caretaker's (usually the mother's) simultaneous communication skills and conversational styles are assessed, with both a play session and a sign language test battery, which includes a 61-sentence expressive test and an open-set adaptation of the Carolina Picture Vocabulary Test (Layton & Holmes, 1985).

For the play session, the parent and child engage in unstructured play with age-appropriate toys and games (e.g. play dough, toy cars, tea set) for two 10-minute play periods. The parent is instructed to play naturally and communicate with the child as she would at home. Each play session is audio-video recorded, and later orthographically transcribed and coded. The results provide information about both the parent and the child.

The results of the communication-styles coding are interesting because they allow us to relate communication style to cochlear implant performance. They also provide direction for intervention. Wallace and colleagues (1994) found that parents who use language that is informative, who respond to the child's utterance and stimulate conversation counteract the risk factor of delayed language development in children with otitis media. The use of language that is directive, non-responsive and non-informing is less effective. These results suggest that parents should be encouraged to be active and assertive conversational partners.

Our work to date suggests that parents and children vary widely in their communication styles and that parents vary in their signing skills (Bedia, Tye-Murray & Spencer, 1995). In our study, videotaped play sessions for 19 pre-operative children playing either with their mother or father were collected. The children ranged in age between 2;2 years, and 7;4 years.

The videotaped samples of parent/child dyads were orthographically transcribed and coded for the following measures: the mode of communication used, assertive-responsive utterance profile and grammatical measures. Grammatical measures included total number of words produced, total number of unique words produced, percentage of errors made in sign, type/token ratio, mean length of utterance in

Table 5.3: Some conversational strategies for adults who interact with young cochlear implant users (adapted from Tye-Murray, 1994, pp 11–50)

---

1. *Allow your child to choose what to talk about, and respond to the communicative attempts*. Observe the child's focus of attention, and try to talk about what your child is doing and topics that interest your child. Make your remarks contingent upon your child's utterances. If your child is primarily non-verbal, respond to the child's facial expressions, gestures and unintelligible vocalisations as if they were conversational turns

2. *Encourage your child to tell narratives and stories, and to give directions*. During conversations, we take extended turns, telling narratives and stories. Encourage your child to tell narratives with such phrases as, 'Tell me more', 'Then what happened?' and 'Who did this?'. Use visual props, such as a quickly drawn sketch, to encourage your child to tell who, what, where, when and why as you refer to the picture

3. *Organise your messages*. An organised message is not verbose and does not have complex verbiage (e.g. the sentence, 'The sweater which we bought last Christmas is still in the box under the bed' is an example of complex verbiage). Important keywords and phrases are repeated, and terminology is precise (e.g. 'The book is on the table' rather than, 'It's over there'). Telegraphic speech, such as the sentence, 'Boy fall on table, got ouch, and cry', is avoided

4. *Speak with clear speech*. Clear speech is characterised by a somewhat slowed speaking rate and good (although not exaggerated) enunciation. Keywords are emphasised, and pauses are inserted at clause boundaries.

5. *Speak positively and avoid critical language*. Critical language is characterised by casting the child in a negative light, or being unduly critical of the child's actions and behaviours. By using positive language and using such words as *can* rather than *cannot* and *do* rather than *don't*, children might be motivated to participate in conversations

6. *Do not over-control your conversations*. Parents who over-control their conversations may ask too many questions, may not respond to their child's utterances, may label excessively (e.g 'Ball. That's a ball. Bat. That's a wooden bat.'), may often correct their child's speech production or language, may recurrently ask their child to imitate their speech and language models and may often change the topic of conversation. Children may respond to these behaviours by becoming passive, helpless or withdrawing from the conversation

---

morphemes, bound morphemes used, and whether messages were signed or voiced, or both.

Each utterance of the child and the parent was also coded according to Fey's coding system (1986, pp 72–3). Assertive conversational acts were labelled as either requestives (utterances that solicit information or actions) or assertives (utterances that label, report facts, state rules or provide an explanation). Responsive conversational acts were defined as utterances that provide requested information, or an acknowledgment of an assertive or performative utterance.

The results were organised to assess mode of communication, parents' accuracy in signing, and conversational styles of parents and child. The findings revealed three important points. First, that parents who reported using simultaneous communication actually used a verbal-only mode 62% of the time with no sign support, thus they may be presenting an incomplete language model to their children in the chosen mode of communication. Second, the parents who did use speech and sign more consistently had children with longer mean length of utterance ($r = 0.436$, $p = 0.05$). Finally, results on the assertive-responsive continuum revealed that parents who had produced relatively large percentages of responsive acts tended to have children who produced longer mean length of utterance.

In summary, this study underscores the importance of providing opportunity for parents to become proficient in their chosen communication mode and encourages parents to foster their children's abilities in becoming active communication partners who can initiate conversation and request information.

Training

The parent-centred training programme is outlined in Table 5.4 (Tye-Murray & Kelsay, 1993). The goals of the programme are to provide instruction about how to maximise children's potential to benefit from their cochlear implants. Parents receive instruction about maintenance of the cochlear implant, effective communication behaviours (including how to repair breakdowns in communication), informal auditory and speechreading training, and language development strategies (Table 5.2). The programme has three components: (1) an introduction to cochlear implant use; (2) a two-day parent seminar (Kelsay et al., 1993); and (3) an eight-week home training programme that includes computerised activities and workbook exercises (Kelsay & Tye-Murray, 1993).

Child-centred intervention

Speech–language pathologists can anticipate that young cochlear implant recipients will require an intense therapy schedule following implantation. Listening and speech skills do not emerge spontaneously as a result of children being exposed to conversation in their environments. A concerted, deliberate rehabilitation effort is required before they learn to utilise the electrical signal from the implant for speech recognition and speech acquisition.

An ideal therapy plan integrates auditory goals with goals for speech production, language acquisition and classroom curriculum. Administrative support from the child's special education programme is essential in casework management. This is because there is a critical need for

Table 5.4: Overview of the Parent-centered Training Program (Kelsay et al., 1993)

Introduction to cochlear implant use (1–2 months post-implantation):
- parents and audiologist develop daily schedule for child to wear the implant
- parents receive training about troubleshooting procedures
- parents learn how speech, language and auditory training can be integrated into daily routines
- parents receive printed materials (Appendices A, B, C) and are invited to use the department's patient library

Parent seminar (10 months post-implantation, for 2 days):
- parents receive instruction about various topics pertaining to implant use
- parents watch audiovideotaped examples of communication breakdowns and repair strategies
- parents participate in group discussions
- parents practise concepts, critique themselves, share experiences and provide support to one another

Home-training programme (10 months post-implantation, for 8 weeks):
- computerised training station consisting of computer, laser videodisc player and touchscreen monitor is sent home
- parents complete computerised exercises and employ repair strategies and other strategies that facilitate effective communication behaviour
- parents complete workbook activities as a complement to the computer training exercises (Kelsay et al., 1993)
- the aural rehabilitation specialist calls parents once a week to answer questions and ensure compliance with the programme

networking between family, classroom teachers, audiologists, speech –language pathologists, and additional cochlear implant and educational team members. Although each child's pattern of progress is individual, the level of therapy should remain high for a prolonged interval, even as long as five years. The speech–language pathologist has the unique challenge of maintaining the child's interest and motivation to achieve goals over years of therapy time.

The key to devising a successful therapy plan begins with assessment. We provide assessment and input for devising goals in three key areas: speech perception, speech production and language comprehension and expression.

Speech Perception

Assessment includes evaluating a child's skills in the areas of both speechreading and recognition of the auditory signal. The assessment battery applies at least three tests: the Audiovisual Speech Feature Test (Tyler, Fryauf-Bertschy & Kelsay, 1991), the Word Intelligibility Picture Identification Test (WIPI) (Ross & Lerman, 1971) and the Repeated Frame Sentence Test (Tye-Murray, 1993). The Audio visual Speech

Feature Test assesses how well a child can utilise five consonantal features of articulation (i.e. nasality, voicing, frication, place of articulation and duration) for speech recognition. The WIPI assesses closed-set word recognition, while the Repeated Frame Sentence Test assesses sentence-level speech recognition skills. The tests are administered in an audition-only, vision-only, and/or audition-plus-vision condition.

One way to organise speech perception training is to frame goals around the type and amount of auditory and visual cues needed to recognise speech (Appendix A). Cues may be organised in a hierarchical order, but goals can be targeted so that they overlap. For example, because /b/ and /m/ differ in manner but are visibly similar, one provides an extra visual cue of placing the fingertips at the side of the nose when producing the /m/ sound. Eventually this visual cue is reduced as the child learns to distinguish /b/ from /m/ using auditory cues. Auditory training programmes that we recommend include those developed by Stout and Windle (1986) and Tye-Murray and Fryauf-Bertschy (1992). For speechreading training, we use the programme described by Tye-Murray (1992b, 1992c). We also send computerised laser-video disc speechreading programmes home with some children, so they complete training exercises in the home during an eight-week period (Tye-Murray & Kelsay, 1993; Tye-Murray et al., 1988). This, of course, requires that the family has access to a laser-video player.

Speech Production

Speech production testing includes tasks that measure accuracy of phoneme production, and intelligibility of words, phonemes and narratives. In addition, we assess children's abilities to produce suprasegmental aspects of speech.

Assessment measures yield a phonetic transcription of elicited and spontaneous speech. These analyses are then categorised by traditional error analysis and phonological error pattern analysis. Traditional analysis provides an inventory of sounds produced as well as a list of deletions, substitutions and distortions. Phonological error analysis provides an inventory of phonological process errors, such as final consonant deletion, cluster reduction and fronting. Based on phonetic inventory and analysis of phonological process errors, possible therapy goals are suggested. Goals may be based on the hierarchy provided by Ling (1976, 1978) and additionally may include a suggestion to target a reduction of phonological process errors, most commonly final consonant deletion and cluster reduction. We encourage the child's speech–language pathologist to increase use of auditory modelling combined with a visual or tactile model. We also suggest the elimination of the visual and tactile models when the child has learned to associate the auditory signal with a specific sound.

Group data from our implant patients provide a basis for comparing results of individual children. Deviations from the average performance act as a guide when suggesting therapy goals. For instance, results to date on the production version of the Audiovisual Feature Test suggest that changes in children's speech production may occur gradually. Information transmission analysis of our data (Eguchi & Hirsch, 1969; Miller & Nicely, 1955; Tye-Murray & Spencer, 1995) reveal how well the child's speech conveyed the features of place of articulation, voicing, duration, frication and nasality. We found that little change occurred before the child had 12 months of experience. For this reason, we counsel children's speech–language pathologists and families to be patient but persistent in encouraging speech skills to emerge. The information from data such as these have also led us to target some sounds earlier than traditional methods suggest. We specifically suggest targeting fricatives earlier, because they occur more frequently within the English language, and are typically perceived and produced better by cochlear implant users compared with hearing aid users.

The Fundamental Speech Skills Test (FSST) (Levitt, Youdelman & Head, 1990) was designed to assess breath stream capacity, elementary articulation, pitch control, syllabification, stress and intonation contour. The results from this test, on our population, suggest that children who use cochlear implants tend to perform better than hearing aid users on these speech parameters relatively quickly. In particular, prosodic speech parameters appear to improve soon. As a result, the child's speech–language pathologist and family are told to look for increases in the child's ability to produce intonation contours and to imitate the melody and rhythm of speech. When these changes become apparent, the speech–language pathologist can explain to parents that these abilities are precursors to the development of specific sounds, and suggest that there will be later gains in speech intelligibility.

Receptive and Expressive Language

The language test battery provides an assessment of receptive and expressive semantic and syntactic skills. The language procedure that we usually apply is the spontaneous language sample analysis. The test protocol calls for a 12-minute language sample to be elicited during a play activity or conversation with the speech–language pathologist (Wisconsin Department of Public Instruction, 1992). This sample is videotaped and later transcribed using an orthographic transcription. The Systematic Analysis of Language Transcripts (SALT) (Miller & Chapman, 1991) provides a measure of total utterances produced by the child in 12 minutes, children's Type–Token ratio, mean length of utterance (MLU), and use of questions, negatives, conjunctions, model auxiliary forms (i.e. could, would, should) and pronouns. The SALT analysis also provides a distribution of incomplete, unintelligible and non-verbal utterances, the number and length of pauses and speaking rate, lists and frequencies of word roots and morphemes, distribution of speaker turns by length of consecutive utterances and types of mazes (fillers, repetitions and reformulations).

The speech–language pathologist on the cochlear implant team compiles the language test results and presents them in a report summary that is available to the parents, school speech–language pathologist and classroom teacher. Included in the report is an inventory of sentence structures that are understood and produced, as well as a measure of mean length of utterance. Specific suggestions for language goals are also made and incorporated into the report. Language goals from our cochlear implant centre emphasise the development of English syntax and semantics. This is partly because children with good language skills are most likely to demonstrate improvement in speech production and speech perception skills.

Implementation of language goals is encouraged through naturalistic language stimulation that occurs in conversation, during story telling or during play. For younger children, vocabulary development is stressed, as well as comprehension and use of conjunctions, pronouns and modals. The use of correct morpheme endings to mark verb tense, plurals and possessives is also an appropriate goal. This is because children who have cochlear implants have an excellent capacity to perceive many bound morpheme markers such as simple past tense /t/ and plurals /s, z/ in English.

In older children, the oral-to-written language technique for language development (as outlined in the series by Cahill and Hrebic, 1990) is sometimes suggested as an option for the school to use. The local speech–language pathologist might videotape a child's short narrative, and then review the story with the child. The child is instructed to transcribe verbatim from the videotape. Such activities offer the child a chance to view, listen and then write his or her own language. Specific language error patterns can be identified by the child with guidance from the school speech–language pathologist and/or classroom teacher. The transcription is made available for revision, editing and final publication in classroom newsletters or child portfolios, and can be used for oral production practice.

Interactions with Educators

School authorities receive reports that provide test results and suggestions for therapy goals after analysing information gained at the annual speech and language evaluation. School personnel are encouraged to call members of the cochlear implant centre staff with questions or comments. Collaborative meetings are sometimes held via telephone or in person to establish information exchange networks. When possible, the cochlear implant centre speech–language pathologist visits the school to observe the child and to provide an in-service training. We offer direct therapy suggestions, consultation and input for the child's goal plan, which is known as the Individualized Educational Plan (IEP). A sample plan that integrates classroom goals with IEP goals is shown in Appendix B.

Rehabilitation for adult cochlear implant users

Some adults require little if any intervention after their cochlear implants are fitted, and/or they do not want it. Other users both need and desire it. Two components of our adult aural rehabilitation programme are speech perception training (auditory and speechreading training) and communication strategies training.

Assessment

The three indices we use when assessing rehabilitation needs or when assessing the efficacy of intervention are the Iowa Consonant Test (Tyler, Preece & Tye-Murray, 1986), the Iowa Sentence Test (Tyler, Preece & Tye-Murray, 1986), and the Sentence Gist Recognition Test (Tye-Murray, Witt & Castelloe, 1995).

The Consonant Test requires the patient to identify 13 consonants in an /aCa/ context. An information transmission analysis (Miller & Nicely, 1955) indicates which features of articulation (e.g. voicing, duration, frication) a client can perceive relatively well and which features a client perceives relatively poorly. The group performance results of one subset of Nucleus patients tested in our centre indicate that, on average, patients tend to utilise the nasality and voicing features relatively well and the place feature relatively poorly. The results also indicate that performance improves over time, especially during the first nine months. The fact that performance changes suggests that patients are learning to use the electrical signal. As such, the potential exists for speech perception training to accelerate and enhance this learning process for adult users. The following example illustrates how a clinician might use group performance data to customise a speech perception training programme. A clinician tests a client and finds that she performs poorly on all of the features. The clinician's first training objectives would focus on helping the client to discriminate and recognise nasality and voicing features. The clinician would not expect the client to make place of articulation distinctions until later in the training programme.

The Iowa Sentence Test comprises 100 sentences spoken by 20 talk-ers. Results of this test provide average data against which other patients are compared. One way that a clinician may use such a test for planning an aural rehabilitation programme is to administer it in both a vision-only and an audition-plus-vision condition. If the client is at or below the norm, the client probably has the potential to benefit from speechreading training. A reasonable goal for the clinician is to move the client's performance up to the mid-range performance of the other clients. On the other hand, if a client falls way above the norm, the clinician might want to focus attention on auditory training and forego speechreading training.

The Sentence Gist Recognition Test is a computer-assisted test with the client seated before a touch-screen monitor. First, a film clip is shown to establish a context for the sentences to be speechread. For instance, one film clip shows two people walking towards a concession stand. In the next clip, a woman with a food service uniform appears and says, 'Would you like some candy?'. Immediately thereafter, a six-split picture screen appears. The client must touch the picture that best represents what the talker said. If they did not correctly recognise the utterance, five repair strategies (repeat, rephrase, simplify, elaborate or say one word) appear on the screen. The client chooses a repair strategy and tries to identify the picture again. If a client touches the say-one-word repair strategy the woman appears and says, 'Candy'. This procedure continues until the sentence is correctly identified or until all six pictures have been touched. Test materials are stored on a laser videodisc that is interfaced with an IBM Infowindow computer and monitor.

We have found a few adult cochlear implant users who perform as well as the average patient on the Iowa Sentence Test where they must repeat words verbatim, but who perform below average on this Sentence Gist Recognition Test. One interpretation of such a pattern of test results is that the client may be more of an analytic speechreader than a synthetic speechreader. That is, the client may listen for the purpose of identifying every word rather than capturing the gist (meaning) of the message. During aural rehabilitation, this patient might be encouraged to relax more when speechreading, and to be more willing to guess about a message.

The majority of clients select the repeat repair strategy when they do not recognise a sentence during the Sentence Gist Recognition Test (see also Tye-Murray, Purdy & Woodworth, 1992; Tye-Murray, Witt & Schum, 1995). Interestingly, this strategy is not the most effective for rectifying breakdowns in communication during real-world conversations (Gagné & Wyllie, 1989). Moreover, use of the repeat repair strategy may lead the patient's communication partner to perceive the patient unfavourably (Gagné, Stelmacovich & Yovetich, 1991; Tye-Murray et al., 1995). A client who selects the repeat repair strategy exclusively during the Sentence Gist Recognition Test might be encouraged to use strategies other than repeat during training.

Training

The speech perception home training programme for adult cochlear implant users provides 12 weeks of training. Each week, patients complete three computerised laser videodisc programmes, one book-on-tape activity and one real-world exercise (Appendix C). To complete each exercise requires 15 to 20 minutes per day. Patients receive a manual that outlines all of the activities. The manual allows for a quick weekly overview of the activities that will be completed, and gives instructions. The manual also provides important tips about how to be a better speechreader and how to incorporate listening practice into daily life events.

Participants take home a computer training station, consisting of a personal computer, a laser videodisc player, a display/touch screen unit and a small Sony Boom Box for completing book-on-tape activities. They complete a one-day orientation at the University of Iowa Hospitals and Clinics, where they learn to operate the equipment and complete practice exercises to guarantee proper use of the manual.

At the end of each week during the training programme, the client mails paperwork from the book-on-tape and real-world activities to the cochlear implant centre. A clinician maintains a log of the participant's progress and returns the paperwork with written comments, thereby providing feedback. Once a week, a clinician calls the client or a member of the client's family to answer any questions or concerns the client may have, and to ask specific questions about the programme and how it is affecting daily communication interactions.

Final comments

We have assumed a narrow definition of aural rehabilitation by describing only speech perception training, speech and language therapy, and parent training. Other services provided at our clinic also fall within the topic of aural rehabilitation. For instance, counselling is an important component of our programme. Some clients experience disappointment after receiving only limited benefits from their cochlear implant, and require counselling and support from the cochlear implant audiologist or psychologist. Some children refuse to wear the cochlear implant or use it as a means to control parental behaviour. The audiologist, psychologist or speech–language pathologist provides counselling to parents about handling such problems. The aural rehabilitation programme also teaches patients or family members to troubleshoot hardware problems and provides information about the use of assistive devices, such as FM trainers.

Acknowledgements

This work was supported by the National Institutes of Health Grants DC00242 and DC00976–01, Grant RR59 from the General Clinical Research Centers Program, Division of Research Resources NIH, and a grant from the Lions Club of Iowa. The audiological data reported in this chapter were collected in an experimental protocol supervised by Dr Richard S. Tyler.

References

Bedia E, Tye-Murray N, Spencer L (1995) Dyad study: the effect of conversational styles on children with profound hearing loss and their hearing parents. Submitted for publication.

Cahill R, Hrebic H (1990) The Stack the Deck Writing Program. Tinley Park, IL: Stack the Deck.

Eguchi S, Hirsch I (1969) Development of speech sounds in children. Acta Otolaryngologica 257(S): 5–43.

Fey ME (1986) Language Intervention with Young Children. San Diego, CA: College Hill Press.

Gagné J-P, Wyllie KM (1989) Relative effectiveness of three repair strategies on the visual identification of misperceived words. Ear and Hearing 10: 368–74.

Gagné J-P, Stelmacovich P, Yovetich W (1991) Reactions to requests of clarification used by hearing-impaired individuals. Volta 93(3): 129–43.

Kelsay DRM, Tye-Murray N (1993) Five Steps to Improving Your Child's Use of a Cochlear Implant. Training Manual. Iowa City, IA: Department of Otolaryngology–Head and Neck Surgery, University of Iowa Hospitals.

Kelsay DRM, Tye-Murray N, Kirk KI, Schum L (1993) Stepping Out: Activities To Do at Home. Training Manual. Iowa City, IA: Department of Otolaryngology–Head and Neck Surgery, University of Iowa Hospitals.

Layton T, Holmes D (1985) The Carolina Picture Vocabulary Test for Deaf and Hard of Hearing. Austin, TX: Pro-Ed.

Levitt H, Youdelman K, Head K (1990) Fundamental Speech Skills Test. Englewood, CO: Research Point.

Ling D (1976) Speech and the Hearing Impaired Child: Theory and Practice. Washington, DC: AG Bell Association for the Deaf.

Ling D (1978) Workbook for Speech Skills. Washington DC: AG Bell Association for the Deaf.

Miller GA, Nicely PE (1955). Analysis of perceptual confusions among some English consonants. Journal of the Acoustic Society of America 27: 338–52.

Miller JF, Chapman RS (1991) Systematic Analysis of Language Transcripts. Madison, WI: Language Analysis Laboratory, Waisman Center.

Ross M, Lerman J (1971) Word Intelligibility by Picture Identification (Test). St Louis: Audiotec of St Louis.

Spencer L (1994). Some ways to nurture children's conversational and language skills. In Tye-Murray N (Ed) Let's Converse: A How to Guide to Develop and Expand Conversational Skills of Children and Teenagers who are Hearing Impaired. Washington, DC: AG Bell Association for the Deaf, pp 51–84.

Stout GG, Windle JVE (1986) The Developmental Approach to Successful Listening. Houston, TX: DAS.

Tye-Murray N (1992a) Conversing with the implanted child. In Tye-Murray N (Ed) Children with Cochlear Implants: A Handbook for Parents, Teachers, and Speech and Hearing Professionals. Washington, DC: AG Bell Association for the Deaf, pp 61-78.

Tye-Murray N (1992b) Speechreading training. In Tye-Murray N (Ed) Children with Cochlear Implants: A Handbook for Parents, Teachers, and Speech and Hearing Professionals. Washington, DC: AG Bell Association for the Deaf, pp 115–35.

Tye-Murray, N (1992c) Communication Therapy for Hearing-Impaired Children and Teenagers: Speechreading, Listening, and Using Repair Strategies. Austin, TX: Pro-Ed.

Tye-Murray N (1993) Aural rehabilitation and patient management. In Tyler RS (Ed) Cochlear Implants: Audiological Foundations. San Diego, CA: Singular Publishing Group, pp 87–144.

Tye-Murray N (1994) Let's Converse: A How To Guide to Develop and Expand the Conversational Skills of Children and Teenagers who are Hard-of-Hearing. Washington, DC: AG Bell Association for the Deaf.

Tye-Murray N, Fryauf-Bertschy H (1992) Auditory training. In Tye-Murray N (Ed) Cochlear Implants and Children: A Handbook for Parents, Teachers, and Speech and Hearing Professionals. Washington, DC: AG Bell Association for the Deaf, pp 91–114.

Tye-Murray N, Kelsay DR (1993) Communication therapy for parents of cochlear implant users. Volta Review 95: 21–32.

Tye-Murray N, Spencer L (1995) Relationships between speech production and speech perception skills in young cochlear implant users. Journal of the Acoustic Society of America, in press.

Tye-Murray N, Purdy S, Woodworth G (1992) The reported use of communication strategies by members of SHHH and its relationship to client, talker, and situational variables. Journal of Speech and Hearing Research 35: 708–17.

Tye-Murray N, Tyler RS, Bong B, Nares T (1988). Using laser videodisc technology to train speechreading and assertive listening skills. Journal of the Academy of Rehabilitative Audiology 21: 143–52.

Tye-Murray N, Witt S, Castelloe J (1995) Initial evaluation of an interactive test of sentence gist recognition (SGR). Ear and Hearing, submitted for publication.

Tye-Murray N, Witt S, Schum L (1995) Conversational interactions between adult cochlear implant users and both families and unfamiliar communication partners: communication breakdowns, repair strategies, and conversational moves. Ear and Hearing, in press.

Tye-Murray N, Witt S, Schum L, Sobaski C (1995) Communication breakdowns: partner contingencies and partner reactions. Journal of the Academy of Rehabilitative Audiology 25:1–27.

Tyler RS, Fryauf-Bertschy H, Kelsay D (1991) Audiovisual Feature Test for Young Children. Iowa City, IA: Department of Otolaryngology–Head and Neck Surgery, University of Iowa Hospitals.

Tyler RS, Preece JP, Tye-Murray N (1986) The Iowa Phoneme and Sentence Tests (Laser Videodisc). Iowa City, IA: Department of Otolaryngology–Head and Neck Surgery, University of Iowa Hospitals.

Wallace IF, Gravel JS, Schwartz RG, Ruben RR (1994) Otitis media, parental linguistic style and language skills of two-year-olds. Child Development, submitted for publication.

Wisconsin Department of Public Instruction (1992)

Appendix A: Organisation hierarchy and sample therapy goals for speech perception training.*

1. Simple contrasts for suprasegmentals

(a) Contrast number of syllables (one versus three syllable words, using picture or word cards as stimuli and dots under the stimuli to indicate number of syllables)
(b) Contrast stress (initial syllable stress versus final syllable stress, using printed words with stressed syllable capitalised, or for children who don't read, circles of different sizes to indicate stressed syllable)
(c) Contrast intonation contours (terminal rise versus terminal fall)

2. Simple contrasts for features of articulation

(a) Contrast sounds that are different in place, manner and voicing (/b/ vs /s/)
(b) Contrast sounds that are different in place and voicing (/b/, /t/).
(c) Contrast sounds that are different in place (/b/, /g/).
(d) Contrast sounds that are different in voicing (/b/,/p/).

Appendix B: Sample integration plan for a primary classroom (1st–2nd grade)

Classroom unit: life cycle of a butterfly

Classroom goals

1. Children will increase sight-word reading vocabulary as they complete daily observation journals of their caterpillar.
2. Children will learn the scientific vocabulary terms associated with the butterfly life cycle including: larvae, cocoon, pupae, metamorphosis, life cycle.
3. Children will sharpen observation and documentation skills by charting the phases of their individual caterpillar.

Child's goals

1. John will differentiate between words with one, two and three syllables given auditory and visual cues, then auditory-only cues.
2. John will increase vocabulary by 5–10 new words per week.

---

*Always begin by using VISUAL and AUDITORY cues, until the child is very consistent, then fall back to auditory-only cues.

3. John will comprehend the concept of plurals, simple past tense, third person singular form and present progressive.
4. John will produce multisyllables with up to four syllable words by marking each syllable with his voice.
5. John will produce /s,z/ in the context of word initial or word final order.

Therapy suggestions to integrate classroom goals with child's goals

1. Play a listening game in which the child will listen to the clinician speaking vocabulary words from the unit which differ in numbers of syllables. The child will identify which word the clinician says by pointing to the correct word. Use index cards with the words broken into syllables and, for children who cannot read, use items or pictures in conjunction with the word cards.

Classroom goals targeted: 1,3
Child's goals targeted: 1,2

2. Using the butterfly unit theme, the clinician writes simple sentences using pertinent vocabulary and includes endings in the sentences. For example:

- My caterpillar is sleeping.
- He eats.
- He is growing.
- He is crawling.
- He grows.

The child can identify endings and underline them or highlight them with a marker. The child can listen and identify between a short or a longer sentence. The child can also pull out words with target sounds and use for production practice.

Classroom goals targeted: 1,2,3
Child's goals targeted: 1,2,3

Appendix C: Speech perception training activities for adults

(A) **Computer programs** (available from our clinic): In this case, these programs are used for auditory training by presenting the stimuli in an audition-only condition.
1. *Analytic training*: A series of traditional drill exercises containing nonsense syllables (i.e. /eebee/ and /eegee/). The exercises are graduated in difficulty and provide practice with analytical speechreading training.

2. *Unrelated sentence training*: 20 sentences spoken by one of 10 different talkers. Clients are asked to select the correct spoken sentence from several pictures. This procedure also provides practice in using repair strategies.

3. *Related sentence training*: Speechreading practice in situation-specific settings (i.e. a shoe store, a doctor's office, a movie theatre, etc. This program allows practice in anticipating difficult listening situations, using repair strategies and correcting inappropriate speaker behaviours.

(B) **Books on tape:** Once a week subjects listen to a short story on audiotape. The length of each story varies from approximately 4 to 10 minutes. Subjects listen to the story once in an auditory-only condition and then answer eight questions about the story. After answering the questions, they listen to the story again while reading the text so that they may correct any misunderstandings.

(C) **Real-world activities:** Once a week subjects complete a real-world activity to receive listening practice in a more realistic setting. For example, one activity requires the client to go to a local store and ask for directions to an item.

Chapter 6
The Management of
Cochlear Implant Children

MARTINE SILLON, ADRIENNE VIEU, JEAN-PIERRE
PIRON, REINE ROUGIER, MICHEL BROCHE, FRANÇOISE
ARTIERES-REUILLARD, MICHEL MONDAIN, ALAIN UZIEL

Introduction

The Montpellier Paediatric Cochlear implant programme began in 1989. Although we provide implants to adults and children of all ages, the majority of patients are children who have either congenital, prelingual or postlingual deafness. Our emphasis is on selecting children for implantation who are under the age of five years. All the patients at our centre have received the Nucleus multichannel cochlear implant.

Description of the centre

The implant centre is composed of a multidisciplinary medical team working in two departments: the ENT Department of the University Hospital of Montpellier and the Audio-Phonology Department at the Saint-Pierre Institute, a children's hospital in Palavas. Surgery, electrophysiology and research are performed at the hospital and the Institute performs some of the selection tests (audiological, speech therapy and psychological assessment), along with implantee follow-up. When at the Institute, the children and their families are provided with lodging.

Description of the team

The team works in close collaboration during all stages of the cochlear implant programme. The team is made up of individuals from different professional disciplines. Two otologic surgeons and an ENT audiologist physician are involved in the selection (medical, audiologic assessment), surgery and medical follow-up of the implanted adults and children. They are also responsible for team coordination. Three speech therapists are involved in selection (speech therapy assessment), re-education directed towards auditory/oral education, and the subjective and objective evaluation of the results. One electrophysiologist carries out the objective evaluations of the auditory nerve and the central auditory pathways by recording the electrically evoked brainstem responses before implantation. He also makes an objective evaluation of the comfort level by electrically evoked stapedius reflex recording during surgery and performs the fitting and adjustments for the speech processor after implantation. One psychologist assesses the motivation of the parents and child before implantation. He prepares the patient for surgery and the postoperative period. After implantation, he evaluates the resulting changes in the child's behaviour. One teacher on our staff is specialised in the management of young deaf children and has an essential role during the follow-up period.

This multidisciplinary medical team is supported by other practitioners during the selection process of children as candidates for implantation. Notably, the radiologist who rules out any morphological abnormalities in the cochlea, a hearing aid specialist who fits appropriate amplification to the patients, and the local teaching and rehabilitation team.

Evaluation of children before cochlear implantation

Children are accompanied by their parents for a 1- to 2-day stay at the implant hospital. During this visit the team undertakes three main tasks: determination of whether the patient meets the selection criteria, provision of information to the patient and the family and preparation of the patient for surgery and the first fitting sessions

Selection

A full assessment is essential before considering cochlear implantation in postlingually deafened adults or children with deafness. The clinical examination will record the precise history of the deafness including the aetiology and age at onset of profound or total deafness. In this way, we attempt to determine whether the deafness is congenital, prelingual, perilingual or postlingual in origin and also its duration. An audiological assessment using pure-tone audiometry and speech audiometry is performed by an audiologist who has considerable experience with childhood deafness. During this session, the benefit of the hearing aid(s) is evaluated. The development and effective use of a sign-based or speech-based communication method is evaluated. A speech therapy assessment considers the child's level of language and psychomotor development. This assessment is also used to determine communication skills and to observe the child's general behaviour. The psychological assessment evaluates the child's cognitive, relational and interaction capacity. It also appraises the parents' motivation and expectations. After these preliminary examinations at the Saint-Pierre Institute, the patients and their families go to the University Hospital in Montpellier to meet the surgeon and undergo cochlear imaging and electrophysiological examinations.

A trial period of at least six months with well-fitted amplification is of primary importance in determining the degree of usable, serviceable hearing in an effort to determine whether the patient obtains any benefit from hearing aids. Thus, cochlear implant candidacy is a complex issue. Multiple physiologic, medical, developmental and psychosocial factors influence the selection. The decision to implant is made during the monthly team meeting where each case is considered and analysed carefully by each member. In the case of congenital or prelingual deafness, early implantation is advised in our centre, usually by the age of 2–5 years.

After the preliminary decision is reached in favour of implantation, it is essential to contact the local teaching and re-education team that routinely follows up the child. In this way, supplementary information is obtained that may influence the final implant decision. Their opinion is always taken into consideration and any information they request is supplied.

Informing Patients and Families

The parents are supplied with answers to the numerous questions they ask concerning implant technology, indications and results. Thus, all members of the team – from the first consultation onwards – provide as much information as possible concerning the working of the cochlear implant and the possibilities of the cochlear implant, whose characteristics will allow the child to develop perception and comprehension of speech. It is important to specify that several months of auditory education will be required.

The parents are informed that the cochlear implant enhances perception of the sound environment, e.g. high-frequency sounds of low intensity, soft sounds such as the noise made by water, the crumpling of paper and so forth. That is, the child will most likely hear sounds in the environment that could not be heard with hearing aids. They are informed that the recognition of words, possibly without lipreading, and the appearance of speech are acquired over time, and are only obtained at least two years post-implantation (Osberger et al., 1991; Frayauf-Bertschy et al., 1992; Cowan et al., 1993; Miyamoto et al., 1993; Shea, Domico & Lupfer, 1994; Uziel et al., 1995).

They are also informed about the limitations of the cochlear implant. The parents must know that the perception and comprehension of speech with the cochlear implant remain difficult in noisy conditions, that communication is difficult when several speakers are involved and that excess distance between the speaker and the implanted patient decreases the comprehension of the message. They are told that music is imperfectly perceived and not always pleasant. However, developments in signal processing are currently producing improvements in this field.

Concerning the risks of surgery, the surgeon informs the family that this operation presents the same risks as a conventional operation on the middle ear (Cohen & Hoffman, 1993; Kileny et al., 1995). The surgeon also explains that delayed complications may occur, such as infection around the cochlear implant, which may require explanation, or device failure. As far as device failure is concerned, our experience is consistent with a 2% rate, as seen in the general cochlear implant population (Kileny et al., 1995). These problems may arise in the first five years and require replacement of the implant. The parents are also informed that a cochlear implant is expected to last for at least 10 years and that it will probably require changing during the life of the child or adult patient.

The consequences of the operation are discussed. The surgeon informs the patient that it is impossible to perform an MRI (magnetic resonance imaging) with a cochlear implant and that it is impossible to use monopolar coagulation during any subsequent surgery, while underlining, however, that solutions exist for these constraints. Finally, the parents are given general information about speech processor malfunctions concerning the microphone, antenna, cables and speech processor. They are told of the constraints related to post-implantation follow-up. At this stage of the consultation emphasis is placed on the expectations patients or parents might have in comparison with the results obtained. It is clearly explained that cochlear implantation does not cure deafness and that different communication aids such as lipreading, cued speech, French Sign Language or other French communication methods they have chosen are to be maintained while the child still manifests the need.

Parents are given the conclusions drawn by the ANDEM (National Agency for the Development of Medical Evaluations) (ANDEM, 1994). This organisation was mandated by the French Ministry of Health to evaluate extending the use of cochlear implants to congenitally and prelingually deafened children. Thus, the team from the Cochlear Implant Center in Montpellier attempts to supply the family and the patients with as much information as possible and answer any questions so that the decision whether or not to go ahead with the implant is taken in full knowledge of the circumstances. This decision is made after time has been taken to reflect, and with agreement of the family and the therapeutic team responsible for the educational and rehabilitation follow-up.

Preparation

This is a very important step in the care of the patient, and family before the cochlear implantation. The different stages they will pass through before surgery and up to the first tuning are explained to them, and particularly to a young child. To do this they are given papers and booklets which, with explanatory pictures, help them understand what will happen.

The parents are told that the child will be hospitalised the day before the operation for final tests to be performed, that the child will be shaved around the ear to be implanted and that the hospital stay will be four or five days. Before the operation, they are invited to come to the cochlear implant centre to meet other implanted children and their families and visit the premises. Thus, the child has an initial contact with the centre's staff and the hospital surroundings. This serves to reduce the worry associated with arriving for the first stay at the hospital. Meeting other implanted children or implanted adults shows the child how to wear the device and what the scar looks like. The child notices the pleasure the other children have in listening with the device and is better prepared to accept it. This preparation reassures the parents who talk at length with other parents and with the implanted adults. During this early contact, a film of the child before the operation is made. Finally, the child is taken to a tuning session to see how, where and with whom the device will be switched on and what has to be done. The same speech therapist in charge of the child is responsible for behavioural tests during device set-up; this saves time and is more effective.

Management of the children after cochlear implantation

The child comes to the cochlear implant centre accompanied by one of the parents three days per month for the first year, then every second or third month (depending on progress made) during the second year and every six months during the third year. Visits are once a year after the third year.

The child and parents are received in a unit made up of eight rooms (parent/child). This living unit allows the families of implanted children to eat their meals together and take advantage of discussing feelings and ideas with other parents. Although this follow-up schedule may appear to be restrictive, it is useful and is well accepted as evidenced by the fact that no absenteeism occurs. During the stay the device is tuned, individual and group speech therapy are given, and parental care is reviewed.

First Fitting of the Speech Processor and Tuning

It should be noted that this requires close collaboration between the speech therapist and the electrophysiologist (Sheppard, 1994). This preliminary contact with the world of sound should not be underestimated or over-dramatised even though this moment has been awaited with impatience by both the family and the child. It is a moment of considerable emotion. The children may show surprise, pleasure and sometimes cry when the high levels of stimulation are sought.

Tuning the speech processor is an important step in using the cochlear implant. It governs whether the patient will adapt rapidly or slowly to the world of sound. The quality of the tuning will allow the child to develop language, and in the adult will lead to a modification in the tone of the voice. Each patient has a specific tuning requirement at any given time, and the stimulation parameters change constantly over the first six months and beyond, until the end of the first year. Other variations due to the general condition of the patient or related to the presence of tinnitus (in adults) or to fatigue may also affect the programming.

The fundamental question posed is to discover the patient's sensitivity to variations in the stimulation parameters. Tests with implanted adults have provided useful information concerning this question as some are able to detect very slight variations in the stimulation, whereas others are only sensitive to more pronounced variations. Different individuals require very different tuning. The dynamic range, i.e. the difference for each electrode between the threshold level (stimulation required to induce an auditory sensation) and the comfort level may vary by a factor of 1 to 20 between different subjects. Thus, it is clear that the precision of the tuning is of significant importance in a subject with a narrow dynamic range because an 'error' would mean that the subject loses precious information. Overestimating the comfort level would induce discomfort in this type of patient, whereas, for those with very wide dynamics ranges, the same 'error' would not have any consequences.

Re-education

Organisation

The child participates in four to six individual speech therapy sessions during the initial stay. The aims of these sessions are to determine whether the device is functioning correctly and to make observations that provide precise information for fine tuning indicated by discomfort, modification of the voice and so forth. Another aim is to assist the child in becoming aware of the world of sounds. Help is given to provide meaning to the sounds perceived. First, the auditory sensation is presented in isolation (using a quiet room and remaining close to the child) but then becomes more generalised in daily life. The numerous sessions give us the opportunity to perform multiple sound tests. The effort we ask the children to make is well accepted as they come to the sessions with pleasure and know that they will find their friends there.

Family participation in the sessions is a considerable advantage. It reassures the parents and they can be shown what reasonably to expect from the implant. Although detailed explanations have previously been given, and the family prepared, expectations are often not concurrent with reality. It is important to re-explain clearly the implant's possibilities and limitations. The parents become aware of the concentration required for hearing with the implant and find it easier to adapt their demands on the child. Often we observe that the child becomes more confident. Usually the parents also see that progress has been made although it may not always be apparent in everyday use; e.g. a reaction to saying the child's name does not often occur before three months post-speech processor fitting.

Participation by the child, parent and speech therapist in games helps the child understand instructions and information that are complex to explain. This exchange also helps us ensure that all the adult's attention is not focused on the child. The child has the time to observe, to understand, to imitate. The parent's attention can be drawn to the child's successes. This means that the members of the family themselves recognise what is important in their own behaviour or in their own interactions and these may be modified or enhanced. We alternate the child's activities and ask for clear responses in order to determine perceptions. More informal games are used to maintain the child's pleasure and spontaneity.

We attempt to establish and encourage real parent–child communication by developing common attention and exchange. The parents become more aware of what the child wishes to express. They observe the child, listen to the child and note that the child communicates and has something to say.

During these regular sessions, the children notice their own progress. The same sound objects that previously were unrecognised now have meaning. They love to listen again to the things they practised at the beginning of their training because they are now on safe ground. The parents may note the child's pleasure and lessen their own impatience or disappointment.

Progression of Exercises

The first step – the detection of sound

The ability to notice the presence or absence of sound is determined using musical instruments, noises and speech. We conduct a series of short games which generate noises that are either of high or low frequency. Of course, we render the child's effort easier by using stimuli that are readily heard with the implant. This approach is not always easy. Exercises must often be changed and we do not expect the child to respond systematically. Often the child observes and does not participate but listens and repeats the game later. The aim is to familiarise the child with hearing and to provide a sense to the sound environment that has exploded into the child's life. We encourage the parents to note the auditory possibilities in the clinic even if the child is unresponsive at home.

The second step – discrimination

An attempt is made to allow the child to differentiate sounds by their tone, their intensity, their duration and their pitch. Visual aids are employed initially but are progressively removed. This step usually lasts six months and is then replaced by more difficult tasks.

The third step – identification

This step is more rewarding for the child, the family and the team. The child starts to apply meaning to what is heard such as indicating which instrument was heard, the type of sound made or the word spoken. The child initially identifies words because they are very different in their length, the number of syllables and/or their phonetic form. Extreme opposites are emphasised for vowels [ɑ and ɪ], [y and ɪ], in the beginning. We avoid the opposition of oral/nasal manners of articulation for consonants but compare stop (or plosive) with fricatives. The oppositions voiceless/voiced are too difficult at this level. We use closed sets of three or four items for these exercises. We then proceed with the identification of two successive words. This involves auditory memory. The perception of short sentences, subject–verb–complement is then undertaken followed by increasingly complex structures.

The fourth step – recognition

This concerns the recognition of a verbal item with or without context. The child is asked to recognise single words in context or in open set, Then the child is asked to do the same tasks with short sentences in context (school, breakfast) or in open set (everyday life). These tasks are adapted to the linguistic skills of the child.

The easiest vowels to distinguish auditorily are used: [y/ɑ/i], then nasals [ɔ̃/ɑ̃/ɛ̃]. The differentiation between [ɑ/ɔ], [i/y], [e/ɛ], [ɑ/ɑ̃], [o/ɔ̃)] are more difficult. As far as consonants are concerned, voiceless plosives [p\t\k] are easily recognised – particularly in the middle of words. At the beginning of words they are often too rapid to be identified. The fricatives [ʃ/s] are easily recognised. The [f] is less easy. Voiced consonants are difficult and the nasal sounds are often identified later. The lateral and retroflex glides [l / ʀ] do not pose too many problems.

The fifth step – comprehension

This consists of training in an interactive communication situation, so it does not differ much from auditory education with conventional hearing aids, except for the particular possibilities offered by the implant. Specially designed materials which take advantage of the ease or difficulties in perceiving vowels and consonants (as described above) may be used. The intonation and prosodic aspects of the voice are emphasised by question–response games, by rhythms and by songs.

All this, of course, is adapted to meet the needs and capabilities of each child. Motivation and emotions may considerably influence perception. A good example of this is that 'mama' is rapidly recognised. Our auditory education always takes account of the child's linguistic possibilities and of the child's particular interests.

Postoperative Evaluations

Another aspect of these individual sessions is objective evaluations. These take place every three months using a series of tests. Table 6.1 describes these. The test results form a picture showing the child's progress and may be used to adapt the rehabilitation approach. Video analysis is very important to monitor progress in cochlear implant users (Tait, 1994).

Characteristics of the Rehabilitation Programme

Group sessions, two during the child's stay, in a special kindergarten for deaf children allow us to assemble several sound elements by creating sketches (play acting) or listening games. The advantage of these workshops resides in the teacher's observation of the children. She sees how they use the implant with the other children in different situations. The group atmosphere also creates true imitation between the children and an awareness of others who wear the same device. They have the opportunity to observe the possibilities offered through the implant as they watch other children react to sounds they hear. The children bond during these activities, something that is very precious at subsequent steps.

A family/team meeting is held at each stay. This takes the form of a discussion, generally after a video has been viewed. This exchange is used for technical discussion concerning the workings of the device (malfunctions, maintenance, possibilities, limitations, perspectives) and discussions concerning educational and teaching choices.

Our centre brings together patients from different regions of France

Table 6.1: Montpellier children's test battery

Tests of perception:		
Perception of nonsenses/syllables	Closed set	High- and low-frequency syllables
Discrimination of duration	Closed set	Discrimination of number of syllables
Discrimination of pitch and onomatopoeic words	Closed set	Three different animal sounds
Syllable rhythm identification	Closed set	Duration and number of syllables
Identification of words	Closed set	12 mono-, bi- or tri-syllable words
Identification of sentences	Six-alternative forced-choice	The sentence is correct if the child identifies any keyword correctly
	Closed set of four items	Sentences consist of subject–verb. Child must recognise the entire message
	Closed set of eight items	Sentences consist of subject–verb complement. Child must recognise the entire message
Integration of visual and auditory input test (lipreading)	Closed set of three items	Uses phonetic discrimination between two monosyllable words
Recognition of short sentences in everyday life	Open set	15 sentences of 4–5 words
Recognition of monosyllable words test	Open set	Lists of 20 words
Speech tracking	Open set	Short stories from picture books
Environmental sounds	Open set of 10 items	
Tests of speech production:		
Onomatopoeic imitation		Everyday life sounds
Repetition of words		20 items (mono-, bi- or tri-syllable words)
Repetition of short sentences		15 items

where educational possibilities are quite varied regarding services for deaf individuals. We take part in intense discussions regarding the use of sign language and cued speech in the education of implanted children. We occasionally invite others to address the group, e.g. technicians along with deaf adults who talk of their experience and broaden the discussions.

A special aspect of our programme is that we also include implanted adults in the rehabilitation process of children. The adults participate in meetings and help us considerably in explaining to parents what is happening to their child. The parents become aware of the reality of deafness and the means by which they can make their child's life easier. The children are interested to see that adults have the same devices as them and, thus, establish an identity with others using cochlear implants. Even the very young children are fascinated by this discovery.

The adult implant users also benefit from these exchanges and can compare their own progress with that of others. They undergo the same follow-up as the children (same frequency, same duration).

They generally come accompanied by their partners or with a family member. Re-education aims to reassure, to decrease impatience, to encourage and motivate the desire to discover the world of sounds. They assess their condition and have the opportunity to note their progress, which is sometimes taken for granted or ignored. Finally, and most importantly, they learn to readjust their expectations, which are often inappropriate, despite explanations and warnings. It is not rare to see disappointment in our adult population. Our role is to give support by demonstrating the progress they have made and by introducing them to people who are a little further ahead in the process.

Another aspect of our programme is the visits by educational teams that work locally with the children or adults. These teams are invited to be present during tunings and speech therapy sessions concerning the child/adult they are following. They meet others of different ages who have been wearing the device for different periods. Contact is made which is then maintained by mail or telephone. The aim is to form an educational cohesion around the child (or adult).

Subjective results

General data are obtained partly from a questionnaire given to the families at each stay (see Table 6.2). The answers to these questions have shown that most of the children demonstrate certain tendencies.

The children all accept the device from the first day onwards whereas some refuse a conventional hearing aid. They wear the device for the entire day and are not inconvenienced by the speech processor or the cables. The children rapidly learn to keep the device clean. They do not like anyone touching the device, and protect it. As an example, one child

Table 6.2: Montpellier questionnaire of children's implant use

1.   Is the child wearing the device?
2.   Can the child put it on alone?
3.   At what time of the day does the child remove the device?
4.   Does the child want the device when getting up in the morning?
5.   Is the child tired in the evening?
6.   Does the child indicate that the batteries have run out?
7.   Does the child play with the antenna, with the setting buttons?
8.   Are some noises bothersome?
9.   How long did it take the child to adapt after the last tuning?
10. Has the child experienced new perceptions since the last stay (music, telephone, speech)?
11. Has the child indicated new noises, does the child ask for explanations?
12. Does the child recognise her name?
13   Has the child's behaviour changed?
14. Does the child show sleeping or appetite disorders?

on a walk with his parents removed the device when coming close to a fountain. He explained that he was afraid of getting it wet.

They take the device and often conduct their own speech tests. For example, they produce sounds such as [ɑ\ɪ\u] and watch the light flashing on the speech processor. In this way, one child showed her parents that the battery was flat. She said [u\u] and showed them that the light did not come on. After using the cochlear implant for two or three years, families report that the children take entire charge of the use of the device. A little girl's grandfather explained one evening that when the girl is tired, she switches the device off, but switches on again if she sees her parents laughing and has the impression that something interesting is going on.

Subjective Results for Speech Perception

Such results are observed in most of the children (Osberger et al., 1991; Fryauf-Bertschy et al., 1992; Cowan et al., 1993; Miyamoto et al, 1993; Shea, Domico & Lupfer, 1994; Uziel et al., 1995). From the start the children derive great pleasure from the perception of speech. They explore the world of sounds by conducting tests with the antenna (transmitter), such as 'I connect, I hear; I disconnect, I can't hear'. Four months post-speech processor fitting, most of the children recognise and reply to hearing their name. They can differentiate between familiar voices of different tones. Perception of the sound environment improves as time goes on and more and more everyday noises are identified (telephone, doorbell, barking dog). At the end of the first year, all the children are able to perceive short, associated words of the subject + verb type. After two years, the children perceive short but more complex sentences and are able to understand longer messages. The auditory memory improves and their semantic field broadens. After three years, the children's perception of language improves their listening capabilities. There is understanding of what is said even if the child is busy doing something else. Long-distance perception improves and the child shows better identification of short sentences presented in open set. The children use the telephone and can conduct a simple conversation with someone familiar, but communication with strangers remains difficult. After four years progress continues to be made as perception is more subtle, more rapid and more efficient. This shows that progress continues even several years after cochlear implantation.

Subjective Results for Speech Production

A broad outline of the children's progress may be described, while bearing in mind that individual variations due to the child and the specific environment are obviously present (Hasenstab & Tobey, 1991; Tobey et al., 1991; Tobey, 1993). Children suffering from congenital deafness and implanted at about 3 years of age and who had previously never spoken start to babble very soon after the initial fitting. Six to eight months after implantation, the vowels show phonetic enrichment with the beginnings of differentiation between [ɑ\o\ɪ]. The child shows better control over voice and is able to modulate it, shout and whisper. One year post-implantation, the children usually take an important step. They are spontaneously ready to repeat words. Their auditory memory is more efficient. Short words are acquired naturally: 'après–attends–allo...'. They start to use the sentence 'maman partie'. Their phonetic enrichment continues with the appearance of the [S]. This sound's intonation is repeated. Their voices are agreeable to hear, with good tonality (sometimes still nasal). The child is increasingly attentive to lipreading and, in this way, more effectively corrects pronunciation.

The second important step takes place about two years post-fitting. Children who have not already started to speak do so now. Their phonetic system becomes increasingly efficient. Plosive sounds such as [p\t\k] are used, nasal sounds such as [m\n], fricative sounds such as [f\s\S] and glides such as [l\ʀ] are used, in most instances. The vowels are used but still with difficulty for nasal subjects. The child is better understood and can now produce three-word sentences, and ask questions. The child communicates verbally in an interactive question–answer game. This rich period continues during the third year as more subtle notions of language take root.

The fourth year corresponds to yet another step as the children show homogenisation of their language. They are easy to understand when saying familiar words. Their pronunciation is correct. Their sentences are sometimes less easy to understand and they still show poor vocabulary and language. At this time we are particularly impressed by the quality of the children's voices, by their melodic and intonation qualities. The children are able to reproduce the characteristics of the accent of the region where they live. The children continue to progress in close conjunction with the stimulation received, the communications aids available (French Sign Language, cued speech) and the educational system in which they are immersed.

Older Children: Implantation in Congenitally Deafened Children over 7 Years

Here the results are different because the child has already constructed a system of communication. Often, two years are required for real progress to be made in the intelligibility of the child's speech. Phonetic alterations concerning nasality or voicing tend to decrease over time. Speech quality remains precarious, but its tone improves with time. Intonation patterns are improved but imperfect. Older children progress far slower than the youngest in terms of speech. Their command of the language is heavily dependent on their level before implantation, even though some children show the emergence of a more natural language after two years; i.e. a language less related to systematic learning. This progress depends on the educational tools chosen and whether or not there is integration with intensive auditory/oral education or within an institution where French sign language is the primary mode of communication.

Objective results

Speech Perception

Support for the subjective findings for speech perception is found in the analysis of videotapes made during every session with the speech pathologist and by results obtained from the administered tests as described in Table 6.1. Figure 6.1 presents the results of the closed-set word identification (chance = 25%), the closed-set sentence identification (chance = 33%) and the modified open-set speech recognition (chance performance approaches 0%). The follow-up assessments were administered periodically at 3-month intervals for one year and then at 6-month intervals. The data in Figure 6.1 represent findings gathered for 53 children who had either congenital or prelingual deafness and were tested between 3 and 48 months post-fitting. The mean age at time of implantation was 4;2. There were forty congenitally deafened children (mean age at implantation: 3 years) and 13 were prelingually deafened children (mean age at implantation: 3;7 years). The mean onset of the deafness was 1;6 years in the prelingually deafened children group. The overall average duration of the deafness was 3;95 years.

Closed-set word at three months and closed-set sentence identification at six months averaged 16.5% and 21%, respectively. Scores for both tests reached 100% accuracy for all subjects by 3 years' experience. The modified open-set speech recognition test was the most difficult test. Children began to achieve scores on the test only after one year of implant experience, with an average in performance of 52.6% by 30 months. Increases in performance were gradual and no plateau in performance was evident even at 48 months. These data reinforce the subjective impressions that children receiving cochlear implants at an early age demonstrate ongoing improvements in perceptual skills.

Psychological Impact Shown by Implanted Children

Unfortunately, there exists no systematic evaluation procedure using standardised methods such as observation lists or clinical questionnaires for this population (Aplin, 1993). Information must be collected in an informal way through contact with the family, the professional caretakers responsible for the child and by direct observation during stays at the implant centre. Progress appears to be greatly dependent upon environmental factors, primarily the family (capacity to accept the child, perception of the handicap in the family and the parents' history) and the

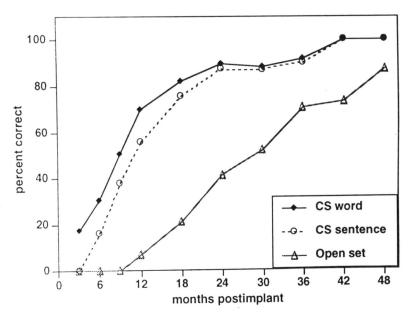

Figure 6.1: Speech perception skills over time are shown. The means are shown for each of the speech perception measures. Closed-set word (closed square) and closed-set sentence (open circles) scores reached 100% accuracy by 42 months experience. Modified open-set speech recognition test performance (triangles) averaged 52.6% by 30 months. Increases in open set showed no plateau in performance even at 42 months post-implantation.

family's ability to form an alliance with a team of professionals. It is important to understand that psychological changes, in both positive or negative dynamics, are dependent on many factors other than the cochlear implant. Although implantation marks an important event in the child's history and an important time for the rehabilitation of the child's deficiency, the event does not make up the child's entire history. The role of interactions in early childhood must also be considered. Finally, there is no standard psychological development, rather individuals evolve in many ways presenting only a few, broad trends as outlined below.

Acceptance of the Prosthesis

The child rapidly incorporates the prosthesis into his/her body image. The device quickly loses the status of a foreign object and is rapidly integrated. As practically 'part' of the body, it is then forgotten (not present in Draw-a-Person).

Cognitive Development

This is difficult to evaluate in the absence of comparative studies; however, it is possible to generalise because of the fact that many of the children who wear a cochlear implant integrate into the normal school environment. This would support the hypothesis that language plays only a partial role in the child's early cognitive development through sensorimotor activities. The use of symbols, verbal or otherwise, marks the development of thought. This is a semantic function. Little by little, language takes a semiotic form. It may, therefore, be considered that the development of language through use of the implant will allow the child to acquire a sense of objectivity and causality, to arrive at socialised thought.

Relational Development

This is increasingly important in the establishment of the functional structures of intelligence. Relative to autonomisation, in early life, vision is the predominant factor in the child's search for information. The deaf child will enter into visual dependency on the mother's face. This dependency leads to retarded autonomisation. The cochlear implant supplies auditory information and can help the child become more autonomous and allow the child to construct a measure of independence. This is confirmed by the parents who are very aware of these changes. They describe this as 'he is no longer hanging on to me', 'he can play alone in his room'. These remarks are an expression of the fact that the deaf child is safe beyond the visual perception of the mother or the person with whom she has identified. Similarly, the parents notice a change in their child's 'character', in particular: the child is more toler-ant to frustration because of increased capacity to 'negotiate'. The situa-tion is no longer 'all or nothing'. The child shows a reduced tendency to resolve conflicts by action. Language slowly replaces screaming and tension, with words substituting for impossible demands on another level.

As far as interpersonal relationships are concerned, the parents report considerable progress in the child's capacity to interrelate as seen by acceptance of another person's point of view, acceptance of collective rules in games, socialised behaviour, etc.

Educational Progress

The special teacher for young deaf children views the child in the educa-tional setting (Geers & Moog, 1991). It is reported that the implanted deaf children are received into groups with other severely hearing-impaired children who wear conventional prostheses. This allows the child to be observed in the context of group activities, in games and in relationships with other children and the immediate entourage. These observations, comparing the implanted and severely hearing-impaired children wearing conventional prostheses, are subjective and general.

There is a rapid acceptance of the new device rather than refusal. The children are proud of the implant, show it to others, take care of the device and very rapidly start experimenting with sound. They show a broad range of perception. During group activities they participate far more and are more attentive. A deaf child generally fixes his/her atten-tion in relation to what is seen (picture, lipreading, cued speech, mimes, gestures) and what is understood from what has been seen. If one of these methods is deficient, the child rapidly loses interest. Thanks to the implant and the fact that the child hears speech, even if the message is not understood, attention is maintained throughout a particular activity. When learning rhymes or poetry, the children take great pleasure in trying to repeat the words spontaneously. They also memorise the words more easily than before implantation. Less tension is noted as far as speech is concerned. The children find it easier to repeat words. Speech becomes more precise and develops spontaneously. Their voices are more melodious. As far as communication attempts are concerned, they use more oral communication. When they wish to express something, they often accompany this with verbal sounds.

Language appears to develop in a more natural manner. Similar steps to those seen in non-deaf children are observed in the implanted chil-dren. The children are in a dynamic acquisition situation. The teacher has less of an impression that the child is laboriously constructing notions, forever repeating the same things. The children memorise information better.

Changes are also seen in behaviour, not only in children but also in the adults who are in the children's immediate entourage. The children feel safe from an affective and material point of view. They are far calmer. Little by little they become less isolated. They approach others more readily. They become more independent. For the parents, this is an important milestone because they feel safer as a result of their child being able to hear them. They feel considerably less disadvantaged. They speak to the children far more, and more naturally. They become more motivated: some parents try to reuse, with more frequency, some aids to communication (for instance, cued speech). This change in the parents, of course, has an additional positive effect on the child's behaviour.

Conclusions

The majority of this discussion has dealt with the process of implanting children and their results after gaining experience with hearing through their cochlear implant. It is clear that significant, positive changes occur after implantation for the children in our programme. The results, of course, vary greatly from child to child, but show that cochlear implantation in young children can be a very important factor in increasing the acquisition of spoken language and its perception. Adults have also benefited from implantation and have provided a baseline of performance with which the children can be compared. They are also excellent role models for the newly implanted child. By encouraging all the members of our implant team and all the implant patients, to interact, regardless of age, an effective and positive re-education programme has been developed.

Acknowledgements

We are very grateful to Dianne Allum for helpful criticisms and for correcting the manuscript.

References

ANDEM (1994) L'implant cochléaire chez l'enfant sourd pré-lingual. France: Ministry of Health.

Aplin DY (1993) Psychological assessment of multichannel cochlear implant patients. Journal of Laryngology and Otology 107: 298-304.

Cohen NL, Hoffman RA (1991) Complications of cochlear implant surgery in adults and children. Annals of Otology, Rhinology and Laryngology 100: 708-11.

Cohen NL, Hoffman RA (1993) Surgical complications of multichannel cochlear implants in North America. Advances in Otorhinolaryngology 48: 70-74.

Cowan RS, Dowell RC, Pyman BC, Dettman SJ, Dawson PW, Rance G, Barker EJ, Sarant JZ, Clark GM (1993) Preliminary speech perception results for children with the 22-electrode Melbourne/cochlear hearing prosthesis. Advances in Otorhinolaryngology 48: 231-35.

Fryauf-Bertschy H, Tyler RS, Kelsay DM, Gantz BJ (1992) Performance over time of congenitally deaf and postlingually deafened children using a multichannel cochlear implant. Journal of Speech and Hearing Research 35: 913–20.

Geers AE, Moog JS (1991) Evaluating the benefits of cochlear implants in an education setting. American Journal of Otology 12: 116–25.

Hasenstab MS, Tobey EA (1991) Language development in children receiving Nucleus multichannel cochlear implant. Ear and Hearing 12: S55–65.

Kileny PR, Meiteles LZ, Zwolan TA, Telian SA (1995) Cochlear implant device failure – diagnosis and management. American Journal of Otology 16: 164–71.

Miyamoto RT, Osberger MJ, Robbins AM, Myres WA, Kessler K (1993) Prelingually deafened children's performance with the Nucleus multichannel cochlear implant. American Journal of Otology 14: 437–45.

Osberger MJ, Todd SL, Berry SW, Robbins AM, Miyamoto RT (1991) Effect of age at onset of deafness on children's speech perception abilities with a cochlear implant. Annals of Otology, Rhinology and Laryngology 100: 883–88.

Shea J, Domico EH, Lupfer M (1994) Speech perception after multichannel cochlear implantation in the pediatric patient. American Journal of Otology 15: 66–70.

Sheppard S (1994) Fitting and programming the external system. In McCormick B, Archbold S, Sheppard S (Eds) Cochlear Implants for Young Children. London: Whurr, pp 140–65.

Tait M (1994) Using video analysis to monitor progress in young cochlear implant users. In McCormick B, Archbold S, Sheppard S (Eds) Cochlear Implants for Young Children. London: Whurr, pp 214–36.

Tobey EA, Angelette S, Murchison C, Nicosia J, Sprague S, Staller SJ, Brimacombe JA, Beiter AL (1991) Speech production performance in children with multichannel cochlear implants. American Journal of Otology 12: S165–73.

Tobey EA (1993) Speech production in cochlear implants. In Tyler RS (Ed) Cochlear Implants. Audological Foundations. London: Whurr, pp 317–16.

Uziel AS, Reuillard-Artieres F, Sillon M, Vieu A, Mondain M (1995) Speech perception performance in prelingually deafened children with the Nucleus multichannel cochlear implant. Advances in Otorhinolaryngology 50: 114–18.

Chapter 7
A Service Network for the Rehabilitation of Cochlear Implant Users

RENÉ MÜLLER, DIANNE J. ALLUM AND JOHN H.J. ALLUM

Introduction

Rehabilitation programmes for cochlear implant users are typically under the guidance of medical divisions of hospitals and clinics because implantation is a medical procedure. The programme at the University Hospital of Basel approaches rehabilitation with an emphasis on educational and audiological issues. It aims to promote the most effective means for patients to utilise information received through an implanted device along with optimal device fitting. The ultimate goal is to provide a service that helps the cochlear implant user become integrated into a hearing community. The rehabilitation is guided by a cooperative arrangement between the hospital and schools for hearing-impaired children. The educators and rehabilitationists are *not* directly employed by the hospital but nevertheless work there.

In Basel, a fundamental cooperation between the clinic and the Riehen School (Gehörlosen- und Sprachheilschule Riehen: GSR), located in a nearby suburb, already existed for fitting high-gain hearing aids. With the advent of implant procedures in adults and children, we saw an opportunity to expand our cooperation into full collaboration to create a cochlear implant programme with shared personnel and facilities.

Background

The precedent for establishing cooperation between a school and a hospital came in the 1950s when the early detection of hearing loss was the major issue. Outside staff of university hospitals – in Zürich, an educator; in Basel, a paediatric specialist – joined the major hospitals and founded the first paediatric audiology departments in Switzerland. From this beginning, the standard and effectiveness of early intervention improved. In particular, the department in Zürich became a source both of development for the approach towards early intervention and for providing public information. The result was that more children were fitted early with hearing aids, and more children were eventually able to be mainstreamed into schools for normal-hearing children. Up to that time in Switzerland, the medical concerns had driven the programme and the ultimate goal of providing long-term goals for rehabilitation did not exist. It was also in Zürich that the need to work with parents brought into existence new professions of deaf educators and educational audiologists. These specialties concerned themselves with the educational and psychological aspects of care for hearing-impaired children (Löwe, 1985; Schmid-Giovannini, 1985; Müller, 1989; Böhler, 1992). Again, the result led to better handling of the hearing-impaired children. However, one problem arose in Zürich because the university children's clinic tended to feel that the support of children outside the hospital setting was not a medical affair. The schools, too, had the tendency to feel that rehabilitation in medical settings was not an educational matter. The question was: Why should the hospital or the school be financially responsible for the support of staff members working outside their respective establishments? The viewpoints were that the medical/technical developments are the major concerns of the hospital, and educational developments are the concern of the schools. Still, both clinics and school departments realised that the new programmes had provided a significant contribution to the successful handling of the psychological and educational aspects associated with hearing-impaired children. Therefore, they ultimately agreed that it was necessary to create a position that would handle the non-medical aspects regardless of the ultimate funding agency. This experience served as an example for establishing a cooperative cochlear implant programme at the Basel University Hospital.

Our cochlear implant programme began in 1986, first with adults and then, in 1991, with deaf children. The expanded programme required an approach where the technical, audiological and medical support went hand in hand with educational, psycholinguistic and psycho-acoustic aspects. From the very first child implanted, the question of educational integration was of paramount importance.

Initially, the programme effectively provided service through the clinical and engineering specialists on the hospital staff. Eventually, the need to reach outside the hospital setting introduced the importance for a stronger input from educators and therapists; i.e. the non-medical aspects. To conceive the programme, we discussed a plan for the holistic treatment of patients where rehabilitation and audiology would be represented strongly in the programme. As long as there was a person who was a member of the hospital staff holding sole responsibility for rehabilitation, the danger existed that the hospital management alone would drive the programme. It was agreed that the Riehen School would provide the personnel within the hospital. This is in contrast with most programmes throughout the world in which the hospital directly employs the rehabilitation or outreach person. In our case, the educational facility employs the person(s) who works within the hospital setting and who is primarily responsible for long-term rehabilitation rather than for immediate speech processor fittings. As mentioned, the position is financially supported by the GSR and the ultimate allegiance of the individual(s) employed in this position is to the educational facility not the hospital administration. For the day-to-day management, logistics and activities, the GSR-employed person, known as a cochlear implant (CI) rehabilitation counsellor, requests guidelines from the leader of the hospital's cochlear implant programme. We also co-sponsored the remodelling of dedicated rooms within the audiology department to provide a work environment for the CI rehabilitation counsellor.

The issue for us was how the close working proximity to each other could best be used to develop a service where we could take into account the continually changing requirements of a growing cochlear implant programme. Further, we had to discover whether or not our aims for the cochlear implant programme were philosophically compatible. To ensure that both medical/technical aspects and educational/therapeutic aspects could find a satisfactory place in the continuous development of our work, the cochlear implant department team of the hospital and the GSR meets every few weeks to set the priorities for short- and long-term goals.

A feedback loop between the medical/technical personnel and those dealing with the everyday lives of the patients is essential. The feedback serves not only as an important measure of how well cochlear implant fitting is progressing but is an ultimate concern of parents striving to provide optimal education for their children. It is also a gauge of what is happening outside the medical environment, which is where cochlear implant users spend most of their lives.

Patient population

Children

In today's environment of changing health care services, a fundamental ingredient for any rehabilitation programme is the understanding that there is always change in terms of personnel and circumstances. This means we must always be in a state of quasi-upgrading. Relating this to our patient load, first, there were postlingual adults, then came the children with dialect-speaking Swiss parents. Most recently, another group of children have joined our clinic and these are the immigrant children of societies composed of those who came to Switzerland for various political and social reasons and have a different mother tongue. They have the special problem of communication where even the mother and father may have different languages. The home language, then, is certainly different from what they hear in the Swiss region they have adopted as home, i.e. the local dialect. Thus, these children have the problem of being in a setting where at least three different languages are spoken. In such cases, the cochlear implant brings up a novel question for rehabilitation. This holds true for the dialect-speaking children, too, because teaching is in high German.

Although there are four separate regions and languages in Switzerland – German, French, Italian and Romansch – for the German-speaking cantons there is the particular problem of distinctly different dialects being spoken from region to region. These dialects differ so greatly from high German, the so-called general language, that many people feel that high German is a foreign language. In many oral programmes for hearing-impaired children, teachers speak in high German but, generally, it is only used in the written form. For the hearing-impaired person, this difference between what may be spoken in the school and what is spoken at home has implications for both socialisation and education. It means that cochlear-implanted children of dialect-speaking parents must learn at least two spoken languages.

Adults

Our larger population is composed of children but the CI rehabilitation counsellor also interacts in the programme for adults. The rationale is that the experience gathered from adults provides an important reference for processor fittings and auditory training. In particular, the fact that postlingual adults are able to communicate details about the signals they hear and about the usefulness of training they receive is very helpful. Rehabilitation for adults usually takes place outside the hospital setting and the rehabilitation counsellor coordinates rehabilitation techniques and the need for further therapy with the local therapists.

The communication tree

We have described the background and rationale for the establishment of the integrated approach to rehabilitation for cochlear implant recipients and the patients whom we serve. The rehabilitation counsellor acts as an interface between the internal and external services we provide. Our analogy is a 'communication tree' with many branches (see Figure 7.1) that reach out to professionals and lay people (i.e. parents or teachers in regular schools) involved with cochlear implant users. There are many aspects that are intertwined and cannot be exclusive of one another:

however, we will deal with the three primary areas, which we call in-service patient care, professional training and outreach patient care.

In-service Patient Care

Care which is provided within the clinical setting is referred to as in-service patient care. Daily activities of the rehabilitation counsellor may include scheduling and record keeping (1 ½ hrs), programming/ processor fitting (1 ½ hrs), testing (1 ½ hrs), counselling (1 ½ hrs) and work on a special project such as materials development (1 hr). During the full week, blocks of time are also allocated for self-education and teaching. Table 7.1 more fully describes the duties and responsibilities of the CI rehabilitation counsellor. The time-intensive involvement of the rehabilitation counsellor diminishes as the children/adults using the cochlear implant gain more experience along with those outside the clinic who work with the cochlear implant user. The tasks of checking the speech processor settings and the evaluation of performance with

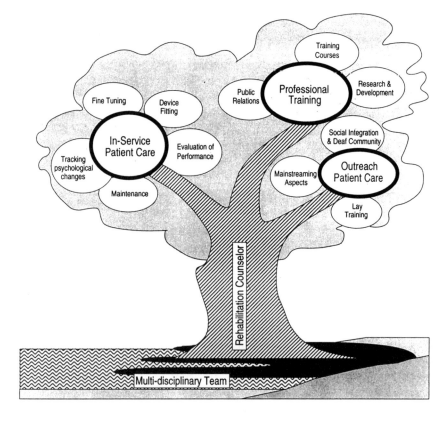

Figure 7.1: The three primary branches of the 'communication tree' showing the interface with the multidisciplinary team (R.J. Müller and D.J. Allum)

the implant continue, but at 3-month intervals for the first year, 6-month intervals for the second year and at yearly intervals thereafter.

Device fitting, maintenance and fine tuning

The hospital programme is networked directly with the schools for deaf children, some of which may be located as far as 200 km from Basel. As of this writing, three separate special education schools cooperate in the fitting of devices for children. Ideally, they could also be used as a resource for checking adults who are local to the school area. Adults, however, obtain all fitting and subsequent adjustments to their speech processor directly at the hospital. Children, who often require observation, multiple short fitting sessions and frequent programme changes, receive their initial adjustments at the hospital and return after 1 month and then every 3 months for the first year and, thereafter, every 6 months. They are also seen at the hospital whenever requested or if

Table 7.1: Components of the duties and responsibilities of the rehabilitation counsellor

Task	Components
Organisation	Scheduling Organise team meetings for selection Equipment maintenance Audiological team
Speech processor fitting	Follow-up programming Clinical partner (fitting children)
Auditory training	Adults Children
Counselling	Pre-selection: information Preoperative: orientation Postoperative: equipment
Teaching	Educators Lay persons Associated professionals
Evaluation	Preoperative Postoperative
Materials development	Evaluation Fitting (games and tools) Training
Data entry	Demographic details Test results
External	Represent the clinic at meetings Present lectures

there is a special need. During the interim periods, a specialist at the school checks the speech processor. Each school has its own programming station and each specialist who does device fitting receives a certificate of training from the Basel programme. This ensures that the psychophysical tasks and orientation to programming are similar. Interaction between the schools and the clinic is facilitated by the rehabilitation counsellor and by reports from the schools about any changes that have been made to a child's programme and why. Such a coordinated approach makes it possible for continuity to exist between the school and hospital programmes so that children receive the best possible care.

Evaluation of performance

A part of the in-service care is the assessment of how the child or adult uses information sent through the implant. Preoperative and postoperative evaluations of a variety of commonly assessed auditory skills for adults (Spillman & Dillier, 1987; Dorman, 1993) and for children (Boothroyd, 1991; Reid & Lehnhardt, 1993; Archbold, 1994; Allum, 1995) are conducted. In terms of the network service, selected educators are trained in the methods of test administration and are able to coordinate with the testing done in the hospital. The final interpretation of the data takes place within the cochlear implant programme at the hospital in conjunction with the rehabilitation counsellor.

Professional training

One of the main emphases of the Basel programme is education. By teaching local professionals about the essential features and postoperative management, the care of those who receive implants in the Basel area is more comprehensive. We think that it is much better for work with the child to take place in school rather than through only a few visits per year to the clinic. Therefore, specific information about the cochlear implant must be given to those who are directly involved with the patients on a day-to-day basis. It should not be only the clinical professionals in the hospital who have the major pool of information because they only influence the patient directly approximately 1% of the time (Lutman et al., 1986). Itinerant teachers, speech therapists and deaf educators should be well informed.

Currently, we provide training courses for educators and therapists. The courses are small, six to ten people, and are composed of those who work specifically with the children. The courses at the hospital have the goal of providing background information about medical, technical and psychoacoustic methods. This enables the speech therapists and teachers of hearing-impaired children to have greater security in knowing how to handle problems when they arise in their local situations. They become more qualified and understand the specific needs of cochlear implant children.

Outreach Patient Care

Throughout Switzerland, there are five clinical facilities that supply cochlear implants to patients in a country which is nearly the size of West Virginia or about one-third the size of England. Most patients come to us from the German-speaking regions, some from the French-speaking regions and some from foreign countries. With a small national programme, where implants number between 35 and 45 per year (one-half taking place in Basel), it is not cost-effective to have a CI rehabilitation counsellor from the joint hospital–GSR programme visit each child's local school. Itinerant educators have a better opportunity to influence rehabilitation in its broader application, a process that usually takes place outside the medical setting, i.e. separate from the clinic. For this reason, outreach patient care must be the result of a coordinated effort between the rehabilitation counsellor, the educational facility attended by the child and the parents. In the case of adults, direct communication with the local rehabilitationists is most effective.

Outreach can be interpreted to mean direct contact by clinic personnel, for training and consultation about cochlear implants, in general, or about guidance for specific patients to those who normally do not deal with hearing-handicapped children. So this branch of the communication tree focuses on the topics that are important for improving the local circumstances at regular schools in a village or city in which a child with a cochlear implant and the family live.

The GSR has long focused its efforts on developing objectives and activities for improving the speech reception skills of hearing-impaired children wearing hearing aids. Now, this is also the case for children wearing cochlear implants. A child must learn to listen to and make use of as much available auditory information as possible. This is the only way to obtain maximum benefit from any device that assists hearing. Specific instruction accelerates this learning and enables the child to develop strategies to facilitate the comprehension of speech. We endeavour to educate lay persons through itinerant teachers from the GSR and through educational courses offered through the hospital.

Networking with teachers of mainstreamed children

Hearing-impaired children in north-west Switzerland are supported by the GSR and by other schools with whom we have a cooperative arrangement. The teachers are mainly responsible for the direct interaction with the children. The building and expanding of normal spoken language is usually the responsibility of the speech therapists or teachers of the hearing-impaired children from special schools. They are also responsible for supporting education if special curricula cannot be provided by the classroom teachers. A special workshop taught through the Basel hospital programme helps the itinerant teachers understand the special needs of cochlear implant children. Such support not only helps the teachers to improve their skills but may even help them to provide normal-hearing children with more favourable conditions for learning.

Teachers in regular schools usually receive no education in instructing hearing-impaired children; therefore, specific counselling and supervision of these teachers regarding the individual circumstances of hearing-impaired children in their classes is essential. The GSR has designed a set of teaching activities that supports listening skills; i.e. teachers learn what to expect a child to perceive through the cochlear implant or hearing aid, or how to identify when children are not responding in a typical manner to assisted hearing. Our itinerant teachers travel to the various schools to assist with educational problems of hearing-impaired children. In particular, interaction with teachers in regular schools is essential because of mainstreaming.

Mainstreaming is a relatively new concept in Switzerland. The process of change in the remediation of the handicapped child is linked with a change from the medical orientation of treatment to the process of social integration. In the past, the opinion of most experts was defined through a medical model, where each child received care as determined by the extent or degree of an organic disability. It followed that the child with its handicap, together with the parents (usually the mother), were personally responsible for taking care of their own needs that arose in regular schools. Today, the individual and the specific circumstances define the opportunities for development of the handicapped person rather than being defined by the organic disability (Eggert, 1995). This means that, for hearing-handicapped children, besides the important aspect of early detection and early intervention, circumstances in regular classes must be adapted in ways that enable the child to share lessons and learning conditions with non-handicapped children (Müller, 1994a and b).

Several investigators concluded that hearing-impaired children and teenagers who receive their education in regular schools go through a well-balanced personality development. In particular, there is no indication that they are more poorly integrated into a normal class than normal-hearing children (Elmiger, 1992). An investigation into the identity and social situations of some 300 hearing-impaired children and teenagers in regular schools, conducted in Zürich, had similar positive findings (Sander & Hildeschmidt, 1993). An often overlooked and completely different question about mainstreaming is how much integration handicapped people want for themselves, and whether they consciously strive to belong to their own subculture. The question is not easy to answer and especially not without having the appropriate conversations with the adults in a subculture who will be greatly affected. Non-handicapped scientists often speculate and describe the plight and condition of the handicapped individual but there are few contributions from those who live their daily lives with a hearing handicap and who have considered or received a cochlear implant. People without any hearing disability send out the message that total integration should be the aim of remediation and that all handicapped individuals should accept this aim. Perhaps they should agree with it, but they do not always do so (Eggert, 1995). The ultimate point for consideration is that teenagers and adults with cochlear implants will never have normal hearing. Therefore, one cannot predict, *a priori*, to which group within the broad spectrum from spoken language communication of normal-hearing individuals to the sign language of a deaf person someone with a cochlear implant will belong. The essence is that the opportunity to choose a social community should be available.

It is not our purpose, here, to dwell on the pros and cons of integrated educational systems. With regard to the work in the cochlear implant department in Basel, realistically, our central clinical–educational facility can only provide a limited number of direct services. This means that a majority of the work should focus on education and support rather than direct rehabilitation. We believe that it is our responsibility to provide a basis of understanding to all those who might come into specific contact with implant users. This would include parents, relatives, special education teachers, teachers in regular schools, speech therapists, hearing aid dealers, paediatricians, educational audiologists and other interested individuals.

Information to parents

Parents also need special attention. They can provide strong support for the integrated training of their child and, therefore, they themselves need special training. They spend the most time with the hearing-impaired child and they are the real experts on their child (Sander & Hildeschmidt, 1993). The cochlear implant programme is working to develop a special training workshop series for parents similar in format to the courses run for professionals. Eventually, the teaching materials should lead to the development of information booklets.

Special issues concerned with developing a clinic–school network

Joint programmes raise a number of issues that university hospitals and special-education schools might not face if either was totally responsible for the child. Typically, in Switzerland, university hospitals are solely responsible for audiologic fitting and medical rehabilitation for cochlear implant patients. The schools, on the other hand, are responsible for educational rehabilitation.

The Swiss invalid insurance and association of health insurance companies have stipulated that reimbursement for device implantation, postoperative fitting and rehabilitation (to ensure appropriate device operation) can only occur through four university hospitals (Basel, Bern, Geneva and Zürich) and one cantonal hospital (Lucerne). Rehabilitation of kindergarten and school-age children with hearing losses is, however, one of the responsibilities of schools for the hearing-impaired, regardless of whether the children are integrated into normal schools or not. Thus, it is clear that a simple way to avoid conflicts of responsibility is for the schools and the university cochlear implant centres to cooperate in the programming and rehabilitation of cochlear implant patients. Some issues that may arise are connected with the organisation and responsibility for speech processor fitting, priority of pre- and postoperative counselling compared with audiologic fitting and testing, and organisation of postoperative testing.

Organisation and Responsibility for Speech Processor Fitting

If an arrangement is made to have the schools for the hearing-impaired children carry out speech processor fitting, two types of cooperation can be envisioned. In the first, personnel from the local schools work within the university clinic under the direct supervision of the clinic's implant team personnel. In this case, it is not necessarily essential that the school's personnel attend a specially arranged course on the fundamentals of cochlear implants because there is continual clinical supervision. It means that speech processor fittings can be learned on the job with adequate feedback from experienced cochlear implant team members. For a more distant school, a different arrangement must be made where a formal educational course, which includes details on processor fitting, is necessary. There also needs to be understanding about the frequency of speech processor fittings to be carried out at the school, and the types of problems that the school should attempt to solve before contacting the clinic. With the advent of modem data communication permitting patient data to be sent back and forth rapidly, it is obvious that this distinction will become less clear in the future. That is, remote processor fitting of child at a school from the clinic could be easily accomplished (Monneron, Ouayoun & Chhum, 1995).

Once an arrangement between clinic and the distant school has been formalised, the question arises as to which groups of patients and which devices should be covered by the schools. It is the mandate of a university clinic to change to or add new or updated devices as they become available or as they show superior performance for patients compared with previously used systems. The clinics will purchase these devices and their fitting hardware and software, perhaps leaving the school with outdated equipment. It is essential that the schools consult with the clinic in determining the pool of patients that they should be servicing and the type of equipment to be purchased. Here, it is necessary to avoid the danger of the cochlear implant companies selling programming equipment directly to the schools because it may happen that the equipment is about to become obsolete, or that equipment may be sold for which no training has been supplied. The latter problem could mean that the school begins working with patients before the necessary training has been obtained. The biggest problem is that university clinics must maintain the ultimate responsibility to the patients for device functioning and proper application. It is normally not within the budgets of schools to purchase programming equipment at regular intervals, or to take courses continually to maintain updated skills in fitting a variety of speech coding strategies and adapting programmes to the very special needs of some patients. The solution, again, is a cooperative, networked service where cochlear implant companies and prospective schools are informed about the role of the university clinic concerning speech processor fitting and then shape their purchasing policies accordingly.

Pre- and Postoperative Counselling

One of the most helpful roles which can be provided by direct cooperation between schools and cochlear implant clinics concerns parent counselling. In most clinics, the role of the clinic team is restricted to preoperative audiologic tests, device implantation and postoperative speech processor fitting. Pre- and postoperative counselling is seldom a priority of the clinic because it is a time-consuming task for which medical or audiological personnel may not be qualified, having received little or no training. This is in contrast with teachers of hearing-impaired children for whom such counselling is inherent in their training and work. Thus, integrating school personnel into the clinic structure has distinct advantages for the school, the clinic, the patients and the patients' families. For the clinic, such counselling can be performed within the preoperative, diagnostic test period that normally takes place during the phase of initial patient hospitalisation and later, during the first speech processor fitting sessions. The results of preoperative counselling can be discussed with the audiological and medical personnel at the team meetings and can help to decide whether recommending implantation to the parents or patient is indicated. For the school, the advantage is direct access to the patients in the clinic environment and involvement in the types of choices patients will have for implantation at the time of the diagnostic work-up. For the patients and their families, the advantage is continuity of care and a better understanding of procedures and possibilities for the future. Ultimately, the knowledge gained by the schools ensures awareness by the teachers concerning the current status of cochlear implants which, in turn, leads to better understanding by parents and a resultant increase in treatment for deaf children who cannot benefit from the use of hearing aids.

Such an arrangement between the school and the clinic is not without its conflicts. First, because the school-employed persons are working within hospital environments, they will have to agree to work under different supervisory conditions, i.e. management structures in schools are more consultative than in hospitals. Second, the holiday structure at schools is long and fixed, whereas those in hospitals are shorter and flexible so that service can be maintained throughout the year. Concretely, speech processor problems and operating-room schedules do not cease during school holidays. Third, when school personnel are involved with speech processor fitting and counselling, they will realise the need to become involved with technical problems for which they will have to be specially trained, and they may need to limit their counselling to a fixed rather than an open-ended schedule. Thus, for the school wishing to work directly within the clinic, there are accommodations to be made to a working style markedly different from that of a school. The clinic, on the other hand, will need to accommodate the remedial methods used in educational settings, provide adequate space and materials, and support the growth of educationally inspired activities.

Postoperative Evaluations

Schools generally work with examination materials that have been developed by a central institution and are in place for a number of years. The examination papers are handed back to the students for the student and the parent to receive immediate and open feedback on test results. Moreover, if two schools are working with the same student, open communication exists about when tests will occur and what the results are. There is a far different situation in the clinic, which reflects the legal requirement for the clinic to protect the patient's right to privacy. Even information given to other institutions, such as those at a national level concerned with evaluating the efficacy of a cochlear implant and improving the patient's quality of life, is always in the form of anonymous patient records. The information transmitted to the patient is generally sparse, unless the patient or parent requests it, in which case it must be provided.

The situation with respect to test materials is also vastly different between clinics and schools. For cochlear-implanted children, a clinic will have to select a group of tests for which years of practice in proving their efficacy to quantify speech perception, recognition and understanding adequately simply do not exist. This means that the university clinic will have to select these materials, test children and modify the materials in an evolving process typical of the scientific environment of a university, but atypical of a school. Although it is possible for the school personnel to be involved in some aspects of the selection of test materials, the scientific method may be strange to school personnel. To avoid possible conflicts over whether test materials should be transmitted to the school or not, university clinics will have to ensure that schools understand both the scientific and medical nature of test materials. It would certainly help resolve the conflict if the university ensured that schools know when testing will occur, even if the preliminary, scientific nature of the tests or associated confidentiality agreements with test designers means that the schools cannot be fully informed about all aspects of test results but are simply given test scores. Eventually, the interpretation of results is shared with parents and teachers alike. It is, perhaps, the immediacy of knowing results that differs between universities and schools.

In the long run, such a joint programme between university and school has the advantage that both schools and clinics can draw on an additional pool of professionals, provide clear and continuous service to the patients and support the use of cochlear implants more effectively. In times when university hospitals and schools are being forced to reduce personnel and cut costs, this represents considerable flexibility in staffing arrangements, service administration and cost-effectiveness of cochlear implantation in both children and adults.

Conclusion

We believe that there is a need for more than a cochlear implant centre, rather a complete cochlear implant support system. It is not only a medical facility that invites patients to the clinic 'from time to time' in order to make various speech processor adjustments and administer some tests. It is a full service that provides direct medical, technical, clinical and counselling services, as well as public relations and education. Even where the concept of a cochlear implant centre is very highly developed, it often provides good support only during the time that the patients/parents and the children are actually in the centre. Our aim is to improve the continual support system/service that must take place outside an institution.

As the population of cochlear implant users and those who are better informed about such devices increases, the need for adaptation will become evident. What seems clear is that the ongoing process of rehabilitation requires the efforts of a large number of differing individuals throughout the cochlear implant user's life. Our goal is to continue with our networking efforts.

We are not in the position to realise this goal without the help and support of a multifaceted and multiprofessional team. It is important for us to show that through our model we are not only intending to guarantee remedial and psychological counselling but also wish to ensure comprehensive follow-up and support. This should evolve from the everyday life situations of the children and take into account the subjective effects of the cochlear implant on the personal well-being of the user, as well as the person's ability to cope with problems that might arise in the family, at school or at work. Our model demands a constant feedback loop circling between medical–clinical–research programmes and educational facilities and social circumstances. On the one hand, this keeps us from becoming one-sided with too much emphasis on the quantitative, objective aspects which do not take into account the impact of our actions on the patients and may only produce interpretations that relate to the person as disabled. On the other hand, it makes it possible to integrate the qualitative changes without neglecting the need to balance the importance of objective information and its implications.

Rehabilitation for cochlear implant users offers a prime opportunity for a strong and close relationship between a clinical facility providing medical and technical support and the educational and training facilities. The Basel hospital–school clinic has a population of both children and adult cochlear implant recipients. It offers more than one type of cochlear implant system and the device-fitting strategies associated with each. Finally, and most importantly, it serves a central function of coordinating diagnostics, surgery, device maintenance services, and ongoing counselling and rehabilitation.

In summary, we have presented a service model for a broad-based cochlear implant support system emanating from the cooperative efforts of a central hospital and schools for the hearing impaired. We have developed new positions that are supported by the school but located within the hospital, an educational programme for professionals and a service programme that reaches beyond the scope of any single facility. Our service to cochlear implant patients is in a continual state of improvement and it would be incorrect to assume that once this network has been completely implemented it will remain the same for the next decade. This service model allows for, and encourages change and adaptation.

Acknowledgements

We would like to acknowledge the work of our colleagues, Danielle Naef Schurch and Angelika Moracchi. We are also grateful for the leadership and support of Professor Rudolf Probst. An important element of our work is the cooperation with the Sprachheilschule in St Gallen, which serves hearing-impaired children in eastern Switzerland, and the Swiss School for the Hard-of-Hearing at Landenhof serving the central region of the country.

References

Allum DJ (1995) Assessing performance in third generation implants in children. Paper presented at the Third International Cochlear Implant Workshop, Würzburg, Germany, 23–24 October.

Archbold S (1994) Monitoring progress in children at the pre-verbal stage. In McCormick B, Archbold S, Sheppard S (Eds) Cochlear Implants for Young Children. London: Whurr, 197–213.

Böhler D (1992) Elternarbeit konkret. Unser Kind ist hörbehindert. Dialog und Praxis. Ein Begleitbuch für Eltern. Meggen, Schweiz: Eigenverlag, Bühlmattstr. 7, 6045.

Boothroyd A (1991) Assessment of speech perception capacity in profoundly deaf children. American Journal of Otology 12 (Suppl.): 67–72.

Dorman M (1993) Speech perception by adults. In Tyler RS (Ed) Cochlear Implants: Audiological Foundations. London: Singular, pp. 145–90.

Eggert D (1995) Der Integrationsgedanke und das Programm einer 'gesunden Schule'. 'Nur die Chance, die nicht gegeben wird, behindert'. Hannover, Universität Hannover, FB Erziehungswissenschaften I., pp 109–32.

Elmiger P (1992) Soziale Situation von integriert geschulten Schwerhörigen in Regelschulen, Diplomarbeit an der Universitat Freiburg, Freiburg, Schweiz.

Löwe A (1985) Hörgeschädigte Kinder in Regelschulen: Ergebnisse von Untersuchungen und Erhebungen in der Bundesrepublik Deutschland und in der Schweiz. Dortmund: Geers-Stiftung.

Lutman M, Archbold S, Gibbin KP, McCormick B, O'Donoghue GM (1996) Monitoring progress in young children with cochlear implants. In Allum DJ (Ed) Cochlear Implant Rehabilitation in Children and Adults. London: Whurr.

Monneron L, Ouayoun M, Chhum S (1995) Self assessment and remote control for the Digisonic cochlear implant. In Proceedings of the 3rd International Congress on Cochlear Implants, Paris, France, 27–29 April, p 258.

Müller RJ (1989) Zur integrativen Beschulung hörgeschädigter Kinder. Unpublished thesis, Heilpäd, Zurich.

Müller RJ (1994a) Ich höre – nicht alles! Hörgeschädigte Mädchen und Jungen in Regelschulen. Heidelberg: Edition Schindele.

Müller RJ (1994b) Wege der Integration – Zusammenarbeit von Schule, Elternhaus und Fachleuten bei hörgeschädigten Kindern. Luzern: Schweizerische Zentralstelle für Heilpädagogik.

Reid J, Lehnhardt M (1993) Post-operative speech perception results for 92 European children using the Nucleus mini system 22 cochlear implant. In Fraysse B, Deguine O (Eds) Cochlear Implants: New Perspectives. Advances in Otorhinolaryngology 48: 241–47.

Sander A, Hildeschmidt A (1993) Kind-Umfeld-Diagnose – ein oekosystemischer Ansatz. St Ingbert, Germany: Werner J Roehrig.

Schmid-Giovannini S (1985) Ratschläge und Anleitungen für Eltern und Erzieher hörgeschädigter Kinder. Zollikon: Heftreihe.

Spillman T, Dillier N (1987) Die Ausnuetzung des Restgehörs durch Hörgerät und Kochleaimplantat: eine Vergleichsuntersuchung mit der MAC-Batterie. Therapeutische Umschau 44: 109-13.

Chapter 8
Managing Educational Issues Throughout the Process of Implantation

PATRICIA M. CHUTE, MARY ELLEN NEVINS,
SIMON C. PARISIER

Introduction

The technological advances made in the field of cochlear implantation over the last decade have resulted in the availability of a device that substantially impacts on the lives of deaf individuals. For the profoundly, postlinguistically deafened adult, improvements have ranged from changes in the quality of life to the ability to use the telephone interactively (Dorman et al., 1991; Skinner et al., 1991). Child cochlear implant users demonstrate marked improvements in their ability to understand speech through auditory means and to produce intelligible speech (Osberger et al., 1991; Staller et al., 1991). Additionally, however, the cochlear implant has made an impact in the classrooms in which these children learn. It has changed the expectations of teachers who have taught the children prior to cochlear implantation. Also, it has introduced other teachers to the concepts of auditory learning through implantation.

Much attention has been paid to the issues regarding candidacy for implantation and speech perception and speech production after implantation (Geers & Moog, 1987; Hellman et al., 1991; Tyler, 1993). However, there has been little information regarding the effects of this device on educational facilities that teach deaf children or how to manage the children as they move through the implantation process. To fully understand the issues involved in educating a child with a significant hearing loss, it is necessary to develop an appreciation for the system in which this task takes place. It is important to obtain an overview of how the school system functions as the site that educates the child. Further, we must understand how the medical facility functions as the site that medically treats the child. This may take some reorientation on the part of professionals evaluating children for cochlear implants as well as teachers who have a child with a cochlear implant in their class-room. As part of this reorientation, the professionals must maintain an approach to rehabilitation based on a balance between science and reality. A view of cochlear implantation that is unrealistic can significantly impede or, in some cases, prevent progress with an implant.

Practically, cochlear implantation is a process and not simply a treatment. As such, it requires the attention of a team of professionals. A multidisciplinary team approach to the management of children with hearing loss is not a new concept (Matkin, Hook & Hixson, 1979; Nevins, 1986). Cochlear implant technology has necessitated a recasting of the concept of the team approach so that the team is *inter*disciplinary rather than *multi*disciplinary. A medical model of deafness is likely to drive the process of implantation because the placement of the cochlear implant is a surgical procedure. A medical model suggests that deafness is a condition to be diagnosed and treated, in this case with a cochlear implant. It requires an extensive time commitment and a partnership between the medical and educational communities rarely seen. It necessitates the interfacing of hospital and school personnel.

The physician is assumed to be the 'captain of the team' in traditional medical models. However, many surgeons may be unfamiliar with the educational needs of deaf children. Thus, what is needed is a truly collaborative team, in which individuals take varied roles of equal importance, alternating in the position of 'expert'. This is in contrast with the traditional medical pyramid with a primary expert at the top and all others viewed as implementers. Team members should be able to explore their individual areas and make recommendations without pressures that view the surgery as a treatment end. Surgeons committed to the perspective of implantation as a process and not a treatment will embrace a team approach to the management of children with implants.

Of critical importance to the success of the process of implantation is the presence of an educator of the deaf on a paediatric cochlear implant team. It is the educational consultant with expertise in the areas of educating hearing-impaired children who can help guide the process of habilitation of the child with a cochlear implant. The consultant serves as a liaison between the medical and the educational facilities.

Educational management of the child with an implant begins during the selection process with observing the appropriateness of the placement, the personnel, the curriculum and the method of communication. How best to perform these observations and what methods foster good communication with the implant team will depend on various geographical, social or cultural constraints. None the less, some method of delivering services to implanted children must be established to ensure successful use of the device. Unfortunately, the choice of a particular service delivery model made by an implant team is often based on economic factors.

Service delivery models

There are several service delivery models that can be used when providing treatment to the child considering a cochlear implant or one who already has an implant. The first of these models incorporates a direct service model where children who receive cochlear implants return to the implant facility (or a facility that is associated with the implant centre) to obtain recommended rehabilitative services. These services are given separately from the child's school and are often geographically distant from their home school district. The second type of service delivery system enlists the services of a speech/language pathologist or audiologist to act as an intermediary with the school system. Although this model has merit in that it uses direct contact with the child's school, there may be differences in training between speech pathologists and audiologists and school-based teachers of the deaf. The differences in training rather than in the child's capabilities may be reflected in the final outcomes. The third type of service delivery model is one in which a particular educational facility becomes a programme that houses a cochlear implant centre within its confines. Special 'cochlear implant schools' which evaluate and rehabilitate these children have identified themselves as having an environment within which children with implants can receive a comprehensive education. In the United States, schools such as Tucker-Maxon in Portland, Oregon and Central Institute for the Deaf in St Louis, Missouri are but two of these cochlear implant schools. Although there are some implant facilities that choose to ignore the educational issues facing children receiving cochlear implants, this is not a model that is recommended or advocated by groups who are committed to implantation. Programmes with no educational component should be avoided by parents who are seeking implants for their children. The last model which addresses the educational needs of children with implants is one that uses the services of an educational consultant. Because this is a model that can service a larger number of children utilising the resources within their own communities, it is the model that receives the most attention in this text.

The educational consultant model

The United States Food and Drug Administration (FDA) guidelines that regulate implant surgery do not dictate the presence of an educator on the implant team. However, the guidelines strongly recommend that the surgeon work with an experienced team of audiology, speech language, rehabilitation, education and psychology professionals (Cochlear Corporation, 1991). An educational consultant working on a paediatric cochlear implant team can determine whether or not a child's local school programme is one that emphasises listening and speaking. This individual is a certified teacher of the deaf with experience in the development of speech, spoken language and auditory skills. In our experience, the role of the educational consultant impacts greatly upon the child's success.

We recommend that the educational consultant make an initial school visit before the child is implanted. This visit becomes part of the evaluation process for candidacy. The purpose of the pre-implant visit is both fact finding and information dissemination (Nevins et al., 1991). Table 8.1 describes the four basic goals of the pre-implant school visit by the educational consultant. The educational consultant arranges for the school visit soon after the child's first appointment at the implant centre.

Because there is still much misinformation about implants and the process of implantation, it is important for the educational consultant to spend some time with school personnel. During this time, the educational consultant provides them with information about the device in general and its potential benefit for the child. Often questions from the child's teachers and other staff drive the nature and level of the information presented in this pre-implant period. For instance, when a child is in a mainstream setting, questions about deafness and language devel-

Table 8.1: Goals and related activities of the pre-implant school visit by the educational consultant

Goal	Activities
1. To disseminate information about the cochlear implant, surgery, and how the implant works	1. Distribute teacher's guide to the implant device 2. Answer questions about candidacy
2. To assess the educational environment of the candidate	1. Record placement type (residential, special class, mainstream) and availability of support services 2. Interview school administrators and personnel
3. To evaluate the child's performance in school environment	1. Observe child in classroom and in special activities (e.g. speech) 2. Examine relevant school records 3. Interview teachers and support personnel
4. To establish a working relationship between implant centre and school	1. Encourage school personnel to voice an opinion on child's candidacy for the implant 2. Create opportunities for informal exchange between local school staff and the educational consultant

opment may be of greater concern to the child's teachers. This is in contrast with questions about the difference between hearing aid and implant technology which may be of more interest to teachers of the deaf and speech–language pathologists.

The pre-implant visit generally occurs after the speech and language evaluation has taken place at the implant centre. This makes it possible for the educational consultant to verify performance observed by the team's speech–language pathologist. It is not uncommon for young children to show greater communication ability in a more familiar, school environment than in the hospital evaluation area. It is important to obtain the child's best performance level because speech and language ability affect candidacy decisions (Parisier, Chute & Nevins, 1994). Interviews with the teacher regarding impressions of the child and the child's overall abilities are vitally important to the decision-making process. The school personnel should be viewed as extended members of the implant team whose input is integral to evaluating candidacy. In addition to observing the child in the classroom and individual speech therapy setting, the educational consultant assesses the overall educational environment of the child's school programme. In this assessment, the educational consultant notes the type of placement (residential vs. day), mode of communication (oral vs. manual) and commitment to speech and audition in the classroom.

Establishing a working relationship

Despite the importance of all the activities designated to occur at the pre-implant visit, the single most important objective is the establishment of a trusting relationship between the implant centre and the school. If the child is, indeed, chosen to be a candidate and receives an implant, the school should, in most cases, be given the lead role in providing rehabilitation after surgery. The work of maximising the impact of the auditory information available through the device will be the responsibility of the local school personnel. Empowering school-based professionals for participation in designing and directing the post-implant rehabilitation programme is not universally accepted. We support this concept, however, because it is a better treatment plan than others when considering long-term use of the implant. Trends indicate that more programmes (both in the USA and elsewhere) are beginning to adopt a model that recognises the valuable contributions of local school professionals as part of the process (Archbold, 1994).

Preparation of school-based professionals to accept the responsibility for post-implant management is directed by the educational consultant. The educational consultant determines the extent of their knowledge base regarding audition and the implant, and their level of skill for incorporating auditory learning into the classroom. In some cases, the school personnel may be knowledgeable about the development of auditory skills with traditional amplification but have had no experience with children who use cochlear implants. In these circumstances, the educational consultant will provide information about the implant device and how it works to combat fear of the unknown technology. At the same time, the educational consultant will reinforce the staff's ability to provide auditory activities in the classroom. In still other cases, the staff may be unfamiliar with the device but also be uncertain about how to develop auditory skills. When local school professionals are open to guidance from the educational consultant, we must offer it in the proper spirit. We believe that this spirit is one of collegial collaboration, not one that is either simplistic or overly formal in nature. The tone set by the educational consultant will influence the nature of the partnership that will be important during post-implant follow-up. When no communication between the clinic, as represented by the educational consultant, and the school takes place in the pre-implant stage, it can seriously affect the post-implant management of the child. This is because feelings of alienation could exist on the part of the school.

The post-implant phase

The post-implant phase is divided into two components: an immediate one that begins at the time of the initial fitting and a second that begins after short-term implant use. The educational consultant attends the initial fitting sessions to observe the early responses of the child. Knowledge of the exact level of responsiveness of the child and the performance which is demonstrated at this time is very useful. The educational consultant makes recommendations to the local school personnel for initial teaching objectives based on the observations.

Characteristics of children at first stimulation

The range of performance that occurs after children have experienced their first stimulation with a cochlear implant can be divided into four groups. Group 1 includes the largest number of children who receive cochlear implants. These children are able to detect a wide range of speech signals (the six sound test [ah, ee, oo sh, s, m] as well as their name) (Perigoe, 1992). This detection is exhibited only in structured tasks with specific listening paradigms (e.g. put the block in the bucket when you hear the sound). The second, and next largest group of children comprises those who are able to discriminate different patterns of speech (e.g. cat versus ice-cream cone). Again, this ability is observed in structured situations. The third group of children exhibits no auditory awareness of sound but wears the speech processor without any complaints or evidence of aversive stimulation. This category includes very young children whose ability to participate in the fitting process was severely limited. However, they have a positive attitude towards wearing the device. The fourth and final group includes those children who refuse to wear the device even when it is turned off. This category of children most often includes the youngest who do not have the linguistic sophistication to understand what is happening. Experience suggests that these are also likely to be children born with normal hearing who later became deafened secondary to meningitis.

Planning initial teaching objectives

The immediate goal of auditory work by school personnel for children in Groups 1 and 2 is to obtain a replication of responses that were seen at the implant centre at the time of the initial fitting. Some children will make this generalisation easily whereas others may have some difficulty in performing the same task outside the structure of the fitting process. A second goal for these two groups is the detection of speech and environmental sounds. We recommend that environmental sound training occur in its naturalistic setting with the aid of the parent. Parents should be trained in ways to make their child aware of the various household sounds and learn how to encourage listening behaviours at home. Detection of speech is practised by using functional words that have a high degree of repetition throughout the course of the day (e.g. calling the child's name).

Children in Group 3 require a completely different approach. These are children whose devices may not be optimally set. Thus, it is the teachers who must observe any overt or covert responses to sound. Continued lack of response would indicate a need for a retuning of the speech processor at the clinic because the original programme was likely a product of the audiologist's best estimation of threshold and comfort levels. Building a cooperative relationship between the school and the implant centre to obtain the best performance from the child is the primary objective for the professionals involved with this group of children.

Objectives for the teachers of children in the final group (those who refuse to wear the device) will focus initially on having the child wear the device consistently. It is likely that the implant centre staff will have established a wearing programme supported by behaviour-modification techniques which can assist the school staff in managing this aspect of implant use. Communication with the implant team is crucial for this group especially if this is the teacher's first exposure to cochlear implants. A child's initial rejection of the device may cause the uncertain teacher more concern than is necessary. However, once the child consistently wears the device, the teachers receive a list of recommendations for the management of this group of children. These and other goals are outlined in Table 8.2.

Table 8.2: Immediate auditory goals implemented following the initial stimulation of the device

If the child:	Then initial teaching objective should encourage:
• detects a wide range of speech signals in structured task	• responding to name • perceiving pattern contrasts (single-syllable words vs. multisyllable words and/or short phrases or sentences vs. long phrases or sentences)
• discriminates different patterns of speech in structured situations	• constant expansion of set of pattern contrasts • carryover of acquired skills demonstrated in structured setting to classroom • introduction to closed-set listening tasks
• wears the processor but shows no auditory awareness	• alerting to presence of speech sounds, especially the child's name • alerting to environmental sounds
• refuses to wear the device	• implementation of a wearing programme • getting the device turned on as soon as possible and begin alerting to speech

A second school visit is arranged by the educational consultant after the child completes short-time use of the implant. The timing of this visit allows local personnel an opportunity to familiarise themselves with the device, observe the child's response to sound and develop questions for the educational consultant. During the post-implant visit, the educational consultant is prepared to review issues regarding the care and management of the device. Specifically, teachers should be shown techniques for performing daily equipment checks. Some level of equipment check can be performed independent of the child. Under ideal conditions the daily check also includes a measure of auditory performance, once the child is capable of responding. For example, the teacher requests the child to raise his/her hand after each auditory-only presentation of the six sound test. As the child's skill with using the implant increases, listening-check tasks can be made more difficult. Despite the fact that home checks take place, a school listening check will ensure that the child will have a functioning device throughout the day. Should the teacher discover that the implant is not functioning properly, she must implement techniques to correct the problem. It is the responsibility of the educational consultant to provide the teacher with this knowledge and that of how to troubleshoot the device.

The educational consultant also provides guidance to the classroom teacher/therapist about the importance of offering an environment that facilitates auditory learning (Ling, 1976) rather than simply scheduling sessions for auditory training. Historically, auditory training called for listening practice in small-group activities. Often these lessons began with the discrimination of non-verbal sounds such as bells, drums and whistles. Listening to speech occurred only after success in identifying these gross noisemakers. Ling (1986) suggested that auditory training results were unsatisfactory because the training seldom related to the child's speech and spoken language development, cognitive level or everyday life experiences. Mischook and Cole (1986) described auditory learning as 'the normal development of a synergistic cluster composed of auditory, speech and language abilities'. They further recommended that auditory learning be best accomplished through 'natural, enjoyable intervention'.

To gain the support of the classroom teacher and the school-based speech–language pathologist in developing an environment that encourages auditory learning, it is necessary to demonstrate some familiarity with the demands and the realities of the school day. The educational consultant's post-implant visit allows for specific recommendations to be made about how to incorporate listening into a particular classroom. After spending time in the classroom and becoming familiar with the classroom's routines, the educational consultant can use real-life examples to identify opportunities for maximising listening. Additional visits are scheduled as required, based on need.

Long-term follow-up

The educational consultant's contribution to the paediatric cochlear implant team parallels the child's educational needs. The presence of the educational consultant on the team ensures that the appropriate services will be available to the children throughout their educational career. This will dictate an ongoing commitment on the part of the facility which initially implanted the child.

There are issues in education that face all children regardless of whether they are hearing-impaired or normal-hearing. These issues may be related to teacher/student relationships or even physical changes in the school building. For the normal-hearing child, a new teacher with a different teaching style or noise from building construction occurring on the school property may be a nuisance. For hearing-impaired children, these types of event may be their downfall. Addressing the child's needs on a continual basis through intervention by the educational consultant will ensure that the child will make the most effective use of the implant in the classroom under a variety of changing circumstances.

One critical educational issue for hearing-impaired children involves decisions concerning movement out of special classrooms. This process shifts the child from a teaching environment in which only hearing-impaired children are taught to one in which there are also normal-hearing youngsters. This is referred to as mainstreaming. The decision to mainstream is usually not based solely on academic standing but must include numerous concerns such as psychosocial development and speech intelligibility. Just as the decision regarding candidacy for implantation should not have been based on a single determinant, decisions regarding mainstreaming also require consideration of many factors.

Although parents often feel that mainstream placement is the main goal for their child, input regarding this decision should come from a variety of sources. Here, once again, the role of the educational consultant is important in assessing the child's appropriateness for the mainstream and the appropriateness of the mainstream setting itself.

The impact that the cochlear implant has made on placement of children in the mainstream is impressive. Chute and Nevins (1994) reported a trend for children with implants to move from self-contained facilities or classrooms towards more mainstreamed settings. Children at their centre were monitored yearly for changes in school placement. While no changes were seen within the first year of implant use, by the fifth year close to 75% of the children were found to have moved out of the self-contained environment.

In addition to placing the deaf child who has a cochlear implant in the mainstream, monitoring the child after placement is also critical. If the implant centre has not adopted an educational consultant model, it is likely that decisions regarding readiness for the mainstream, choosing a mainstream placement and monitoring the child in the mainstream placement will be made without participation of any implant centre personnel. Failure to participate at this stage of the child's educational career may jeopardise the gains accomplished and invite mismanagement when support for the child is most crucial. However, it is a naive expectation to believe that comprehensive pre-mainstreaming evaluation ensures later social and academic success. For the process to be completely successful, ongoing monitoring by the educational consultant of the child in the school placement will increase the potential for the child's success in the mainstream setting.

Whether it is for success in the mainstream or success in the self-contained classroom, the child who uses a cochlear implant must be carefully managed. Issues of management do not begin and end with the surgical implantation of the device but rather grow and change with the child. The education of hearing-impaired children and, specifically, those with cochlear implants has heightened the awareness of many issues facing special education today.

Deaf education in the future

Trends in the field of deaf education indicate that we are about to reach a crossroads (Moores, 1990, 1991, 1993). Many programmes may identify themselves with the movement of the deaf community towards adoption of American Sign Language as the primary language of instruction and a bilingual, bicultural approach for managing the whole deaf child in the United States. This movement is real, and many schools are adopting policies that favour this philosophical orientation. Cochlear implant technology is also changing the philosophical orientation of another group of parents and educators – those who value speech, spoken language and preparing a child for competition in a hearing society. Cochlear implantation has heightened attention to the importance of audition for all children with residual hearing. This technology may make the development of intelligible speech a more reasonable and reachable goal for deaf children.

Facilities committed to a comprehensive implant programme must ensure that the educational issues are managed properly throughout the complex and ever-changing process of implantation. Attending to the needs of the whole deaf child, rather than simply the audiological aspects of the hearing loss, will result in a comprehensive management plan emphasising the important role of education in contributing to future academic and economic success of these children.

References

Archbold S (1994) Implementing a paediatric cochlear implant programme: theory and practice. In McCormick B, Archbold S, Sheppard S (Eds) Cochlear Implants for Young Children. London: Whurr, pp 25–59.

Chute PM, Nevins ME (1994) Educational placements of children with multichannel cochlear implants. Paper presented at the meeting of the European Symposium on Paediatric Cochlear Implantation, Montpellier, France, 26–29 May.

Cochlear Corporation (1991) Package Insert. Cochlear Corporation, 61 Inverness Drive East, Englewood, CO80112, USA.

Dorman M, Dove H, Parkin J, Zacharchuk S, Dankowski K (1991) Telephone use by patients fitted with Ineraid cochlear implant. Ear and Hearing 12: 368–69.

Geers AE, Moog JS (1987) Predicting spoken language acquisition in profoundly deaf children. Journal of Speech and Hearing Disorders 52(1): 84–94.

Hellman SA, Chute PM, Kretschmer RE, Nevins ME, Parisier SC, Thurston LC (1991) The development of a children's implant profile. American Annals of the Deaf 136: 77–81.

Ling D (1976) Speech and the Hearing-impaired Child: Theory and Practice. Washington, DC: AG Bell Association for the Deaf.

Ling D (1986) Devices and procedures for auditory learning. Volta 88: 19–28.

Matkin N, Hook P, Hixson P (1979) A multidisciplinary approach to evaluation of hearing-impaired children. In Audiology: An Audio Journal of Continuing Education Tape No. 7. New York: Grune & Stratton.

Mischook M, Cole E (1986) Auditory learning and teaching of hearing-impaired infants. Volta 88: 67–81.

Moores DF (1990). Deja-vu. American Annals of the Deaf 135: 201.

Moores DF (1991) The school placement revolution. American Annals of the Deaf 136: 307–8.

Moores DF (1993) The winds of change. American Annals of the Deaf 138: 315.

Nevins ME (1986) Multidisciplinary assessment of the hearing-impaired child. Panel participant at the Texas Speech/Language and Hearing Association Annual Convention, Austin, Texas, April.

Nevins ME, Kretschmer RE, Chute PM, Hellman SA, Parisier SC (1991) The role of an educational consultant in a pediatric cochlear implant program. Volta 93: 197–204.

Osberger MJ, Chute PM, Pope M, Kessler KS, Carotta CC, Firszt J, Zimmerman-Phillips S (1991) Pediatric cochlear implant candidacy issues. American Journal of Otology 12 (Suppl.): 80–88.

Parisier SC, Chute PM, Nevins ME (1994) Pediatric cochlear implants: surgical and rehabilitative issues. In Lucente FE (Ed) Highlights of the Instructional Courses. St Louis, MI: Mosby, pp 145–54.

Perigoe CB (1992) Strategies for the remediation of speech of hearing-impaired children. In Stoker R, Ling D (Eds) Speech production in hearing-impaired children and youth. Volta 82: 71–84.

Skinner MW, Holden LK, Holden TA, Dowell RC, Seligman PM, Brimacombe JA, Beiter AL (1991) Performance of postlinguistically deaf adults with the Wearable Speech Processor (WSP III) and Mini Speech Processor (MSP) of the Nucleus multi-electrode cochlear implant. Ear and Hearing 12: 3–22.

Staller SJ, Dowell RC, Beiter AL, Brimacombe JA (1991) Perceptual abilities of children with the Nucleus 22-channel cochlear implant. Ear and Hearing 12(4): 34S–47S.

Tyler RS (1993) Cochlear Implants: Audiological Foundations. California: Singular Publications.

Chapter 9
Auditory Pre-training and its Implications for Child Development: The Importance of Early Stimulation in the Deaf Child

ALICIA HUARTE IRUJO, MAITE MOLINA, MANUEL MANRIQUE

Introduction

Paediatric audiological treatment and the education of the child with hearing difficulties are usually more successful the earlier the problems are tackled (Loewe, 1992). Many authors emphasise the importance of auditory stimulation in the early years of life (the critical period) which has definitive consequences for language acquisition (Holm & Kunze, 1969; Rubel et al., 1984).

In the human being, the limits of this critical period and the precise nature of acoustic stimulation which can determine normal development have been defined by Ruben (1986), Curtiss (1889) and by the quasi-experimental studies based on the observation of wild children (wolf boys) who are deprived of all verbal communication during early childhood (Itard, 1921). The first boy, discovered at the age of eight, was never able to acquire more than 10 words. The second, discovered during puberty, only learned to communicate by using signs.

According to Chouard et al. (1983) and Uziel (1991), the critical period for the acquisition of language lies between birth and the age of four to six years. This critical period for early development corresponds to a phase of special neuronal flexibility in which auditory sense perception is essential for the normal development of the cerebral cortex (Hubel & Wiesel, 1965; Movshon & Van Sluyters, 1991). Under normal conditions, 50% of the human brain takes on its structure before the age of 3, and 80% before the age of 8. This emphasises the importance of carrying out early stimulation, particularly in cases where any sensory handicap, such as hearing loss, is present.

The development of auditory stimulation in the child forms part of a whole and so it is important to stimulate all the aspects which contribute to the child's maturation (Aimard & Abadie, 1992). The child needs to be stimulated in order to achieve balanced development which embraces physical, neurological, psychological and social factors. This development depends, on the one hand, on what the child inherits from the parents, which is genetic; and, on the other hand, how the child is conditioned by the environment in which it develops. This means that we can consider the child's overall development as being the product of heredity enhanced by the stimulation received.

From gestation to around the age of eight, the enrichment of the brain is a direct consequence of the connections made between neurons. It can be described in the following manner. The five senses – sight, hearing, touch, taste and smell – act as a channel or means of entry for external stimuli, such as a voice or a smell, to reach the neurones and discharge small doses of positive energy into them. Each charged neuron automatically joins up with its neighbour, thus creating networks or circuits along which new stimuli later circulate. Therefore, the more stimuli there are, the greater the number of neuronal circuits and the better the cerebral development. 'Exercising the senses does not only mean making use of them, it means learning to manage them well. It means learning, so to speak, to feel because we only know how to touch, see or hear to the extent that we have learned how to do so' (Rousseau, 1990).

From the moment of birth, the child learns. The child does so by observing, listening to sounds, smelling, tasting, touching, doing things, moving, imitating and repeating. All of these activities presuppose stimulation and motivation (Gimeno, Rico & Vicente, 1986).

All sensory information is essential for the initiation and development of mental functions in the child, given that cerebral activity depends essentially on sensory stimuli. So, the brain is not capable of feeling, reacting and thinking normally if it is in a sensory vacuum. Comenio suggests that 'there is nothing in the mind which has not been first in the senses' (1992).

Early stimulation is the best means of awakening children's brains. *We must teach them to hear.* This process of development is severely affected in children who have congenital or prelingual deafness. The repercussions on the child's psychomotor and linguistic development and on the personality are well known (Gajick et al., 1985; Lafon, 1985; Launay & Borel-Maisonny, 1989; Morgon, Aimard & Daudet, 1991). In such cases, it is even more important to take early action to provide stimulation.

All hypoacusic children benefit from auditory stimulation. However small the residual dynamic ranges may be, it is important for the auditory channels and cortical areas to receive signals and for their development to be encouraged. This is because the auditory system not only has the function of hearing but is also used for structuring time and space (Lafon, 1985).

None the less, auditory education should not be regarded as a purely passive process in which sound stimulation is enough to bring about normal development. Such stimulation in the child should be thought of as an active process in which professional support should be complemented by the child's motivation to learn to hear because hearing is essential for keeping in touch with the outside world (Peña, 1988).

In the preliminary learning phase, auditory pre-training is intended to awaken the child's sound perception, with its variations in frequency, intensity and duration. These apparently simple objectives are of vital importance when it comes to fitting cochlear implants in young hypoacusics children. It should be kept in mind that the sooner a properly programmed cochlear implant is fitted, the better we can fulfill the objectives of early stimulation.

Rationale for auditory pre-training

Starting from the basis that objective audiological tests such as the EABR (evoked auditory brainstem response) and stapedial reflex measurements do not replace the conventional forms of behavioural audiometry (McCormick, 1993; Kileny et al., 1994), an auditory pre-training protocol has been devised which facilitates quicker and more effective programming of the cochlear implant.

Auditory pre-training is aimed primarily at prelingual children who have had no experience with sound. Usually these are children aged between two and six years who need to become conditioned to sound and undergo auditory learning so that the cochlear implant can be programmed. This conditioning plays an essential role in the progress of all types of learning, as socialisation is impossible in a person who is incapable of conditioned gestures and reactions. One of the greatest difficulties in programming the cochlear implant in children is precisely their lack of conditioning regarding sound. It is, therefore, necessary to carry out auditory pre-training which aids in the detection of problems and helps achieve greater reliability in the adjustment of electrodes during programming.

The observations of the speech therapist and the audiologist who carry out the programming, as well as the interaction with the child in the course of this process, are aspects which are important to evaluate. Not all children react in the same way to acoustic stimulation. For this reason, it is very helpful for the child to be properly conditioned and to be able to adapt to the different types of games to which the child is exposed when the objective is to achieve responses to auditory stimuli.

Objective of pre-training

In the programming of the cochlear implant, which is carried out three or four weeks after surgery, the hearing threshold and the comfort threshold are determined for each of the electrodes. To make this task easier, auditory pre-training is performed. The objectives are: (1) to achieve correct sound conditioning by training the detection of sound (presence/absence of sound), the discrimination of intensity (a lot/little noise) and the identification of intensity (there is no/there is a little/there is a lot of sound); and (2) reinforcement and support of the basic required vocabulary.

Programme of activities

A programme of play activities must be drawn up which is adapted to the individual child according to individual characteristics and then organised systematically. We must not forget the importance of early stimulation and the child's own development (Thompson, 1982). In accordance with the child's own characteristics, the exercises are carried out with visual support. This is gradually eliminated in favour of the child's auditory perception if the child obtained some benefit from the hearing or vibrotactile aids. This enables the child to acquire a skill which is assimilated so that it can be applied to purely acoustic stimuli.

How to achieve correct sound conditioning

Detection: Presence or Absence of Sound – There is/is no Sound (see Figure 9.1)

When faced with a sound stimulus, the child indicates the presence of sound by means of an action. Therefore she should be able to listen for a sound and also learn how to wait for one. This period of waiting for a sound is particularly important, and the sound stimulus should not be presented at regular intervals as this could spark a false response. The stimulus should be introduced in a variable manner, so that it takes the child by surprise, thus avoiding incorrect automatic responses.

At the outset, the sound stimulus should be presented visually in order to draw the child's attention and create a certain security. Then the visual support is gradually eliminated so that we can see how the child is responding to the vibrations and acoustic stimuli. All these exercises can be given using several forms of games. The first is referred to as

Figure 9.1: Presence of sound/absence of sound. colour the stars when you hear and see the sound

psychomotor back-up, where the child performs an action when receiving a sound stimulus such as jumping into a hoop, making arm movements, lying down on the floor, rolling a ball, hiding, etc. (Boulch, 1984). The second is using graphic back-up; that is, using a selection of pictures, placing stickers whenever a sound stimulus is detected, sticking coloured paper to make a picture, punching something, sticking plasticine balls, cutting something out and so forth. Finally, there are a variety of other games because we must not forget the importance of the child's own initiative, motivation at any moment, and creativity of the speech therapist. If the child is very active, restless and full of fun, the activities must revolve around the child's own interests; for instance, pushing over a tower of beakers, shooting indians on horseback with a toy pistol, throwing toys into boxes, throwing a ball into a basket, making towers and so forth (Gladys, de Viller & Mueller, 1988).

Discrimination of Intensity: A Lot of Sound/a Little Sound (see Figure 9.2)

It is useful to associate these exercises with a large number of elements that help the child assimilate what is being taught; for instance, some kind of gesture must always be used to express the idea of a lot of sound

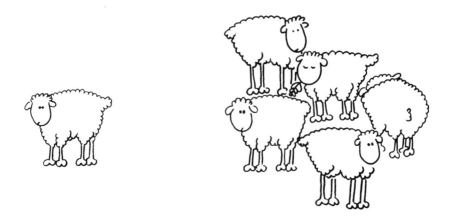

Figure 9.2: Soft noise/loud noise. Place stickers on the sheets when you hear and see the soft noise (one sheep alone) or loud noise (many sheep)

or a little sound. Thus, using the same categories of games, the exercises recommended are all performed with visual back-up. An example of a game with psychomotor back-up is when cards containing a few and a lot of pictures are placed on the floor and the child jumps on the card which corresponds to the type of sound stimulus. If we want to make this more entertaining and exciting, the game can be made more difficult by putting something on the child's head and having the child cross her arms, hop, etc., so as to gain greater motivation. It is also useful to play the same game the other way round: the child plays a soft sound, for example on the drum, and the speech therapist jumps on the card that indicates little sound. We can also make the child follow a drumbeat (fast/slow rhythm). Using graphic back-up, the child draws on a card that either contains a few pictures or one with more elements depending on whether a low-intensity sound or a more intense one has been detected. Other suggestions for games would be using different constructions made out of beakers, boxes, lego, etc., placed at different heights depending on the intensity of the auditory stimulus. When the child hears the sound, she puts a doll in the place where it belongs according to the intensity.

During the sessions it is important to give back-up in the form of lipreading, gestures and facial expression in order to achieve greater motivation in the child and a higher degree of communication. Better communication should help to ensure that this activity is not seen as 'boring'.

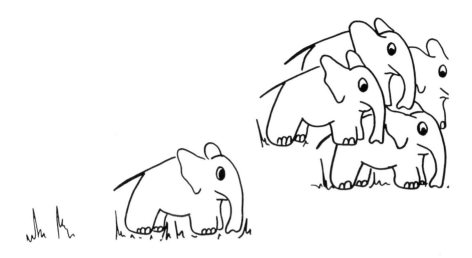

Figure 9.3: No sound/soft sounds/loud sounds. Punch the picture, if you hear and see no sound, soft sounds or loud sound

Identification/Intensity – No Sound/Soft Sounds/ Loud Sounds (see Figure 9.3)

Once the child has absorbed these three concepts, we combine the three options: no sound, soft sounds, loud sounds. Thus, the exercises described above are carried out with psychomotor, graphic and play support, with a direct application to the concepts of sound, low-intensity sound and high-intensity sound (comfortable sound stimulus).

Reinforcement and support of the basic vocabulary required

The child should learn certain words by gesture, lipreading or other means of communication to achieve good communication with a view to the future programming of the cochlear implant. This minimum vocabulary can be summed up in the following list: nothing; a little; a lot; can you hear?; does it hurt?; yes; no. We usually divide the list of words that the child knows into whether they are words, signs or lipreading. We also group them according to whether they are articulated and/or actively used.

Other Complementary Exercises

All the exercises described above should be accompanied by dramatisations and games into which sound elements are introduced: objects which fall, objects which make a noise when struck, objects which make a noise when broken and so on. All this helps the child to learn to detect the presence of sound. We then have to indicate to the child that the sound exists by means of gesture or expression.

We can also perform other complementary exercises which help to condition the child to sound. These are: (1) exercises requiring attention: following objects with the eyes, appearing and disappearing games; (2) exercises which stimulate the visual and auditory memory: games involving relationships, classifying similarities, opposites, associating images, sequencing pictures, etc.; (3) bucco-facial exercises: using the mouth, the lips, the tongue, the teeth, blowing, facial expressions (smile, sadness, crying, laughing), articulation, contrasts between tension and distension of the orofacial muscles, and other body language (spontaneous gestures, looks); and (4) exercises which stimulate pre-language, such as working on all the aspects which aid language stimulation by reinforcing knowledge of the body, notions of space and time, audio-visual perception, audio-visual memory, psychomotor skills, coordination, vocalisations and onomatopoeic sounds (Boada, 1986).

The team

In very small children, both sound conditioning and hearing measurement are confined to the observation of their reactions to acoustic stimuli. The child can blink, change facial expression or behaviour, move, etc. Not all such reactions are obvious, and may often be difficult to interpret and verify. The collaboration of all the people involved in the child's education and surroundings must, therefore, be called upon. During this phase, many people are needed in the conditioning process, which can be regarded as teamwork carried out jointly by audiologists, speech therapists, teachers and relatives. The professionals who work on this pre-implantation phase are the same people who continue with the task after implantation.

The team of audiologists performs the programming of the cochlear implant. They are responsible for supervising and devising the specific guidelines to enable the child to participate in the task of programming the cochlear implant.

Direct contact must be established with the child's speech therapist and teachers, either through personal interviews or by telephone, in order to guide the pre-training process. Auditory pre-training should be carried out in the conditions in which the child 'senses' best. It is very useful to employ a series of technical devices such as individual prostheses, linear amplifiers, amplifiers with sound adjustment, vibrators and so on.

Auditory education is an education of the sense perception and works by encouraging listening and analysis of what is heard to make the child take an interest in the world of sound. Regarding communication, the deaf child does not construct oral language spontaneously. It is difficult for the child to work out what the sound forms represent and to establish a relationship between them and their meaning.

Surroundings and family back-up are important. The family should be informed about hearing loss, and should take an active part in the process of stimulation and education. They are responsible for continuing the work which is done in the speech therapy sessions. They should do so by means of play to reinforce the concepts handled in the sessions without attempting to substitute the work of the speech therapist.

Structuring the sessions

The therapist should create an attractive, dynamic and well-planned environment for the sessions and should bear the following factors in mind during each session. First, use the surroundings to encourage the child. The aim of planning the environment is to organise it in such a way that it increases the child's interest as well as the need to communicate by stimulating the child's demands and by rewarding communicative exchanges. In this way, the non-verbal context is planned so that the materials and activities function as both discriminatory and reinforcing stimuli.

The chances of children communicating and participating in the activities are greater when the objects or activities around them specifically interest them. We must observe what kinds of object(s) attract them most and where they look when faced with a variety of objects. Pre-training should ideally be carried out with a single toy, and the other objects should be hidden. Whenever the child's interest in an object diminishes, we can change to another type of game or activity with the same objectives. Participation is also facilitated when there is an object in the surroundings which the child wants, but cannot get without help; when we create the need to require more of something; when *we* have the materials necessary to carry out an activity; when something unexpected happens or there are surprising reactions. Children generally learn certain routines and expect that they will always be the same. We can create situations which to some extent shatter the child's expectations; for instance, by doing something absurd like putting socks on our hands as if they were gloves. During all these activities, it is important to achieve interaction with the child by 'listening' to the child and watching attentively to create a climate of positive interaction. We should aim to create positive emotions by means of a relaxed physical appearance, by staying close to the child and maintaining eye contact in order to establish shared attention.

Further ideas to keep in mind are to select the correct objectives according to the child's stage of development; to respond to the child's own initiatives; to reinforce the child's communicative attempts or verbal utterances, with the aid of the therapist, and with access to the material in which the child is interested. Further, closely observe the child; get to know how the child communicates to ensure that the session is dynamic and motivating according to the child's own interests and, finally, encourage feedback.

Materials

It is important that materials chosen for use during the period of conditioning to sound awaken the child's motivation, are dynamic and suitable for the child's age, are easy to manipulate and can be used in different ways. The equipment can be classified under the headings of psychomotor skills, play, disposable material, sound material, educational murals and stories. A list of toys and objects is given in the appendix to this chapter. To find out whether the child is conditioned to sound, a series of evaluative norms can be used to confirm that the objective has been achieved (see Table 9.1).

Conclusions

We have provided pre-training to 80% of our prelingual children who were between the ages of 2 and 6 years and who have received cochlear implants at our centre during the last three years. In those children who received no preparatory training, the team took longer and had to make a greater effort to achieve a thorough programming of the different electrodes of the cochlear implant, and the adjustments for programming were less accurate. The objective of training the chil-

Table 9.1: To find out whether the child is conditioned to sound, a series of evaluative norms can be used to confirm that the objective has been achieved

1. Does the child respond to an auditory stimulus?	If so, with or without visual stimulus?
2. What type of stimulus does the child respond to?	Environmental stimuli, stimuli created in an artificial context (instrument)?
3. What type of technical help has been used?	Vibrotactile/auditory prosthesis/others.
4. Level of attention, direction of gaze	Non-existent/poor/adequate
5. Period of waiting prior to an auditory stimulus	Non-existent/poor/adequate
6. Imitation of gestures	Non-existent/poor/adequate
7. Verbal production	Non-existent/poor/adequate
8. Do you consider that the child has had sufficient training?	Yes/no
9. Do you think that the child has assimilated the concept?	Yes/no
10 Observations:	

dren to detect the presence or absence of sound was achieved by all the children, but the concept of soft and loud sounds was harder to put across, as it is more abstract.

Our experience has led us to conclude that such children need to receive auditory pre-training so that the programming of the cochlear implant can be adjusted more effectively. For us, the maturity of the child was in direct relation to the degree of conditioning to sound: the longer the pre-training phase where the child was given auditory stimulation prior to programming, the better the adjustment of the different electrodes of the cochlear implant.

References

Aimard P, Abadie C (1992) Intervención precoz en los transtornos del lenguaje del niño. Barcelona: Editorial Masson.

Boada H (1986) El desarrollo de la comunicación en el niño. Barcelona: Anthropos.

Boulch J (1984) La educación por los movimientos. Buenos Aires: Paidos.

Chouard C, Meyer B, Josset B, Buche JF (1983) The effect of the acoustic nerve chronic electric stimulation upon the guinea pig cochlear nucleus development. Acta Otolaryngologica 95: 639–45.

Comenio JA (1992) Didactica Magna. Madrid.

Curtiss J (1989) Issues in the language acquisition relevant to cochlear implants in young children. In Owens E, Kessler DK (Eds) Cochlear Implants in Young Deaf Children. San Diego: College Hill Press, pp 293–306.

Durivage J (1984) Educación y Psicomotricidad. Mexico: Trillas.

Gajick, Ramos S, Perez C, Catala C, Mora A (1985) Habla y audición. Método verbotonal: Editorial Naullibres.

Gimeno JR, Rico M, Vicente J (1986) La educación de los sentidos. Madrid: Santillana.

Gladys B, de Vila M, Mueller M (1988) Manual de juegos. Buenos Aires: Bonum.

Holm VA, Kunze LH (1969). Effect of chronic otitis media on language and speech development. Pediatrics 43: 833-39.

Hubel DH, Wiesel N (1965) Binocular interaction in striate cortex of kittens reared with artificial squint. Journal of Neurophysiology 28: 1041–59.

Itard JM (1921) De l'éducation de l'homme sauvage on des premiers développements physiques et moraux du jeune sauvage del'Aveyron. Paris: Goujon.

Kileny PR, Zwolan TA, Zimmerman-Phillips S, Telian SA (1994) Electrically evoked auditory brain-stem response in pediatric patients with cochlear implants. Archives of Otolaryngology, Head and Neck Surgery 120: 1083–90.

Lafon JC (1985) El niño deficiente auditivo. Barcelona: Editorial Masson.

Launay CL, Borel-Maisonny S (1989) Transtornos del lenguaje, la palabra y la voz en el niño. Barcelona: Editorial Masson.

Loewe A (1992) Estimulación temprana del bebé sordo. Buenos Aires: Editorial Panamericana.

McCormick B (1993) Paediatric Audiology 0–5 Years. London: Whurr Publishers.

Morgon A, Aimard P, Daudet N (1991) Educación precoz del niño sordo. Barcelona: Editorial Masson.

Movshon JA, Van Sluyters RC (1981) Visual neural development. Annual Review of Psychology 32: 477–522.

Peña J (1988) Manual de logopedia. Barcelona: Editorial Masson.

Rousseau JJ (1990) El Emilio. Madrid: Editorial Alianza.

Rubel EW, Born DE, Deitch JS, Durham D (1984) Recent advances toward understanding auditory system development. In Berlin CI (Ed) Hearing Science: Recent Advances. San Diego: College Hill Press, pp 109–57.

Ruben RJ (1986) Unsolved issues around critical periods with emphasis on clinical application. Acta Otolaryngologica 429 (Suppl): 61–64.

Schaffer CE and O'Connor M. (1983). Manual de terapia de juego. Mexico: Manual Moderno.

Schwartz S and Miller JH (1988). The Language of Toys. New York: Woodbine House.

Thompson B (1982) El libro de presecolar. Mexico: Editorial Diana.

Uziel A (1991) Les implants cochleaires chez l'enfant: acquisitions et controverses. Review of Laryngology 112: 319–23.

Appendix: types of materials for use during pre-training

Psychomotor skills:

- Modules made of polyurethane foam, lined with brightly coloured towelling
- Blocks (balance, jumping, dragging)
- Hoops and bricks of unbreakable polypropylene
- Balls and beachballs for work with psychomotor skills
- Ropes
- Equipment for making rhythms: keys, handballs, whistles (see Durivage, 1984)

Play:

- House
- Book of handicrafts: cutting, sticking, punching
- Domino cards with fruit, people, colours, months, numbers, etc.
- Puppets (to give puppet shows, awaken the child's interest)
- Balloons
- Whistles
- Toy animals (set of farm yard animals small enough for the child to handle)
- Picture cards: sports, villages, food, the market, animals, etc.
- Building bricks: duplo, clipo, macro-bambino
- Wooden puzzles, associations (vowels)
- Jigsaw puzzles, the house, the town, etc.
- Idea-association games, memory games, domino set with numbers, words, colours, hours
- Abacus
- Games based on the observation of crafts
- Cooking and housekeeping games

- Games involving time sequences
- Threading beads
- Stackable pyramids, cubes (see Schaffer and O'Connor, 1983)

Disposable materials:
- Stickers
- Punches
- Paints, finger painting
- Plasticine
- Blackboard, coloured chalk
- Coloured card
- Tissue paper

Sound material:
- Sound, tape recordings
- Box of objects that make sounds, for developing psychomotor skills and for blowing
- Musical instruments: rattles, bells, tuning forks, recorders, xylophone
- Dolls which make noises

Educational murals and stories:
- Sequences of images
- Imitation of sounds: onomatopoeic games
- Cards of sequences
- Phonetic lotto (see Schwartz and Miller 1988)

Chapter 10
Components of a Rehabilitation Programme for Young Children Using the Multichannel Cochlear Implant

SHANI DETTMAN, ELIZABETH BARKER, GARY RANCE, RICHARD DOWELL, KARYN GALVIN, JULIA SARANT, ROBERT COWAN, MARISA SKOK, ROD HOLLOW, MERRAN LARRATT, GRAEME CLARK

Introduction

Rehabilitation with young hearing-impaired children may be defined as a teaching/learning process where the role of the clinician is to facilitate acquisition of listening, speech and language in a normal developmental order. This is often referred to as habilitation. It differs from rehabilitation for adults, which is the process by which lost communication skills are reacquired. It is worth discussing the role of the cochlear implant as a tool in this process. For the adult with acquired hearing loss, the cochlear implant might be expected, in part, to facilitate rehabilitation by restoring the auditory sense. The aim is to facilitate speech reception and provide the adult with a speech feedback loop. For a child receiving the cochlear implant, the aims are more complex. The device needs to provide speech perception abilities to facilitate the development of the entire linguistic system, to develop a range of speech sounds, to enable speech monitoring via auditory feedback and to access shared knowledge of the world.

Range of approaches for the education of deaf children

Historically, the education of the deaf has involved two main methods: the oral/aural approach and the signing approach (Clark et al., 1991).

The approach known as oral/aural relies on the use of listening and lipreading cues. The signing approach uses a gestural code for language (Markides, 1988). Within these two key methods there are different emphases. These may be considered along a continuum from visual to auditory perception. Figure 10.1 illustrates the different communication systems used at present in Australia.

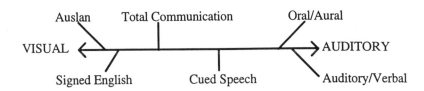

Figure 10.1: The range of communication/rehabilitation approaches used with deaf children from highly visual input to highly auditory input

Cole (1992) gives an excellent introduction to the philosophical differences behind visual intervention versus auditory intervention for hearing-impaired children. One view is that the hearing-impaired child has a reorganised cognitive and psychological system, due to the hearing loss, and therefore requires visual coding of language. An opposite view is that the hearing-impaired child has normal cognitive function and organisation but requires 'adequate' auditory and linguistic experiences to develop optimally. Language learning, according to this model, is expected to follow the normal developmental order. The preferred approach for the education of the deaf, held by the authors of this chapter and others, advocates providing 'adequate' auditory and linguistic experiences by improving aspects of the normal mother/child interaction and the normal environment. Cole (1992, p. 14) suggests providing 'embellishments' of the normal situation by sitting closer to the child, using an interesting voice, and increasing the frequency and consistency of interactions. An additional embellishment, used in our approach, is to analyse carefully the auditory components of the everyday linguistic input used by the primary caregiver (usually the mother). The linguistic input used in play interactions and everyday routines is modified so as to provide increasingly difficult auditory contrasts and to provide the ordered steps in listening, speech and language.

The influence of technological improvements on rehabilitation approaches

Improvements in audiometric technology in the 1940s made it possible to assess the hearing of infants and fit wearable hearing aids to young children. Up to 95% of children who had previously been labelled as 'deaf' before the 1940s were found to have useful residual hearing (Hardy, 1965). It was at this time that the oral approach, consisting primarily of lipreading training, became known as the oral/aural approach. The new definition took into consideration the use of hearing aids to facilitate communication. The Acoupedic Program was formulated in 1974 by Doreen Pollack (1984). Her efforts resulted in a set of guidelines for teaching how infants could be educated to use aided residual hearing.

Further improvements to hearing aids and the advent of cochlear implants allowed even more young children to access language through their audition. Throughout the 1980s, recommendations for the rehabilitation and education of children using cochlear implants were published (Selmi, 1985; Neinhuys et al., 1987; Tyler, Davis & Lansing, 1987). Nienhuys et al. (1987) recommended 'an ongoing diagnostic teaching approach' and individual, daily one-hour sessions throughout the cochlear implant programme. Ling described the need for training and testing the young child with a cochlear implant at four levels of auditory function: detection, discrimination, identification and comprehension (Ling & Nienhuys, 1983).

Factors affecting performance with the cochlear implant

Wide variability in speech perception performance for adults with the cochlear implant exists due to such factors as age at implantation, aetiology, number of active electrodes, choice of single- or multichannel implant and duration of profound hearing loss (Blamey et al., 1992). Factors that cause variability in children's speech perception performance include: cognitive immaturity, linguistic delay, auditory inexperience (Boothroyd, 1991), delayed and/or deviant speech production, motivational factors and the choice of educational approach (Dowell, Blamey & Clark, 1995). Luxford and others (1987), in a discussion of results for children using the House single-channel implant, described four main factors which had an effect on implant performance: onset of deafness, age at implantation, education and therapy settings accessed by the child and the child's mode of communication. In general, it was reported that the best performers included those who were deafened later in childhood or were implanted at an early age. Also those attending mainstream educational settings and participating in auditory-verbal therapy programmes improved more quickly on listening tasks (Luxford et al., 1987). A study of 100 children and adolescents (aged up to 19 years) using the Nucleus multichannel implant investigated the factors that were associated with open-set speech performance (Dowell, Blamey & Clark, 1995). Because of the variety of tests used with children of different age-groups, the speech perception scores were divided into seven categories of speech perception ability from detection and discrimination to identification tasks and open-set comprehension. Eleven variables were investigated: age at onset of hearing loss, duration of profound hearing loss, age at implantation, experience with the cochlear implant, the amount of preoperative residual hearing, number of electrodes in use, mode of stimulation, dynamic range for electrical stimulation, whether the hearing loss was congenital or acquired, whether the course of hearing loss was acute or progressive and whether the educational placement used oral or total communication. This study showed that children who had more experience with the device postoperatively (P <0.001), a shorter duration of hearing loss (P <0.001) and more preoperative residual hearing (P <0.001) were in the higher categories demonstrating better speech perception performance. In addition, children with a progressive course of hearing loss (P <0.001) and those in an oral education setting (P <0.05) were also in the higher categories. In this study, there were no significant differences between the children who had an acquired hearing loss and those who had a congenital hearing loss. Also, in this study there was no significant difference between the oral and the Total Communication groups with respect to the amount of preoperative residual hearing or the length of profound deafness. In other words, the children in the total communication settings were not, as a group, more profoundly deaf nor deaf for longer than the oral group of children (Dowell, Blamey & Clark, 1995). Based on these data, it could be argued that the educational setting itself appears to have some effect on the development of speech perception abilities for cochlear implant users. Other studies confirm these findings and give strong support to the argument that an oral rehabilitation programme is important to optimise young children's performance with the multichannel cochlear implant (Reid & Lehnhardt, 1993; Staller, Beiter & Brimacombe, 1994; Dettman et al., 1995).

Overview of our current programme for children under five

The components of our programme for children under the age of five are given in Figures 10.2 and 10.3. The preoperative programme (Figure 10.2) shows an approximate time course of 3–6 months. The components of the postoperative programme are listed in Figure 10.3. A description of all facets of the preoperative and postoperative programme has been given previously, (Rickards et al., 1990; Clark et al., 11991; Osberger et al., 1991)

Choice of Approach

It is likely that no single educational approach will be effective for all children using cochlear implants. The full range of educational approaches (Total Communication, oral/aural and auditory/verbal) used

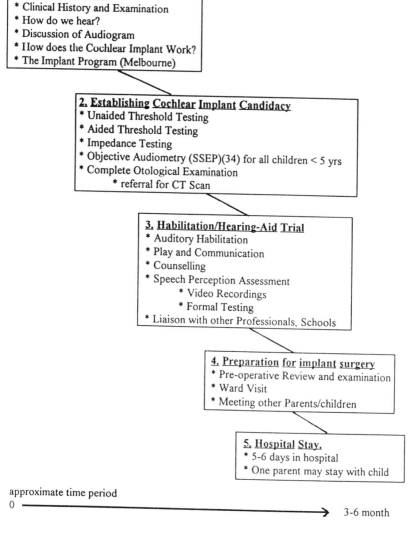

1. Initial Discussion
* Clinical History and Examination
* How do we hear?
* Discussion of Audiogram
* IIow does the Cochlear Implant Work?
* The Implant Program (Melbourne)

2. Establishing Cochlear Implant Candidacy
* Unaided Threshold Testing
* Aided Threshold Testing
* Impedance Testing
* Objective Audiometry (SSEP)(34) for all children < 5 yrs
* Complete Otological Examination
    * referral for CT Scan

3. Habilitation/Hearing-Aid Trial
* Auditory Habilitation
* Play and Communication
* Counselling
* Speech Perception Assessment
    * Video Recordings
    * Formal Testing
* Liaison with other Professionals, Schools

4. Preparation for implant surgery
* Pre-operative Review and examination
* Ward Visit
* Meeting other Parents/children

5. Hospital Stay.
* 5-6 days in hospital
* One parent may stay with child

approximate time period
0 ————————————————————→ 3-6 month

Figure 10.2: Preoperative rehabilitation: components of the rehabilitation/hearing-aid trial: auditory rehabilitation, play and communication, and counselling are described in the text

with hearing aid wearers is likely to be required for cochlear-implanted children. Both Cued Speech and Auslan are not recommended at present for implanted children at our clinic. The use of Cued Speech has declined in popularity in Melbourne. Auslan uses a different syntactic structure from English and has no spoken equivalent. This means that it is impossible to speak and sign Auslan at the same time. As there is no auditory component in the communication, the choice of Auslan does not appear to be consistent with the choice of a cochlear implant for a child. The approach of first choice, at present, includes aspects of the

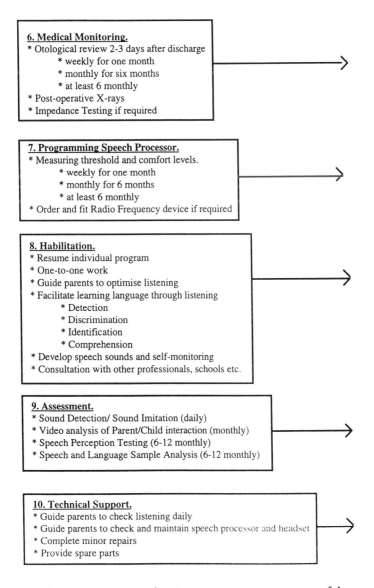

Figure 10.3: Postoperative paediatric programme: components of the postoperative habilitation programme are given in the text below

auditory/verbal and oral/aural methods. The expectation is that young children learn language and speech by first learning to listen.

Frequency of Training using a Unisensory Input

It could be argued that a rehabilitation programme for a child using a cochlear implant should not be any different from the approach used for a child using hearing aids. However, the signal provided by the implant is likely to be very different from any sound that the child has heard before and may require an initial phase of adjustment. For the child with a profound hearing loss using hearing aids, the detection of high-frequency consonants may not be within the child's audible range. Traditional rehabilitation methods have utilised visual and tactile means to teach these sounds as well as emphasising the vowel formant transitions to aid consonant discrimination. In contrast, children using a multichannel cochlear implant can detect all high-frequency speech sounds so that these can be incorporated into audition-alone activities, embedded into words, phrases and sentences, as well as trained in isolation.

The cochlear implant is an auditory device. To best optimise its use, one-to-one training with an auditory, unisensory component appears to be necessary. Brown and others (Brown & Yaremko, 1991) have gone so far as to suggest that a rehabilitation approach without unisensory input is 'useless'. Tye-Murray (1992) has suggested that at least 10–15 minutes a day should be devoted to formal speech perception training and that informal follow-up throughout the day should occur. However, proponents of the auditory/verbal approach would suggest that listening is a way of life and should be integrated into every aspect of the child's day. For the young child, auditory learning is motivated and facilitated by everyday routines and play interactions. The child associates sounds and language when being fed, dressed, cuddled, sung to and in play interactions (Mischook & Cole, 1986).

The frequency of individual sessions may vary for those in Total Communication settings where it may be necessary to specify at least one activity per day that is completed without the visual cues of lipreading or sign language. The frequency of individual sessions also varies greatly for families who, owing to their distance from the clinic, family commitments and attendance at other early intervention services, cannot attend the weekly cochlear implant clinic sessions. The cochlear implant clinician needs to establish an optimum programme for each family in order to merge the child's prior communication skills with the new auditory input provided by the cochlear implant. During sessions at our clinic, approximately one-half to two-thirds of each rehabilitation session is completed using only audition. An individual weekly programme of one-to-one sessions with the child and one or both parents is completed. A typical session is outlined in Table 10.1.

Table 10.1: A typical one-hour individual session may include these seven components

---

1. Discussion with parent (5 min)
   - Review weekly aims, note any new speech sounds, new responses, new words, etc.
2. Sound detection. AUDITION ALONE (1–2 min)
   - 'm', 'or', 'ar', 'ee', 'oo', 'sh', 's' and other sounds
3. Sound imitation. AUDITION ALONE (2–3 min)
   - Sounds and words relevant to child's current goals
4. Structured task. AUDITION ALONE (10–15 min)
   - Introduce listening, language, speech or auditory memory targets
5. Language interaction. NATURAL ORAL/AURAL INTERACTION (approx. 30 min)
   - Less structured activity loaded for target structures
6. Auditory selection/comprehension. AUDITION ALONE (5 min)
   - Perception of target words as the toys are packed away
7. Set new goals with parent (5 min)

Skills Necessary to Facilitate Auditory Learning

The clinician working with a hearing-impaired child requires a knowledge of the following areas associated with normal-hearing children: (1) hierarchies for listening development; (2) developmental order of language acquisition and speech sound acquisition, including suprasegmental aspects; (3) a knowledge of acoustic phonetics and how to apply this to speech and language acquisition. The clinician should also have had experience in behaviour management/reinforcement schedules and in methods used to modify mother/child interactions. When a child has a cochlear implant, additional knowledge about the function of a cochlear implant and its speech processor are necessary. It is also useful to know about the speech processor programme, including number of electrodes, frequency boundaries and dynamic ranges, all of which might influence the child's discrimination abilities.

Parent as Facilitator

The cochlear implant clinician's role is to facilitate auditory learning, provide access to a range of auditory cues and guide parents to develop language actively in their child. Bloom and Lahey state, 'the facilitator's task is to provide experiences that clearly demonstrate certain concepts while providing the linguistic forms that code these concepts at a time when the child is attending to both' (1978, p. 573). The clinician provides the parent with some guidelines. First, the child's attention needs to be engaged by the parent, or the parent should follow the child's lead. Second, the child and parent need to share a common topic or referent. Third, play activities need to be selected that have maximum auditory contrasts. In this way, the child is likely to succeed in discriminating between sounds during play. The clinician then assists the parent in gradually introducing an ordered set of auditory contrasts within natural play. When children are listening well, they will teach themselves language and speech production skills. This process is in contrast with what is commonly referred to as 'auditory training'. The choice of words is quite deliberate. The clinician facilitates a natural developmental process for the hearing-impaired child that corresponds to the way that normally hearing children learn language. The parent is the primary agent of change. Experienced clinicians will agree that we cannot make a young child say a particular sound until that child is ready to contribute spontaneously. In addition, providing lists of syllable strings for training or lists of same/different words does not appear to correspond with the way that normally hearing children learn to communicate. Auditory training has an emphasis in teaching sounds and sound contrasts and implies that the teacher is the primary agent of change. This may be appropriate for the school-aged child when post-cochlear implant re-habilitation addresses remediation of skills. That is, improving specific areas of listening, speech, and language deficit and/or delay.

Our experience indicates that some young implanted children are able to sort out the relevant auditory cues from normal language models. They require increased repetition and an optimum signal-to-noise ratio but are able to discover the rules of communication for themselves. Other young implanted children will need to have listening and language steps provided for them. The cochlear implant clinician needs to evaluate the child's progress and intervene where necessary.

For older children who already have a language system, the rehabilitation programme concentrates on matching the new auditory input provided by the implant with existing communication skills. This requires selection of activities that are cognitively appropriate and functional for the child. Discriminating between alternative forced choices is unlikely to be motivating for long. On the other hand, selecting a game activity 'just for fun' is not likely to guide the child through the necessary steps to achieve her optimum listening potential. The clinician assists the parent to maximise the child's listening. Some children implanted at an older age may only be able to learn to use auditory cues to aid lipreading. Others have been able to develop open-set listening skills sufficient to learn new language through audition and to use the telephone. Liaison with teachers becomes important for the school-aged child as well as individual work with the child and parents. Some aspects of the pre- and postoperative rehabilitation programme are described in detail below.

Preoperative rehabilitation during hearing aid use

The primary aim of the preoperative period is to investigate the child's ability to acquire speech and language through the auditory modality. If the child demonstrates satisfactory progress with conventional hearing aids, the clinician may suggest that ongoing rehabilitation is required rather than cochlear implantation. However, this decision is rarely clear cut. As mentioned earlier, there is evidence to suggest that those children who show good use of low-frequency hearing preoperatively will be among the top performers with the cochlear implant (Dowell, Blamey & Clark, 1995). Three areas of preoperative intervention may be described: auditory rehabilitation, play and communication, and counselling.

Auditory (Re)habilitation

In the preoperative period, the clinician investigates the child's use of hearing aids and radio-frequency devices. Modifications to the hearing aid fitting such as the mould, gain or type of aid are made, if required. Using the hearing aid, the child is trained to complete play audiometric tasks, responding to verbal stimuli. To facilitate postoperative programming of the speech processor, it is preferable that the child be able to complete a response following a stimulus, increase waiting time (to reduce false positives) and cooperate by sitting at a table for increasing periods of time. The young child is encouraged to play stimulus-response games daily with the parent. The child, using hearing aids, is encouraged to respond initially to visual and 'whole' body cues as the adult says 'Go!'. Next, facial gestures, such as raised eyebrows, are used with the stimulus sound as the clinician says 'Go'. The child then responds to the sound although the adult's mouth is partially obscured with card or hand. Finally, the child responds to the sound when no visual cues are present. Simple speech sounds utilising the loudest low-frequency vowels are used initially. In Australian English, this includes: 'bar, bore and buh, buh' (as in bus). If the child has successfully learned this task, the adapted Ling (1976) sound test can be used to establish which phonemes the child can detect: 'm', 'or', 'ar', 'oo', 'ee', 'sh' and 's'. Environmental sounds and musical instruments are not used as stimuli for the following reasons: speech sounds may be of a shorter duration than non-verbal sounds, speech sounds may be processed in a different brain hemisphere than musical sounds, speech sounds have greater range and variability, and speech sounds should be imitated by the child to improve auditory/vocal feedback skills (Ling & Ling, 1978).

Another task during preoperative rehabilitation is babble imitation. The young child is encouraged to imitate a speech model on demand, as soon as possible after the spoken model. Often a hand cue is required to prompt the child to imitate. The clinician says an interesting sound, parent imitates, then child imitates. A range of different speech sounds are used. Preoperatively, these vary in syllabic pattern and use only loud, low-frequency vowels: e.g. 'buh, buh, buh' versus 'bar'. This sound check may include low-, mid- and high-frequency sounds, familiar words and simple questions that are within the child's linguistic and auditory range. The parent is encouraged to carry out this task daily with the child.

Another task called 'Item Selection' has been well described in auditory-verbal programmes. In general, after some toys have been introduced and talked about, the clinician asks: 'Give me the...' or 'Point to the...'. This can be another useful daily sound check to monitor listening progress. While some young hearing-impaired children will not attempt this until the age of three or four, it is possible to model this task and ask the parents to select the specific toy, thus reducing pressure on the child. The aim of this task is not only to evaluate progress but to facilitate the child's own confidence in audition-alone tasks. The choice of toys should include maximal auditory contrasts, initially, to ensure success. The aim is not to 'teach' the names of the toys but to facilitate the skill of listening.

Play and Communication

We encourage play development. The child's use of toys and social behaviours are examined using well-known normative data for the development of cognitive tasks (Westby, 1980). The child's developing play skills are discussed but are not, on their own, determinants of candidacy for the cochlear implant procedure.

The parent/child interactions are considered during this preoperative phase. The parent and child are videotaped at regular intervals, as they play with a range of materials. The toys are chosen to elicit a range of pre-verbal and early language structures and to allow the interaction to be as open-ended as possible. That is, a specific puzzle or book is not chosen as this may limit the interaction to these concrete items. Activities such as water play, play dough and building blocks allow for greater range of play ideas. The parents' successful attempts to engage the child are highlighted and discussed. Negative comments about the interaction are never discussed directly with the parent. Appropriate methods of engaging the child, following the child's lead and reinforcing the child's communication attempts are modelled. Occasionally, the parent views the videotape with the clinician to prompt discussion.

Analysis of the videotaped sample using the Tait and Wood analysis procedure (Tait, 1987, 1992) is completed for all children who are too young to complete formal speech perception, speech and language tests. This provides a baseline measure of pre-verbal behaviours. Aspects of emerging pre-verbal language such as turn-taking, eye contact and auditory comprehension are analysed. These data are used to guide clinical aims and to evaluate the efficacy of cochlear implantation for young children.

In cases where the hearing loss is acquired, the clinician's role is to guide the parents in maintaining existing speech and language skills. Speech production deterioration and voice changes following meningitis have been described in the literature (Binnie, Daniloff & Buckingham, 1982). With adequate amplification and intervention, it may be possible to halt or reduce the loss of communication skills. This will depend, however, on prompt referral to the cochlear implant clinic at a time when the parents are only just beginning to understand the hearing loss.

Finally, the preoperative period provides an opportunity for the child to gain some success and confidence in dealing with new people in new surroundings. It allows the children to develop familiarity with the clinician and the clinic routine. For the older children, this period may help them to understand the long-term commitment needed to enter the cochlear implant programme. For some parents, it is important to deal with the logistics of attending the clinic punctually for weekly intervention. Taking into consideration that the child's behaviour in the clinic environment does not always reflect the behaviour in the home, occasionally additional time is needed to discuss the management of behavioural problems and tantrums. The hearing aid may be used to seek attention as the child pulls it out and throws it across the room. Occasionally referral for social work intervention and/or expert family counselling is required.

Counselling

Information regarding the cochlear implant and the speech processor are provided. The range of hearing thresholds that would be expected are described and compared/contrasted with the child's existing hearing aid responses. The expected time course and long-term commitment to attending weekly intervention are detailed.

Some parents may still be coming to terms with their child's hearing abilities and may require additional counselling. Of particular concern may be the family of a child recently deafened by meningitis. There is a need for prompt referral for CT scans to evaluate the possible effects of ossification occurring within the cochlea. Ossification may become apparent on CT scans two to three weeks after the labyrinthitis has resolved. However, it is at this time that the parents may be unable to deal with new information. Some teachers and professionals have criticised the cochlear implant clinic for proceeding with X-rays and preoperative assessments if the family are not accepting the hearing loss. It is possible, however, that significant bone growth could reduce the success of subsequent cochlear implantation. At workshops organised by our clinic, parents of children deafened by meningitis were asked if they felt they should have proceeded more quickly or more slowly through the preoperative programme than they did. All, in hindsight, expressed the view that they would have preferred to proceed more quickly.

We encourage new candidate families to meet other families who have already made the decision for implantation. The Cochlear Implant Parents Support Group includes the families of children in the preoperative and postoperative phases of the programme. They organise themselves to meet approximately four times per year. The families arrange a week-long camp once per year and have a group picnic in December. In addition to contact with this group, the clinician may arrange a meeting between the parents considering the implant and one other family. The families are matched, when possible, so that the hearing-impaired children are at a similar age and have similar cause and course of deafness.

The preoperative period provides the opportunities to investigate the parents' long-term goals for their child. Decisions regarding mode of communication – oral or Total Communication – probably reflect the first contacts that the parents have with other professionals and other hearing-impaired children and adults. Communication is not an isolated ability, but consists of a number of skills that respond differently to different rehabilitation approaches. Parents whose personal values emphasise language and cultural aspects may choose a system which appears to access language cues; that is, Total Communication. Parents whose personal values emphasise the ability to speak may tend to choose an oral system (Musselman, Lindsay & Wilson, 1988). Almost all parents attending the cochlear implant clinic for the first time express their own decisions regarding mode of communication and educational preferences. In the Melbourne clinic, both oral and Total Communication settings are represented. Approximately 60% of a group of 80 children were from oral programmes, and the remaining 40% were from Total Communication programmes. Only five children (6%) have changed their communication mode based on subsequent performance with the cochlear implant. Two children changed from oral to Total Communication because their need for augmentative communication was noted. Two children changed from Total Communication to oral settings because their listening and language performance improved markedly one year post-implant. One child changed from a Total Communication setting to an oral setting, but then required a Total Communication signing interpreter after three years to assist with more difficult language concepts within the classroom.

Of relevance to preoperative rehabilitation is that the parent may be caught in the middle between two professionals who have differing opinions. The cochlear implant clinician may be discussing research results that suggest that young children, with a short duration of profound deafness, in oral programmes appear to be among the best users of cochlear implants. The teacher or early intervention agent may be suggesting to the parent to provide an early language model via sign language. If the parents have already made their decision regarding communication, the cochlear implant team does not aim to change this. However, if no direction in communication has been established, we would recommend an oral approach with a strong auditory emphasis for all young cochlear-implanted children who have no additional handicaps.

Conclusion of the Preoperative Period

Throughout this period of intensive rehabilitation, all relevant information about the child's progress is given to the parents. This allows them to make an informed choice about proceeding with the cochlear implant. Information about the surgery, hospital stay, risks of the procedure and the hospital consent form are discussed. The child's current listening, speech production and language skills are discussed with reference to the amount of residual hearing. It is at this point that the cochlear implant team may make a recommendation whether to proceed with the cochlear implant or not. If the parents decide to proceed with the cochlear implant for their child, a surgery date is planned and the child and family are prepared for the hospital stay. The child is hospitalised for 5–6 days. The operation occurs on the day following admission and takes approximately three hours. Approximately 2–3 days following discharge from hospital, the child is reviewed by the otologist. A decision is then made by the surgeon as to when the speech processor can be fitted. This is usually two weeks following the surgery but may depend on the child's recovery. Subsequent otological review occurs weekly for a month, monthly for six months and at six-monthly intervals thereafter.

Postoperative speech processor programming

Speech processor programming is an aspect of postoperative rehabilitation that is discussed here only briefly. The level of stimulation required to programme a threshold level and a comfortable level for the 22 channels of the Nucleus device is determined. All channels that produce a useful hearing sensation are included in the child's speech processor programme. Although a useful indication of the child's programme can usually be obtained in the first session, it may take a few weeks to complete the individual programme. Typically in the first month after the operation, all weekly sessions are used to programme the speech processor. As the child begins to demonstrate detection of the full range of speech sounds, for example, the adapted Ling sound test, rehabilitation sessions may alternate with programming sessions. Programming then occurs monthly for approximately six months, then at six-monthly intervals.

Postoperative rehabilitation programme

The clinician's role in the postoperative programme is to facilitate the transition from detection and discrimination of the new auditory input to identification of speech input and subsequent auditory comprehension.

Sound Detection

The child is encouraged to perform a sound detection task at the beginning and end of all programming sessions. This, as in the preoperative programme, requires the child to place a peg in a board, race a car down a ramp, push a candle into play dough or various other activities in response to a sound. In addition to the adapted Ling sound test, many other sounds are included for their different spectral and timing features. These may include: buh-buh-buh, ch-ch, t-t-t-t, ee-or-ee-or. A first lexicon of words may also be used, once again with the aim of eliciting responses from the entire spectral range with various time and intensity cues. These words may include: bye bye, no more, up-up-up, 1-2-3-4, and family members' names.

Sound Identification through Imitation

As soon as the child demonstrates a readiness to imitate on demand, this task is used to check that the speech processor is working. The parent presents the child with a range of sounds, babble and words each day to check quickly that the speech processor is working and is set on the correct sensitivity setting. The child imitates. The entire task should take no longer than one or two minutes. There may be certain sounds that are not yet present in the child's phonetic repertoire. The child may imitate the correct number of sounds and correct pattern and this will indicate that the sound has been heard even if the child is unable to produce it accurately. If the child can imitate a range of sounds that differ in loudness then the dynamic ranges programmed in the speech processor are likely to be appropriate. The sound detection and sound imitation tasks should be presented daily by the parent.

Sound Discrimination

Many of the ideas for the first steps in learning to listen are taken from the work of Simser (1989) and Romanik (1990). These are excellent resources for rehabilitation. Here, we describe discrimination of syllabic cues and spectral cues including vowel and consonant contrasts.

Syllabic cues

Within the context of natural play, the young child is exposed to a number of auditory contrasts. Initially, play is concerned with toys that differ in syllabic pattern. A number of activities are suggested, such as:

• Water Play or Race Track	round and round and round, STOP
• Making a slide	up-up-up, down/wheeee
• Blowing bubbles	blow, pop-pop-pop
• Blowing candles	oooh-be-careful, hot
• Toys in water	bub-bub-bub (for the boat)
	ar (for the aeroplane)
	ch ch ch, oooo (for the train)
• Play dough	roll-it-over, roll-it-over, STOP
	cut cut
• Bathing dolly	rub rub rub, wash wash wash
	brush brush brush her hair/teeth
• Making 'musical' instruments out of cardboard and paper (real instruments are not used as it is preferred that the child listen to and respond with speech input)	bang bang (for the drum) too-de-loo-de-loo (for the flute) ting a ling (for the triangle)
• Nursery rhymes	Round and Round the Garden and others

The language used within this play always includes syntactically correct phrases; however, the key word may be repeated more often. An example follows: 'Round and round and round, STOP. There goes the *car* round and round and round, STOP. He stopped at the light. Off we go again, round and round and round, STOP.' The syllabic pattern associated with the toy is often learned first as there is a high degree of auditory redundancy. The sound–toy associations may then gradually be shaped toward the usual name for the toy by using both the name (car) and its syllable pattern (round and round and round, STOP) equally. An example is: 'There's the *car*. You drive the *car*. Round it goes. Ooops, the *car* stopped at the light. That's your *car*.'

Spectral cues

The next level of auditory contrasts may be introduced when the child begins to select the appropriate toy after hearing the adult refer to it and/or spontaneously imitates the syllabic patterns. Activities may be selected that differ in vowel and consonant information while maintaining the same syllabic pattern. The play activities are selected on the basis of ordered auditory contrasts. A suggested order follows:

- Vowels contrasted with consonants
- Vowels and diphthongs with widely different timing, intensity and formant cues may be contrasted next
- Vowels with similar formant cues contrasted
- Consonants with varied place, manner and voicing cues contrasted
- Consonants with minimal differences (i.e. rhyming words with similar manner, place or voicing cues) contrasted last (adapted from Romanik, 1990).

The position of the sound contrast within the word needs to be considered; that is, initial, medial or final position. In addition to the auditory contrasts, the clinician should consider the order of development of various semantic categories (e.g. colours, shapes, sizes), syntactic categories (e.g. nouns, verbs, prepositions) and auditory memory skills. The keywords need to be embedded at the start, middle and ends of phrases. Finally, the clinician needs to set daily and weekly goals with the parents. It is necessary for the clinician to communicate the goals to the parents in small and achievable steps. Gradually the parents should be able to set goals independently for their child. Some suggested activities for each sound contrast are detailed in the appendix. Only the keyword examples are given which should be embedded within natural phrases.

Comprehension

Children learn language by first determining the meaning intended in communication, independent of the language forms. The first 'looking' response to a referent is often the earliest evidence of auditory comprehension. The child appears to understand that a response is required but is unsure what to do. As early as the first week after fitting the speech processor, there is an expectation that the child will attend to questions such as 'Where's Mummy?', 'Where's your eyes, nose, etc?'. If the child does not respond, the adult provides the answer for the child. 'There she is [pointing and looking]. There's Mummy.' The child soon learns the expected scenario; that is, a question requires a response. Typical activities are suggested below that can occur each time the parent walks into the child's room:

- Looking at mobile   Where's the clown? Blow, blow, make them go around
- Looking at kitchen clock   Where's the clock, tick-tock-tick-tock

- Playing in lounge room   Where's puss puss? Mee-ow
- Looking toward window/door Where's the puppy-dog? Woof-woof
- Looking toward ceiling   Where's the light? Turn it on/off

The child soon begins to turn and point to these items as they are mentioned many times in the day. Question forms may become more complex and the child typically starts to imitate the question, rather than answer. Activities that require auditory closure may be introduced at this point:

- Looking at books, toys   What does a cow say? Moo
                                  What does a cat say? Mee-ow
                                  What does the baby say? Waa-waa-waa
- Filling in the gaps   (adult says) Ready, set...(child says)
                                  GO!
- Counting   (adult starts) 1, 2, 3, ...
                                  (child continues) 4, 5, ...
- Nursery rhymes   Adult starts, child continues next line

In order to assist the child in answering the question rather than imitating it, a third person may be needed to model the response. Comprehension activities regarding a small group of choices or objects may be used next:

- Following instructions   Stand up, sit down, touch your nose
                                  Put the car and the train in the box

- Attributes (these can vary in   Which one is blue?
  semantic and syntactic   Which one has four legs?
  complexity and length)   Give me all the things that go in water?
- Story sequences   Putting pictures in order,
  (context known)   recalling stories.

Comprehension activities eventually can include a greater number of objects, more attributes and more key elements to expand auditory memory. Finally, comprehension activities may include an open set of objects and remote events:

- What am I?   I am something in this room. I am
                                  pink. I have four legs. You can sit on me...
- Story sequences   Recalling sentence material in correct
  (context unknown)   order
- Looking at books, pictures Answering questions, having a
                                  conversation audition alone
- Revising topics from   Spelling lists
  school curriculum   Class presentations

Conclusion

This chapter has briefly described the components of the current rehabilitation programme for children under the age of five who use the 22-channel cochlear implant in Melbourne. A combination of auditory/verbal and aural/oral methods is the first choice of approach for young cochlear-implanted children. Suggested activities have been described that elicit the normal developmental hierarchies for listening, language and speech production. Further reference to Romanik (1990), Simser (1989) and Caleffe-Schenck (1990) is recommended in order to develop individualised programmes for cochlear-implanted children.

References

Binnie CA, Daniloff RG, Buckingham HW (1982) Phonetic disintegration in a five-year-old following sudden hearing loss. Journal of Speech and Hearing Disorders 47: 181–89.

Blamey PJ, Pyman BC, Gordon MB, Clark GM, Brown AM, Dowell RC, Hollow RD (1992) Factors predicting postoperative sentence scores in postlinguistically deaf adult cochlear implant patients. Annals of Otology, Rhinology and Laryngology 101: 342–48.

Bloom L, Lahey M (1978) Language Development and Language Disorders. New York: Wiley.

Boothroyd A (1991) Assessment of speech perception capacity in profoundly deaf children. American Journal of Otology 12 (Suppl): 67–72.

Brown C, Yaremko R (1991) Special considerations of cochlear implant in children Australian Journal of Communication Disorders 19: 25–30.

Caleffe-Schenck N (1990) Auditory Training Program Handbook. Englewood, CO: The Listen Foundation.

Clark GM, Dawson PW, Blamey PJ, Dettman SJ, Rowland LC, Brown AM, Dowell RC, Pyman BC, Webb RL (1991) Multiple-channel cochlear implants for children: The Melbourne Program. Journal of the Otolaryngology Society of Australia 6: 348–53.

Cole EB (1992) Listening and Talking: A Guide to Promoting Spoken Language in Young Hearing-impaired Children. Washington, DC: AG Bell Association for the Deaf.

Dettman SJ, Barker EJ, Dawson PW, Blamey PJ, Clark GM (1995) Vowel imitation task: results over time for 28 cochlear implant children under the age of eight years. In Clark GM, Cowan RSC (Eds) International Cochlear Implant Symposium in Melbourne 1994. Annals of Otology, Rhinology and Laryngology 104 (9, Part 2, Suppl.166): 321–24.

Dowell RC, Blamey PJ, Clark GM (1995) Potential and limitations of cochlear implants in children. Annals of Otology, Rhinology and Laryngology 104(9, Part 2, Suppl. 166): 324–27.

Hardy W (1965) Communication. Acta Otolaryngologica 206 (Suppl.) 36: 95–97.

Ling D (1976) Speech and the Hearing Impaired Child: Theory and Practice. Washington DC: AG Bell Assocation for the Deaf.

Ling D, Ling AH (1978) Aural Habilitation: The Foundations of Verbal Learning in Hearing-impaired Children. Washington, DC: AG Bell Association for the Deaf.

Ling D, Nienhuys TG (1983) The deaf child: habilitation with and without a cochlear implant. Annals of Otology, Rhinology and Laryngology 92: 593–98.

Luxford WM, Berliner KI, Eisenberg LS, House WF (1987) Cochlear implants in children. Annals of Otology, Rhinology and Laryngology 96 (Suppl. 128): 136–38.

Markides A (1988) Speech intelligibility: Auditory-oral approach versus total communication. Journal of the British Association of Teachers of the Deaf 12(6): 36–141.

Mischook M, Cole E (1986) Auditory learning and teaching of hearing-impaired infants. In Cole E, Gregory H (Eds) Auditory Learning. Volta 88 (Suppl): 67–81.

Musselman S, Lindsay PH, Wilson AK (1988) An evaluation of recent trends in preschool programming for hearing-impaired children. Journal of Speech and Hearing Disorders 53: 71–88.

Neinhuys TG, Musgrave G, Busby PA, Blamey PJ, Nott P, Tong YC, Dowell RC, Brown LF, Clark GM (1987) Educational assessment and management of children with multichannel cochlear implants. Annals of Otology, Rhinology and Laryngology 96 (Suppl. 128): 80–82.

Osberger MJ, Dettman SJ, Daniel K, Moog JS, Siebert R, Stone P, Jorgensen S (1991). Rehabilitation and education issues with implanted children: Perspectives from a panel of clinicians and educators. American Journal of Otology 12 (Suppl): 205–12.

Pollack D (1984) An acoupedic program. In Ling D (Ed) Early Intervention Programs for Hearing Impaired Children. San Diego, CA: College Hill Press, pp 181–253.

Rance G, Rickards FW, Cohen LT, Burton MJ, Clark GM (1993) Steady state evoked potentials: a new tool for the accurate assessment of hearing in cochlear implant candidates. In Fraysse B, Deguine O (Eds) Cochlear implants: new perspectives. Advances in Otorhinolaryngology 48: 44–48.

Reid J, Lehnhardt M (1993) Post-operative speech perception results for 92 European children using the Nucleus Mini System 22 cochlear implant. In Fraysse B, Deguine O (Eds) Cochlear implants: new perspectives. Advances in Otorhinolaryngology 48: 241–47.

Rickards FW, Dettman SJ, Busby PA, Webb RL, Dowell RC, Dennehy SE, Nienhuys TG (1990) Preoperative evaluation and selection of children and teenagers. In Clark GM, Tong YC, Patrick JF (Eds) Cochlear Prostheses. London: Churchill Livingston, pp 135–52.

Romanik S (1990) Auditory Skills Programme for Students with Hearing Impairment. Special Education and Focus Programmes Division, NSW Department of School Education, Australia.

Selmi A (1985) Monitoring and evaluating the educational effects of the cochlear implant. Ear and Hearing 6 (Suppl 3): 52S–59S.

Simser J (1989) Auditory Verbal Therapy. Taken from conference proceedings Learning to Listen. Auditory Verbal International, 305 Merchants Bank Building, 6 South 3rd St, Easton, PA 18042 USA.

Staller SJ, Beiter AL, Brimacombe JA (1994) Use of the Nucleus 22 channel cochlear implant system in children. Volta 96: 15–39.

Tait M (1987) Making and monitoring progress in the pre-school years. Journal of British Association of Teachers of the Deaf 11: 143–53.

Tait M (1992) Video analysis: a method of assessing changes in pre-verbal and early linguistic communication following cochlear implantation. Paper presented at the First European Symposium on Paediatric Cochlear Implantation, Nottingham, UK, 24–27 September.

Tye-Murray N (Ed) (1992) Cochlear Implants and Children: A Handbook for Parents, Teachers and Speech and Hearing Professionals. Washington, DC: AG Bell Association for the Deaf.

Tyler RS, Davis JM, Lansing CR (1987) Cochlear implants in young children. ASHA 29: 41–49.

Westby C (1980) Language abilities through play. Language, Speech and Hearing Services for Schools 10: 154–68.

Appendix: Sound discrimination of spectral cues. Suggested activities for contrasting vowels and consonants

Vowel strings versus consonants:

Activities	*Language/sound contrasts*
Playing with the doll	sh (going to sleep) versus wake up!
Alarm clock (speech sounds are	t t t t (ticking) versus ding-a ling-a ling
used, not the clock itself)	t t t t versus cuckoo–cuckoo
Toys, blocks, containers	in versus underneath
Colours	red versus yellow
	blue versus purple

Vowels versus other vowels:
More difficult contrasts are chosen as the child demonstrates success

Play dough	cut cut cut versus push push push
Toy cars, airplanes	'brmmm' versus 'ar'
	'mm' versus 'ar'
Colours	red versus green
	green versus blue
Making a clock face	tick tock tick tock
Drawing a watch on your wrist	
Making playground toys	see-saw-see-saw
out of cardboard	
Hospital play	ee-oo-ee-or
	(for the ambulance)
Farm animals	quack quack (for the duck)
(by sound association)	clip-clop-clip-clop (for the horse)
	hop hop (for the rabbit)
	woof woof (for the dog)
Farm animals (by name)	cat, cow, duck, dog

Consonant contrasts:

Consonant contrasts and rhyming words are among the most difficult auditory contrasts

Making a snake	(slithering) 'sss' versus (asleep) 'sh'
Face/body parts	eyes versus ears
	toes versus nose
Zoo animals	donkey versus monkey
Toys, blocks, containers	in versus on
	behind versus beside

Chapter 11
Achieving Auditory Speech Perception Skills In Profoundly Deaf Children With Hearing Aids and Cochlear Implants

JEAN S. MOOG, ANN E. GEERS

Introduction

The term profoundly deaf is commonly applied to children with unaided pure-tone-threshold averages (PTA) of 90 dB or greater. We have been using powerful hearing aids with profoundly deaf children for many years at the Central Institute for the Deaf (CID). Although most of these children cannot understand very much speech through listening alone, what they are able to hear through their hearing aids is often sufficient to be of benefit both for speechreading and for learning to produce speech with good intelligibility. Many of these children have the potential for normal or near-normal language and academic development with appropriate intervention (Moog & Geers, 1985; Geers & Moog, 1989a). This potential is greatly affected by small amounts of residual hearing that can be trained to interpret a degraded speech signal.

A number of studies have demonstrated that the development of speech and language skills in profoundly deaf children is related to the degree of residual hearing and auditory speech perception ability (Geers & Moog, 1989b, 1992; Boothroyd, Geers & Moog, 1991). The more speech a child can perceive, the easier it is to teach her to understand and produce it. However, the most important contributor to progress in learning spoken language is early oral education and dependence on speech as a primary communication mode (Geers & Moog, 1989a). Without appropriate training and early intervention, small amounts of residual hearing do not appear to contribute to the development of spoken language (Geers & Moog, 1992).

Some children are so profoundly deaf that they receive no measurable benefit from auditory training with hearing aids and depend primarily on speechreading and the help of highly skilled teachers to teach them to understand and produce spoken language. It is children in this group who stand to benefit most from cochlear implants. These children were the focus of an intensive investigation at CID which has been reported in detail in a monograph edition of the *Volta Review* (Geers & Moog, 1994a). This chapter describes the accompanying rehabilitation programme that allowed these deaf children to capitalise on small amounts of audition for producing and understanding speech.

The CID auditory learning programme

Description of the School Programme

All of the children enrolled in the CID school programme receive rigorous auditory and spoken-language instruction throughout the day. They are also involved in auditory lessons for short periods every day. However, in addition, they use their listening skills in all activities throughout the day so that listening is an integral part of everything they do. This immersion in spoken language may be the most important factor influencing the degree to which a deaf child develops auditory skills and spoken language skills. Our auditory learning programme consists of audiologic management, a curriculum of listening skills, and emphasis on listening and talking in all activities throughout the day. This programme is based on over 80 years of experience teaching deaf children to talk, including hundreds of children with hearing aids and over 60 children using the Nucleus-22 cochlear implant.

One important aspect of auditory learning is effective audiologic management to keep children's sensory aids working, and working at their very best. With cochlear implants, as with hearing aids, unless the device is working, there is no way for the child to get maximum benefit from it. We believe it is important for teachers to learn how to monitor sensory aids as well as learn how to evaluate speech perception performance of the children they are teaching. Teachers should feel comfortable about their knowledge of sensory aids although audiologists are available on a full-time basis to help children with hearing aids and cochlear implants in our school.

A task which is clearly within the domain of the audiologist is the programming of the implant. For children with cochlear implants, a critical factor is that the quality of the speech processor programme has a profound effect on the child's access to sound and the quality of sound received. However, teachers and parents can learn to do 'sound checks' with the child and to recognise when the child does not respond as expected. Any of the following may be indications of a technical problem with the implant itself: a change in the child's responsiveness to sound, a change in the quality or intelligibility of the child's speech or a change in the child's general behaviour, such as having a difficult time paying attention or withdrawing from group activities. In addition, the child may report that the implant produces sound that is intermittent or of poor quality. If these kinds of problems are observed, it is very important that the child be seen by the implant audiologist to determine whether the cause is with the device, and to remedy the situation. A child is not getting maximum benefit from the implant if it is not operating at maximum level. Furthermore, if not attended to, the problem may become worse and the child may begin to resist wearing the implant or change the loudness setting to compensate for the unsatisfactory auditory signals. In our experience, most technical problems have been with faulty microphones or processors, broken ear hook or cords, and rechargeable batteries. These kinds of problems can easily be remedied and, if attended to, the child will have improved access to sound through the implant.

Speech Perception Instructional Curriculum and Evaluation (SPICE)

The Speech Perception Instructional Curriculum and Evaluation (SPICE) (Moog, Biedenstin & Davidson, 1995) is a listening skills curriculum that was developed to provide a guide for teachers working with severely and profoundly deaf children. The objectives focus on developing listening skills without lipreading. The primary purpose of developing 'listening-alone' skills is to heighten the child's attention to the acoustic cues so that ultimately these cues will aid in speechreading. The organisation of items listed on the SPICE rating form (see Table 11.1) suggests a sequence in which speech perception skills are likely to be acquired and this makes it useful for: (a) specifying the child's present ability to perceive speech; (b) planning instruction in auditory skills; measuring and recording progress; and (d) reporting to parents.

Principles for developing the SPICE curriculum

The principles used in developing the SPICE curriculum are the same as those appropriate for any auditory training programme.

Table 11.1: SPICE curriculum instructional programme goals

1. Detection:
   GOAL A: Detect speech in a lesson setting
   GOAL B: Indicate onset and termination of speech

2. Suprasegmental perception: duration, stress and intonation:
   GOAL A: Discriminate between two stimuli differing in duration, stress
            and/or intonation
            ('Daddy is driving the green car' vs. 'Stop' or 'Hippopotamus' vs. 'Dog')
   GOAL B: Identify among three stimuli differing in duration, stress and/or
            intonation
            ('The chicken says peep, peep, peep' vs. 'Watch out!' vs.'Cow')
   GOAL C: Identify among four stimuli differing in duration, stress and/or
            intonation
            ('Humpty Dumpty sat on the wall' vs. 'Happy birthday to you' vs.
            'Twinkle, twinkle little star' vs. 'I'm a little teapot, short and stout')
   GOAL D: Differentiate stimuli with similar duration, but differing stress and
            intonation
            ('Turtle' vs. 'Football' or 'Oh no! The balloon popped' vs. 'The girl likes
            to eat cheese')
   GOAL E: Identify among sentences differing only in duration of key words
            ('The dog is sitting on the table' vs. 'The kitten is sitting on the chair')

3. Vowel and consonant perception:
   GOAL A: Identify six sounds
            -o-, ee, oo, s, sh, m
   GOAL B: Identify words differing in vowels and consonants
            bike, moon, cup, peach
            doughnut, rainbow, jump rope, suitcase
   GOAL C: Identify words differing in vowels
            boat, bat, bait, bite
   GOAL D: Identify words differing in consonants
            cake, whale, game, paint

4. Connected speech:
   GOAL A: Identify key words in sentence context
            Put the spoon on the table
            Put the fork on the table
            Put the knife on the table
   GOAL B: Identify practised sentences
   GOAL C: Converse using picture context
   GOAL D: Converse about a familiar topic
   GOAL E: Connected discourse tracking

- *Tasks are first presented through lipreading and listening.* Directions, explanations and initial trials are given using a combined visual and auditory presentation in order to assure that the student understands the task. When the student has demonstrated the ability to do the task using both lipreading and listening, the stimulus is presented using audition only. If the student is unsuccessful after two to three repetitions of the auditory stimulus alone, visual cues are added until the correct response occurs. The correct response should be followed immediately with another presentation of the auditory stimulus alone. This back-and-forth accommodation, adding visual cues as needed, helps the child acquire the ability to perform the task and engage in the activity using only audition.

- *Speech is expected as a step in conducting the activity*. Once the student has identified the stimulus, whether a sound, a word, a phrase or a sentence, the student is expected to say the sounds or the words. Requiring the child to say the words can be helpful in learning to recognise them when they are heard and provides essential practice for speech, as well. Second, associating speaking with listening makes clear to the student that one purpose for listening is to be able to use the auditory information to improve speech production. It is important to remember that practice in speaking is necessary for the perception advantage from the sensory aid to be translated into improved speech intelligibility.

- *Stimuli are presented in random order*. Sets of stimuli are always presented in random order and with a conscious effort to avoid giving the child cues of any kind. Children are adept at watching for the slightest cue from the teacher about which choice they should make. For example, if the teacher inadvertently looks at the object being named just before saying it, the child may observe that and select the right item even if the words could not be identified auditorily. Even when random presentation is observed and subtle cues to the correct response eliminated, it must be remembered that if the child has only two objects from which to choose, she will make the correct choice about half of the time simply by guessing.

- *Sets can be manipulated to create tasks of appropriate difficulty*. In order to produce realistic listening tasks which are challenging but within the child's ability to succeed, the teacher can manipulate the sets in which the stimuli are presented. Sets can be manipulated in a variety of ways such as: (1) size of the set; (2) degree of contrast among items in the set; and (3) related contextual cues. Therefore, effective manipulation requires analysis by the teacher of not only acoustic characteristics of the stimuli but also of linguistic and situational components.

The size of the set in which the stimuli are presented is one factor affecting the difficulty of the task. For example, it is easier to identify words in sets of two or three than in sets of five or six. Generally, objectives for lessons are assessed and activities presented in closed or limited sets. An objective may be made more difficult by expanding the set, either making it a larger closed set or changing it to a 'limited set' as described below. Objectives may be made less difficult by closing the set; that is, making the set smaller.

A 'closed set' means that there are a specified number of stimuli and the student knows what is included in the set. For example, a child might be expected to identify body parts out of the following closed set: arm, leg, hair, knee, face. A 'limited set' is one in which natural situational and/or contextual cues define the set, but the number may be unspecified. For example, telling the child that you will be naming parts of the body demonstrates using the context to limit the set but does not provide the precise set from which the child can choose. 'Open set' is the term used when contextual cues are absent. Having a child listen to a list of words or to phrases or sentences with no cues as to what those words, phrases or sentences might be, is an example of an open-set presentation.

In the beginning, the closed sets are small and as the child gains proficiency in listening and in understanding words, the size of the set is increased. Thus, objectives are made less difficult by reducing or closing the sets and are made more difficult by expanding the sets. Gradually expanding the set helps the child in learning to transfer auditory skills developed in closed sets into functional use in natural situations. Of course, young children with limited attention spans and limited auditory memory will, at first, need to choose from small sets. Very young children will even need to be taught the skill of making choices and pointing to them before they will be able to participate in these types of activities. As soon as possible, however, the teacher should begin to increase the number of choices available to the child.

Degree of contrast among stimuli in the set is another factor affecting difficulty of the task. As the child gains facility in making discriminations among words or phrases with large acoustic differences among them (e.g. long vs. short speech patterns), the set can be modified to include words or phrases requiring finer auditory discriminations (e.g. speech patterns with similar duration but different stress).

Another factor affecting the difficulty of the set is the presence of contextual clues. In limited-set tasks, the situational and contextual cues are minimal, but there are still differences in levels of difficulty. For example, for a child who is learning to answer questions involving information about self or family, initially the questions could be limited to names of family members, ages of siblings, favourite activities or the family pet. Thus the child would know in advance which questions to expect. As the child gained facility, the topic might be expanded to include questions about the family vacation and descriptions of other activities at home. Here the child would not know the questions in advance. Similarly, telling a child that the topic being discussed is a particular character in a television show provides more cues about the topic than asking questions about the whole episode.

Teaching strategies for implementing the SPICE curriculum

As a teacher works with a child, it is important to pay attention to the kinds of errors a child makes in order to analyse what aspects of the task are confusing the child. For example, if the stimuli include hat, shoe, shirt and pants, the child may confuse shirt and shoe because shirt and shoe both start with [sh]. On the other hand, the confusion may be between hat and pants because both of these contain the same vowel. If shirt is confused with shoe, the teacher might remove shirt or shoe from the set so a discrimination between them is not required. However, to provide practice making this difficult discrimination between shirt and shoe, the set could be reduced to only those two to help the child focus on the vowel differences and the final consonant in shirt. If the confusion is between hat and pants, similar procedures could be used.

Although developing listening skills requires effort from the child, activities that are interactive and interesting can keep the tasks from being tedious. In addition to varying the activities, we also recommend varying either the child's response or the reinforcers used. Some examples of this are varying objects that can be put on the picture named, putting pictures or objects in a mailbox, putting objects in a dump truck and letting children dump them at the end of the session or stringing beads into a necklace. Working diligently and then achieving success is a combination that produces high motivation and ultimately results in optimum learning. Therefore, it is very important to structure the tasks so that the child will experience success. In order to do this, the teacher must have in mind the features a given cochlear implant transmits or that the child can perceive through a hearing aid, the factors that affect the difficulty of the task, the auditory skill level and the linguistic level of the child. As in any teaching, the pace of the activity should be kept fast enough so that it is not boring, but slow enough for the child to succeed; difficult enough to be challenging, but not so difficult that success is out of reach.

Organisation of the SPICE curriculum

The SPICE provides a sequence of lesson objectives for listening-alone tasks and a variety of activities are suggested for reaching each of the objectives. These activities are designed primarily for children in the 3- to 12-year-old age range and most can be adapted for the linguistic abilities of any child. The suggested activities are provided as examples and are intended to stimulate teachers, audiologists and speech–language pathologists to come up with many more.

The SPICE has helped teachers gain a better understanding of what the children can hear through their implants or hearing aids. Having a sequential listing of objectives has been helpful to teachers in planning instruction. Although the specific examples used in the SPICE are provided in English, the overall principles are the same in any language and only the words need to be changed to reflect the acoustic targets.

The SPICE is organised in terms of goals as listed in Table 11.1. The goals are organised into four categories: detection, suprasegmental perception, vowels and consonants, and connected speech. Detection is the first level to be developed. At this level the child demonstrates awareness of speech, typically in response to his or her name and to speech in some context.

Suprasegmental and vowel–consonant goals are developed in parallel. The suprasegmental section lists skills which require the child to differentiate speech sounds according to their patterns. The stimuli differ from each other in terms of duration, stress or intonation, or some combination of these. When beginning practice in suprasegmental perception, it is easier for the child to discriminate when there are gross differences in duration, stress and intonation (*babababa* vs. *up* or *shoe* vs. *butterfly*). The specific goals and objectives are organised to proceed from gross differences to finer and finer differences. The set size proceeds from discrimination in sets of two to identification in sets of three or more.

The vowel and consonant perception section requires the child to differentiate among stimuli that have the same duration, stress and intonation, and differ only in vowels and consonants (*cake* vs. *fish* or *hotdog* vs. *cupcake*). Once the student has progressed through about half of these word-identification tasks, work is begun in the connected speech section. Typically, children are able to begin working at the connected-speech level once they are able to identify words auditorily from among sets of 6–8 words.

The connected speech section addresses the perception of words in the context of phrases and sentences, rather than single words. The first skills developed in connected speech require the child to identify sentences relying primarily on one or two keywords within a sentence context. Skills progress to understanding and conversing about pictures and familiar topics and then to imitating and comprehending connected sentences in the context of a story. Success at this level is dependent not only on speech perception abilities but also on linguistic abilities.

As a child acquires the skills listed on the SPICE, practice should be provided in more natural situations throughout the day. As with all teaching, developing the skills in a lesson is one aspect, but the ultimate goal is for the child to use the skill for communicating. The skills developed through activities listed in the connected speech section are intended to help the child transfer skills learned in lessons to natural situations. In addition, teachers can present familiar material through listening alone in classroom activities as children demonstrate the ability to benefit from this type of learning (see Figure 11.1).

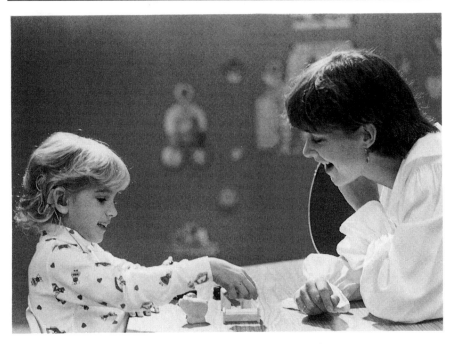

Figure 11.1: Testing speech perception performance with the ESP

Sensory aids comparison studies

The effectiveness of the CID auditory learning programme is documented in a longitudinal study of 39 very profoundly deaf children over
three years in a daily auditory and speech training programme (Geers &
Moog, 1994a). Thirteen of these children used Nucleus 22-channel
cochlear implants, 13 used Tactaid VII tactile aids in addition to hearing
aids and another group of 13 children continued to use powerful hearing aids. Each implanted child was carefully matched at the beginning of
the study to a child in each of the other two sensory aid groups in their
age, hearing, speech production skill, language performance, non-verbal
IQ and family support. At the end of three years it was apparent that children in the cochlear implant group had made significantly greater
progress in their acquisition of auditory speech perception (Geers &
Brenner, 1994), speech production/intelligibility (Tobey, Geers & Brenner, 1994) and language/communication skills (Geers & Moog, 1994b;
Nicholas, 1994). In fact, by the end of two years, performance of the
group of children with implants had shown such dramatic improvement
that an additional hearing aid control group of profoundly deaf children,
matched in age to the children with cochlear implants, but with at least
15 dB more residual hearing, was selected from the CID school population. In this chapter, the speech perception benefits of a cochlear
implant are presented in comparison with two profoundly deaf groups,
those with little or no residual hearing and those with some ability to
hear amplified speech.

In order to illustrate the advantage of 15 dB more hearing for a profoundly deaf child and the use of a cochlear implant to help children gain this advantage, performance of children who had used a multichannel cochlear implant for three years (CI) was compared with two groups of hearing aid users: those with PTAs between 90 and 100 dB (HA+) and those with PTAs greater than 100 dB HL (HA−). All three groups had used powerful hearing aids since their hearing loss was first identified in infancy. All three groups received daily auditory and speech training in an oral programme where they depended on spoken language for communication both at school and at home. The purpose of the comparison was to demonstrate that children with PTAs in excess of 100 dB HL who receive cochlear implants can achieve auditory and speech skills that are comparable to those of children with PTAs between 90 and 100 dB HL. Without an implant, children with losses greater than 100 dB make limited progress in acquiring speech perception skills, even with the same intensive oral training on a daily basis

Table 11.2: Description of subject characteristics for sensory aid comparison study

| Group | n | Age (yrs; mos) | | PTA (dB HL) | |
		Mean	Range	Mean	Range
CI	13	8;10	5;8 to 14;2	118	103 to 125
HA+	13	9;0	5;5 to 14;1	96	90 to 100
HA−	13	9;2	5;1 to 15;5	110	101 to 123

The average age and PTA thresholds of the three matched groups of children are summarised in Table 11.2. The groups did not differ significantly in age, but the HA+ group exhibited significantly better PTAs than either the CI or the HA− groups. Speech perception ability was measured with the closed set CID Early Speech Perception (ESP) test (Moog & Geers, 1990) and the Word Intelligibility by Picture Identification (WIPI) test (Ross & Lerman, 1971) and the open-set Phonetically Balanced Kindergarten (PBK) list. The ESP consists of picture cards, including 12 spondees and 12 monosyllables (see appendix for Figures). Both of these tasks require the child to recognise words on the basis of spectral rather than just temporal cues, but the monosyllable task is more difficult because the words differ only in vowel sounds (e.g. boat, boot, belt, etc.). The more difficult WIPI test presents words out of a choice of six rhyming items (e.g. leaf, street, meat, teeth, feet, beet) and requires the ability to identify consonant sounds. The most difficult test, the PBK, requires the child to listen to a list of 25 monosyllabic words and say each word as it is presented. Results, expressed as mean percentage correct scores, are plotted in Figure 11.2 for the three comparison groups (CI, HA−, HA+). In all cases, there is no significant difference between performance of the CI and the HA+ group, but both the CI and the HA+ groups scored significantly above the HA− group.

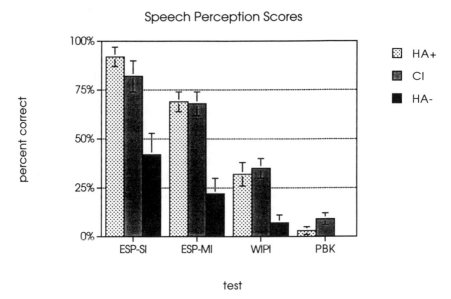

Figure 11.2: Average percentage correct scores (with standard errors) on the spondee identification (ESP-SI) and monosyllable identification (ESP- MI) subtests of the CID Early Speech Perception Test, the Word Intelligibility by Picture Identification (WIPI) test and the Kindergarten Phonetically Balanced Word List (PBK) obtained by children with PTAs between 90 and 100 dBHL who wore hearing aids (HA+) and children with PTAs greater than 100 dBHL who wore cochlear implants (CI) or hearing aids (HA–)

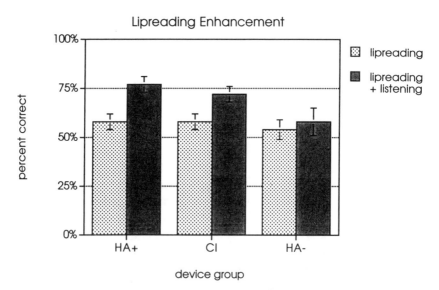

Figure 11.3: Average percentage correct scores (with standard errors) on lipreading-only and lipreading-plus-listening speech reception obtained by children with PTAs between 90 and 100 dBHL who wore hearing aids (HA+) and children with PTAs greater than 100 dBHL who wore cochlear implants (CI) or hearing aids (HA–)

The degree to which a sensory aid improves face-to-face communication is even more important than auditory-only speech perception for these profoundly deaf children. Children were tested on their ability to understand sentences in a lipreading-only condition and in a lipreading-plus-listening condition with their devices (hearing aids or cochlear implant) turned on. Results are shown in Figure 11.3. There is no significant difference between the CI group and either the HA+ or the HA– group in the lipreading-only condition. However, in the lipreading-plus-listening condition, the CI and HA+ groups both had significant enhancement (14% and 19% above lipreading-only scores, respectively) whereas the HA– group scored significantly lower (only 4% above lipreading-only performance).

Conclusions

Two important contributors to successful acquisition of spoken language by a prelingually deaf child are the amount of auditory benefit provided by a sensory aid and the child's participation in an educational programme that has been carefully designed and implemented with auditory goals in mind. Such a programme teaches the child to access the information available through the sensory aid. If use of spoken language as a primary means of communicating is a goal for a deaf child, then careful fitting of hearing aids or a cochlear implant must be accompanied by an equally carefully managed rehabilitation programme.

References

Boothroyd A, Geers AE, Moog JS (1991) Practical implications of cochlear implants in children. Ear and Hearing 12(4, Suppl.): 81–89.

Geers AE, Brenner C (1994) Speech perception results: audition and lipreading enhancement. Volta 96(5): 97–108.

Geers AE, Moog JS (1989a) Factors predictive of the development of literacy in profoundly hearing-impaired adolescents. Volta 52(1): 69–86.

Geers AE, Moog JS (Eds) (1989b) Evaluating speech perception skills: tools for measuring benefits of cochlear implants, tactile aids and hearing aids. In Owens E, Kessler D (Eds) Cochlear Implants in Children. Boston: College Hill Press, pp 227-45.

Geers AE, Moog JS (1992) Speech perception and production skills of students with impaired hearing from oral and total communication education settings. Journal of Speech and Hearing Research 35: 1384–93.

Geers AE, Moog J (1994a) Spoken language results: vocabulary, syntax and communication. Volta 96(5): 131-48.

Geers AE, Moog JS (1994b) Effectiveness of cochlear implants and tactile aids for deaf children: the Sensory Aids Study at Central Institute for the Deaf. Volta 96(5): 232.

Moog JS, Geers AE (1985) EPIC: A program to accelerate academic progress in profoundly hearing impaired children. Volta 87: 259–77.

Moog JS, Geers AE (1990) Early Speech Perception Test for Profoundly Hearing-Impaired Children. St Louis: Central Institute for the Deaf.

Moog JS, Biedenstein J, Davidson L (1995) Speech Perception Instructional Curriculum and Evaluation (SPICE). St Louis: Central Institute for the Deaf, p 221.

Nicholas J (1994) Sensory aid use and the development of communicative function. Volta Review 96(5): 181–98.

Ross M, Lerman J (1971) Word Intelligibility by Picture Identification. Pittsburgh: Stanwix House.

Tobey E, Geers A, Brenner C (1994) Speech production results: speech feature acquisition. Volta 96(5): 109–29.

Appendix

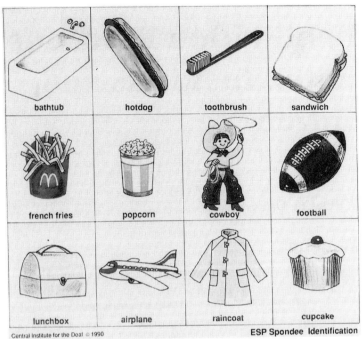

A Stimuli for the standard version of the Spondee Identification subtest of the CID Early Speech Perception Test

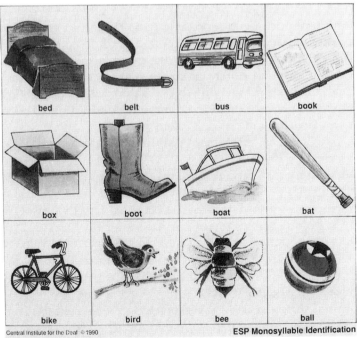

B Stimuli for the standard version of the Monosyllable Identification subtest of the CID Early Speech Perception Test

Chapter 12
Rehabilitation Procedures Adapted to Adults and Children

ERSILIA BOSCO, DEBORAH BALLANTYNE, MARIA TERESA ARGIRÒ

Introduction

The development of the cochlear implant programme at the III ENT Clinic of Rome University 'La Sapienza' stems from the interest of our research team which was set up in 1980 to study, evaluate and rehabilitate individuals with hearing impairment. The multidisciplinary approach was chosen to deal more effectively with the complex problem of providing treatments that would be tailored to the true needs of each hearing-impaired patient. In 1993, the study was extended to include a cochlear implant programme. Initially, the programme began with the rehabilitation of postlingually deafened adults. At the time of writing in 1995, it also embraces and treats pre- and perilingual deafness in both adults and children. By December 1994, our centre had conducted 159 initial examinations of potential cochlear implant candidates and 62 complete evaluations for meeting the selection criteria (see Figure 12.1). The evaluation process included complete medical and audiological assessment, hearing aid trials, evoked potentials, HRCT scans of the cochlea, psychological examination and electrical promontory stimulation (Bosco et al., 1995).

Unfortunately, in Italy, not many patients manage to receive a cochlear implant even if they meet the selection criteria because, to date, reimbursement is not provided by the National Health Service. Furthermore, even from region to region, provision for financial assistance can vary and is often limited to a small number (e.g. preference for children rather than adults, low income bracket, etc.). Hence, financial problems such as these inevitably restrict the number of people who ultimately will receive such a device in Italy.

The initial fitting session takes place 5–6 weeks after surgery and during the first year the patients come in for fitting sessions at three, six and 12 months, though children obviously require more frequent visits.

ADULT COCHLEAR IMPLANT SELECTION PROTOCOL

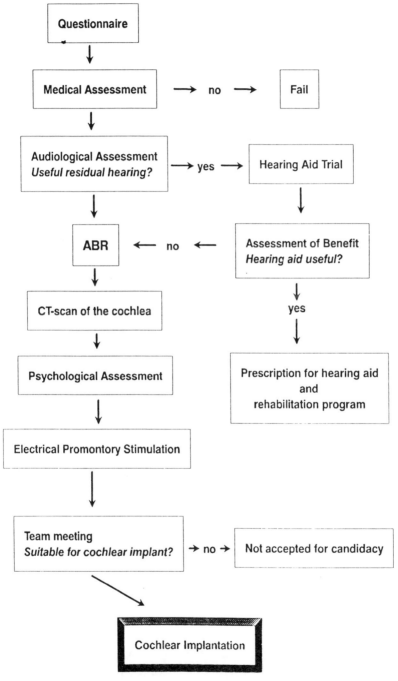

Figure 12.1: The procedures applied to the selection of adults for cochlear implantation

Rehabilitation in adult subjects

Structure of Sessions

The rehabilitation sessions follow specific structural characteristics. There are three sessions per week, each lasting 50–60 minutes and one of these is a group session of 60–80 minutes with two clinicians who are always present (speech therapist/psychologist, phoniatrician/ psychologist, speech therapist/phoniatrician and/or audiologist/ psychologist). In this way, the patient is exposed to different speaking voices and styles of communication. This also enables us to place emphasis on specific aspects of rehabilitation: acoustic training, articulation, breathing, exchange (communication) modes, reinforcement, motivation and so forth. Furthermore, more than one clinician helps avoid excessive involvement in the patient–clinician relationship.

At the beginning of each session, one of the clinicians explains the aim of the session. The materials to be used and the sequence of activities in each session are organised in relatively flexible work units. A diary account of each meeting is kept by one of the clinicians in which specific difficulties, misunderstandings and patient observations are noted. At the end of each meeting, one of the clinicians makes a summary of the work done, underlining the positive aspects. The coordinator, in our case the clinical psychologist, arranges meetings with family members to discuss progress and difficulties encountered by the patient. When necessary, meetings are arranged between the parties (patient/family) to set up alternative communication patterns. Also, as needed, the phoniatrician/speech therapist organises breathing and other exercises to improve control of voice output and speech articulation.

Characteristics of the Sessions

A highly significant negative correlation is seen to exist between the duration of hearing loss and performance in implanted subjects (Clark et al., 1987). For this reason, our rehabilitation programme for adults is structured to minimise the negative effects on central processing which usually derive from a long period of sensory deprivation. The rehabilitation protocol (Bosco, Argirò & Filipo, 1993) which has been developed for use in our implant programme is based on four basic concepts: personalisation, graduality, continuity and significance.

Personalisation

Personalisation refers to the many aspects of the patient which influence the individualisation of the rehabilitation process and its materials. This means that the speech materials, the composition of each single rehabilitation unit, the types of communication exchange, the duration of training sessions and the types of reinforcement used are all taken into account as they relate to the requirements and difficulties of each individual patient.

The sociocultural status is reviewed because it can affect both rehabilitation procedures and the level of materials to be applied. This aspect includes many variables such as the profession, language competence, level of sentence construction and type of syntax used, experience with reading, writing and so forth.

Cognitive skills are estimated. The attention span of the subject is important because it is essential during the rehabilitation process to avoid counter-productive fatigue or boring, repetitive tasks. The person's skill with cognitive organisation, with particular attention to style and the possible forms of rigidity (inflexibility) are considered in order to enable rehabilitation exercises to be explained in an understandable and easy-to-remember manner for the subject. Individual personality traits are considered; for instance, we have noticed that frequent changes in mood have been observed, mainly in extroverted personalities. Overall communication skills include, in particular, the use of gestural expression, lipreading abilities, use of contextual clues and the use of space during communication.

Finally, age at implant and age at onset of deafness are considered. The age of the patient is clearly an important variable not only for children but also for adults. In our experience, the elderly are more sensitive to mistakes and tend to generalise negative events. Age at onset of deafness influences rehabilitation at all levels because it facilitates the planning of suitable work units and the making of adequate proposals for acoustic and phonatory assessment and training.

Graduality

This refers to the process of ordering exercises from easy to difficult; that is, developing 'progressive' materials. It became necessary to scale both the difficulty of the single work units within the rehabilitation protocol and the complexity of the tasks to be faced in each situation.

The most basic training is an introduction to the care and maintenance of the equipment. All subjects learn how to handle the device in terms of such things as changing of batteries, raising and lowering volume and sensitivity controls, choosing the most suitable processing strategy, using the telephone receiver and so on.

In each session, speech materials of increasing difficulty are applied to highlight temporal organisation, intensity discrimination, redundancy cues, phoneme discrimination, and syntactic and semantic complexity. Short exercises on the suprasegmental and paralinguistic aspects of the spoken word are included. This is because we found them to be very useful in training subjects to pay attention to aspects that provide information on the emotional status and intentions of a speaker. The various listening modes (with/without lipreading; closed/open set) are represented in each session, naturally at varying levels of difficulty. Even the instructions given to the subject relative to practising comfortable listening in various circumstances are graded in difficulty ranging from a quiet room at home with one member of the family, in the kitchen while preparing a meal, in the car and so forth.

The materials and the listening situations that are assigned to the patient should be difficult enough to encourage up interest and also to act as positive reinforcement. If tasks are too difficult they will tend to be frustrating, thus bewildering the subject and causing anxiety. When the attention level lowers, new, enjoyable exercises should be employed (games using imitation and vocal expression, movement exercises and other less stressful tasks).

Continuity

Rehabilitation sessions are organised at regular intervals over a continuous stretch of time. Any interruptions must be discussed with the patient. Apart from favouring a serene and well-organised relationship between the two parties (implant patient and rehabilitation team), the regularity of the sessions enables us to divide the tasks into manageable units and to verify quickly what the subject has managed to learn during the previous session.

Significance

Each session should hold significance for the patient. From the patients' point of view, this means they are helped to become aware of having made even minor progress in the detection, discrimination and recognition of acoustic and verbal stimuli or, at least, in their general ability to communicate at some level.

Patients are encouraged both to make use of words or expressions which are typical of their own surroundings and to learn the meaning of new words. Postlingual subjects are asked to collect nursery rhymes and songs remembered from childhood. An attempt is made to sing some of them with the therapist. The choice of excerpts to be used for the speech tracking tasks (Owens & Telleen, 1981; Fenn & Smith, 1987) is based both on the syntactic and grammatical characteristics of the extract and on the *interest* that the particular topic has for the patient.

Group Sessions

One in every three sessions is held with other implant wearers who have been deaf for the same length of time. This has proved to be very useful.

The sessions liven up noticeably and the subjects are able to compare notes about their progress, experiences, difficulties and so on. In such group sessions, patients are encouraged to express feelings, personal considerations and experiences in relation to the effect that the new sensory perception has created. This enables them to express their feelings and ideas to a group of people who will, most certainly, understand them. Furthermore, in these group meetings, each subject is asked to suggest some exercises to the other members. The interaction also stimulates them to improve their voice production relative to both quality of utterance and articulatory precision. It is up to the clinicians to avoid excessive competition and to explain the reason for different performance (i.e. abilities of the different patients), when necessary.

Work Units

Each session begins by asking the patient to describe, in an informal manner, their listening experience in and outside home surroundings; new experiences and personal impressions described by the patient are never underestimated. Often, unexpected progress is made and the patient can offer useful observations for the organisation of the following session. After having laid out the basic plan for the specific work unit, combinations of the following sequences, based on the levels reached by each individual, are put into practice.

Development of speech discrimination skills

This entails training with/without lipreading in closed and open sets. It should be noted that all speech materials presented in a closed-set format are always read aloud first by the clinician and then by the patient, in order to provide a dual training task: acoustic and phono-articulatory.

At the beginning of the rehabilitation programme, the basic variable is the temporal organisation of speech. Thus, lists of mono-bi-tri-syllabic words, graded from easy to difficult levels, containing simple (CV) and more complex (CVCCV) structures which cover the whole range of possible syllabic structures in the Italian language are used. However, it should be taken into account that in Italian there are very few meaningful monosyllabic words. Furthermore, even when present, they are not nouns but prepositions, articles, pronouns, adverbs and specific forms of declined verbs.

We employ lists of words with different emphasis on intensity, such as: Loud/Soft–Soft/Soft/Loud; Soft/Loud–Loud/Soft/Soft; Soft/Soft/Loud–Loud/Soft/Soft; Loud/Soft–Soft/Loud/Soft; Loud/Soft/Soft–Soft/Loud/Soft. Lists of bisyllabic words for phoneme discrimination have been developed. These words present the various phonemes in an initial or medial position. Lists of words with phoneme contrasts are presented where each difference in phoneme content gives a different meaning to the word (e.g. matto–gatto–ratto; rullo–rutto–russo).

Lists of common sentences are presented for both questions and statements in order to train the subject on intonation patterns (Vuoi il caffé?; Grazie, no!; La cena è pronta.). Specific lists have been drawn up for listening-and-speaking tasks based on intonation patterns using both single words and whole sentences: suprasegmental word tasks (carico–caricò; capito–capìto–capitò); and suprasegmental utterance tasks (Sei riuscito a vederla – Sei riuscito a vederla? – Sei riuscito a vederla!). These latter sentences are identical from a segmental point of view but change according to intonation and the introduction of pauses (e.g. Come posso fare io da solo? – Come? Posso fare io da solo?). From a functional point of view, intonation is an essential source of modulation and is needed in order to convey the type of utterance that is being made (statement, question, exclamation), to indicate the pragmatic value to be attributed to what is being said (joking, ironic, serious) and to highlight the parts of the utterance which the speaker intends to emphasise so that the listener can understand the sense more clearly.

Another type of exercise uses sentence lists associated with a game called 'Change without changing'. This is the basis for training paralinguistic aspects of language: the same sentence is listened to and repeated by the patient, changing speed of repetition, voice intensity and/or type of pauses (silence and full pauses). These exercises are carried out in a playful manner, thus allowing the subject to make use of all possible extra-auditory cues.

Phoneme confusion matrices are employed in order to verify improvement in phoneme recognition. When a specific phoneme is found to be repeatedly difficult for a given patient, it is given special attention and is introduced into word lists where it is presented alternatively in the initial, medial and final position. Full sentences containing these words are also used so that the task does not become too boring.

Speech tracking

This is a method employed for training subjects in the perception of continuous discourse (De Filippo & Scott, 1978). Graded extracts, based on the linguistic and cultural levels of each patient, are read aloud in units (words, phrases or sentences) by the therapist. The patient is asked to repeat the unit after the clinician and is not allowed to go on to the next unit until the previous one has been expressed correctly. Scores are recorded as a WPM (word per minute) index which is obtained by dividing the number of words repeated correctly by the number of minutes employed. Hence, it is a compound measure of speed for communication as it takes into account transmission time, correction time and response time. Variations in the index offer useful information relative to the effectiveness of verbo-acoustic communication abilities when using the cochlear implant. The ultimate aim of this procedure within the context of the rehabilitation protocol is to reach, where possible, the correct repetition of the extract without the aid of extra-auditory cues. However, for statistical purposes, tracking is also used before and after implantation during audiological assessment, with the same method but applying extracts which are graded by difficulty in random order.

Patient/therapist conversation

Simple conversation is made relative to everyday situations, recent happenings and interesting news. We always attempt to stimulate the patient by dealing with subjects that are challenging but at the same time personally meaningful.

Brief conversation between two therapists

This exercise requires that the patient listen attentively and then participate, if possible, in the conversation. The patient is asked to repeat the sentences contained in the therapist's conversation. If the patient has reached a relatively good level of understanding, even if lipreading is used, the patient is invited to take part in the conversation.

Listening to music and/or singing songs

The patient is asked to listen to music or a song in a relaxed manner. When possible, the patient may attempt to reproduce the rhythm of the music, first together with the therapists and then alone. Sometimes, the patients are even asked to sing, following the written text.

Auditory perception tasks

Bisyllabic nonsense syllables are presented in closed- and open-set groups. The patient is asked to identify and/or repeat what is heared. Very low levels of extrinsic redundancy (phonemic only) are included. For speech discrimination tasks, familiar words and sentences are presented in closed- and open-set groups but with a higher level of extrinsic redundancy (phonemic, semantic and syntactic).

Training for use with telephone

Listening and communication strategies include keyword codes and use of written materials such as lists of questions. The questions are asked by the clinician over the phone to the patient, initially as written and then in randomised order. The patient is asked to identify which question has been asked. The next level of exercise is a telephone conversation about a familiar subject. The ultimate aim of this type of training is to reach, where possible, a totally functional use of the telephone.

At the end of each session, the clinicians go over the work units used in the session, help to organise work to be done at home and discuss possible doubts.

Patient's Handbook

A 'Rehabilitation Handbook' is created for each patient. The cochlear implant wearer is encouraged to carry out the various exercises which include sections on general information (practical information for the correct use and handling of the device), suggestions for improving personal listening strategies and aids for increasing communication abilities (use of observation, body language and ways to decrease the detrimental effects of surrounding noise).

The section on listening tasks is quite large and includes: sound detection (list of 150 sounds which the subject must gradually learn to perceive, initially with the help of a member of the family); discrimination of words of different length (mono- vs. trisyllable (ma/cinema); mono- vs. bisyllable (ma/tema); bi- vs. trisyllable (tema/cinema); discrimination of words of different length that are placed at the end of a sentence (il nuovo film è veramente bello/bellissimo); discrimination of sentences of different length using familiar words such as the days of the week, months, names, etc. (Sabato vado al cinema/Domenica vado al cinema con Mario); stress-in-sentence tasks (QUELLA è la mia giacca blu/Quella è la MIA giacca blu, Quella è la mia GIACCA blu/Quella è la mia giacca BLU) and question/statement tasks (Maria va al mare/ Maria va al mare?).

There are also reading exercises with graded difficulty; vowel discrimination tasks (male–mele–mole); consonant discrimination tasks (gatto–matto–ratto) and suggestions for tracking exercises which should be done with and without lipreading. Training for telephone use includes: positioning of the telephone receiver, familiarity with the various signals and communication strategies.

The tasks described in the handbook are fairly similar to those used during the various rehabilitation sessions, so that the exercises can be easily understood by the patient. The materials, however, differ sufficiently so they do not become boring. This form of homework requires the cooperation of a friend or relative. The families of our implant patients have always supported our initiatives with enthusiasm. Now and again, some patients have come up with new material invented at home. In fact, this handbook proves to be useful as a guideline to discipline and to motivate the patient towards directed training even when at home.

Discussion

Various interesting questions have arisen in the course of our clinical experience. An interesting finding, apropos of our patients and contrary to reports given by other cochlear implant users (incidentally, using alternative stimulation strategies) during the months immediately after implantation, is that we did not witness any 'plateau effect'. In our opinion, such an observation should be taken as a lack of significant progress with use of the device and could be attributed, in part, to the device (coding strategy), but more specifically to the context of our rehabilitation. That is, we consider the detail and care with which the work units have been graded. Their frequency, along with the optimal use of positive reinforcement tactics, undoubtedly contributes to the favourable outcome of rehabilitation. Still relative to the 'plateau effect', the psychological advantage offered by immediate positive results is undeniable. In our experience, a plateau is never effectively reached because the subjects' potential manifests a non-linear growth function even after having reached levels predicted on the grounds of data available prior to surgery. In this process, many factors come into play, including physical, physiological and psychological interactions.

Another interesting observation was that all patients manifest a certain degree of difficulty in using integrated senso-perceptive schemes. Rossi (1994) describes how all inputs coming from the various sensory organs pour into the specific primary cortical areas where they are memorised and compared with already stored information. In turn, this sort of information can also be compared with heterosensory data, at a level with the adjacent secondary cortical areas. Once decoded information from all the sensory channels goes to the posterior tertiary areas where central integration takes place and it produces a representation of what each organ has perceived in that specific moment. In deaf subjects, what cannot be heard directly and perceived at a higher level as a result of the hearing loss is integrated, at least partially, by visual inputs (lipreading). Studies are being carried out (Robertson & Irivine, 1989; Ryals, Rubel & Lippe, 1991) as to how the renewed auditory input is perceived and integrated at higher levels and as to whether the auditory information, which has been missing for a long time, might, at least on a temporary basis, contribute to disrupting the pre-existing organisation of senso-perceptive schemes. At present, in our centre, a study is being conducted by carrying out Positron Emission Tomography (PET) techniques before and in various stages after implantation, in order to obtain comparative data over time which might be able to explain such phenomena.

During rehabilitation, discrimination of keywords was made easier by pronouncing various series of acoustically and/or semantically similar items until recognition of the target word was complete.

For example, with acoustic similarity, a target word such as *campione* would be presented in four stages as follows: **ca**/ne – **camp**/aga – **campi**/ – **campione**. Semantic similarities, on the other hand, are presented as follows: where the target word is Tiger, for example, it is described as being an animal – fierce – yellow and black stripes – to be found above all in India. Collins and Lofts, in their revision of Ceylon's spreading-activation theory of human semantic processing (1975), show how names of concepts are stored in a lexical network; that is, organised along lines of phonemic and orthographic similarities, and that the semantic network is organised along the lines of semantic similarity. The oral exercises mentioned above have been useful in avoiding both the interference which written materials exerted on auditory perception and the fixation of incorrect recognition schemes.

Another observation is that variability in performance appears to be linked directly with the duration of hearing loss, with the level of education and with the quantity and quality of rehabilitation received. A certain degree of variability also was noticed for the same patient during the individual rehabilitation sessions and was associated with rapid changes in mood. The variability did not seem to be linked directly to the results obtained in that particular session but to factors external to the rehabilitation itself. However, in such situations, we attempt to reassure patients that we understand their state of mind, not by making general statements as to how well they are getting on but by giving them concrete evidence of their progress with the implant in relation to previously mistaken tasks.

As a final comment, it is necessary to balance the relationship between the patient and the clinicians in the rehabilitation team. As in all long-term relationships of this kind, patients can fall into a state of dependence, excessive faith in their newly acquired competence, intense emotion, and dangerous contrasting and/or distracting attitudes.

Rehabilitation in children

Overview

The children implanted in our department differ from one another mainly in relation to the age at onset of deafness and age at implantation. For this reason, the rehabilitation procedures applied to each of these children must be modified according to their intrinsic characteristics (Bosco et al., 1994). Our experience with adults taught us the importance of dealing with the subject as a whole and confirmed the need for a multidisciplinary team. In the children's cochlear implant programme, the team differs from that used for adults in that it introduces other specialists dedicated to working specifically with children.

Any prosthetic, rehabilitative procedure applied to the deaf child

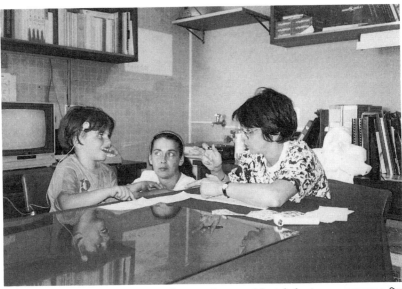

Figure 12.2: Eliciting responses from a 5-year-old girl during processor fitting (reproduced with permission.)

will necessarily have a direct influence on the child's future psychological and educational development. Therefore, it is essential that the team involved should not only know about the child's hearing but also about how she behaves in differing circumstances taking into consideration that child's various perceptive and cognitive potentials along with details of her emotional and socio-family conditions (see Figure 12.3) (Downs, 1987; Bosco, 1991; Hellman, Chute & Kretschmer, 1991).

It should be stressed that even before applying the implant, a great deal of time needs to be spent with the children to set up a valid interpersonal relationship and to observe and assess their behaviour in various situations (at home with relatives, at school with other children and teachers, in play situations alone and with peers). During the whole rehabilitation process, regular meetings are set up with relatives and teachers specialised in sensory handicaps to achieve a number of aims. First, to offer information and methods that can help to develop communicative modes that are adequate for the changed senso-perceptive condition of the child. Second, to encourage the expression of doubts and uncertainties by all involved, offering a friendly ear and giving advice when possible. Third, to obtain updates from teachers on progress in schooling, such as selective attention with the device under various listening conditions, re-integration of hearing with other senso-perceptive schemes, language development both written and spoken, awareness of the children in relation to their changed condition, as well as practical and emotional problems linked to the device. Fourth, to introduce a member of our team into the school staff meetings (relative to the

SELECTION PROCEDURE FOR CHILDREN

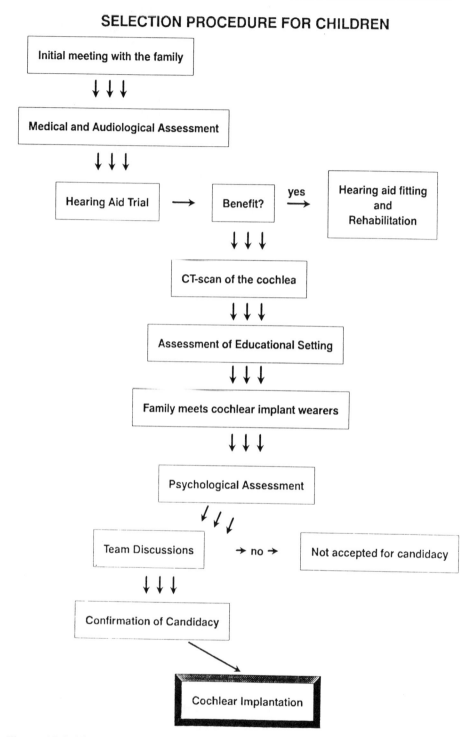

Figure 12.3: The process through which children and their families go when considering cochlear implantation for the child

class in which the child belongs) in order to involve all the teachers who come into contact with the cochlear implant wearer.

Every three months, group meetings are held between relatives and families of all our implanted children, guided by the psychologist, in order to enable the parties to 'socialise the experience'; that is, to encourage the exchange of emotions and experiences which would otherwise remain unexpressed.

The local speech therapists who will be dealing with the child all undergo a period of training in our department to acquire familiarity with all implications of this new form of prosthesis, to involve them in the various stages (selection, fitting, rehabilitation) and to make them self-sufficient in their responsibilities within the rehabilitation procedures. This training is implemented even when the local therapists have ongoing and continual interaction and integration with our clinic.

In the following section, we will discuss our experience with teenagers and children. Owing to our philosophy of attempting to create a *trait d'union* between adults and children where clearer reference (baseline) patterns can be used for future experience, we chose to begin with adolescent subjects before applying the device to young, prelingually deafened children.

Experience with Teenagers

Considering that adolescence represents a delicate phase in the child's development during which unsolved childhood conflicts and problems can all be represented (Freud, 1968; Canestrari, 1990) and any major change can lead to disruption and disharmony in future development from all points of view, the subject's personality should be studied in great depth.

The main characteristics of the rehabilitation programme used for these children, taking into account the intrinsic differences that exist between them, are as follows: two local sessions per week (teenager plus speech therapist) during which time we make use of the local therapist who works with the child following the training period in our department. This is essential if continuity is to be maintained. Further, there are two sessions per week held in our department (teenager plus two members of the rehabilitation team): one in which the child receives individual attention and the other in which children participate together.

Individual sessions

Sign language, in our country it is Italian Sign Language (LIS), may be needed to help comprehension and memorisation of the spoken word. However, in our case, one teenager was only familiar with a few elements of LIS which he eventually began to recognise auditorily and reproduce verbally. We used sentence structures typical of spoken Italian and new terms and elements were only presented in spoken and written modes (without LIS). For basic language development, emphasis may focus on movement and on the figurative elements of language in order to create situations which will give immediate significance to the acoustic message. The largest emphasis, however, will be on the pragmatic aspects of language. Each new word is anchored to a concrete situation. Attention is placed on the transition from keyword sentences to nuclear sentences and ultimately to expanded sentences.

Long-term deafened teenagers learn how words can be used as an instrument for thought and as a tool for discovering new relationships between the different elements. For a 13-year-old girl who had fairly good global communication ability but poor language skills, speech discrimination was the main focus of rehabilitation. Pragmatics were still a major focus in the individual session even though it was obvious that words still had a meaning for this girl who had been a hearing aid wearer from onset of deafness to 6 years of age. The use of terms and sentences occurring in school provided relevant and useful materials from which exercises could be designed, i.e. mathematical terms, idiomatic expressions in English and so forth.

Voice production in these teenagers may be unclear and scarcely understandable. Many exercises are needed, including those in which one makes use of a mirror for the control of articulatory functions. Teenagers learn that voice can be a useful and pleasant tool for communication. In some cases, the teenager can eventually manage to self-correct mistakes as a result of making use of newly acquired auditory feedback.

Group Sessions

The sessions in which the teenagers are together should be of average difficulty for each child. An example is when having ascertained that one is better at distinguishing temporal and frequency cues, and that the other is better at constructing sentences, play situations can be created in which the relative strengths of each child are combined. The sessions are stimulating and enjoyable inducing the children to work together without creating excessive competition. After a period when successful rehabilitation goals have been reached, perhaps by a year after implantation, it is possible that rehabilitation will need to be reorganised to take into account changing individual needs. This means a reduced number of sessions within the department, more work at school and at home and less need for common sessions. However, children should continue to meet during fitting sessions which continue on a regular basis at the clinic.

Younger Children

In our clinic, the rehabilitation of prelingually deafened children is carried out by a speech therapist. She is an expert in the treatment of profound deafness and, for the rehabilitation of cochlear implant wearers, uses a method based on musical rhythms created by Zora Drezancic (1982a, 1982b, 1989). The following is a brief outline of this method, but the reader is advised to consult references for further details.

The fundamental basis (baseline) is a knowledge of the possibilities and the limitations of the child and that there is active cooperation by the parents. Parents take part in all sessions (two per week) in order to learn the exercises that the therapist uses with the child each time. The exercises are in game form. The materials are personalised, i.e. developed by the parents and the therapist together. The parents are taught how to present the exercises at the most suitable moments of the day and for how long. Stress is placed on the playful and varied nature of the exercises.

The use of multisensory models is applied within a structure where voice production is the primary characteristic for spoken, modulated and singing modes. Using a series of games, auditory, tactile, visual and motor stimuli are presented to the child in an interactive mode. The aim at this stage is to favour conditions for the natural acquisition of language similar to those in which the normal-hearing child learns to hear, listen and speak. This is accomplished by demonstrating that different impressions relevant to all sensory channels can be derived when the human voice plays a predominant role.

The basic multisensory models are represented in this method by rhythmic structures which coincide with those relative to speech. For example, Ta-Te corresponds to simple bisyllabic words (càde, pìno, bìro); Ta-TeTi corresponds to a more complex structure as in multisyllabic words where the accent is on the antepenultimate syllable. These rhythmic structures are presented in four increasingly difficult stages which make use of the voice, coordinated with arm and hand movements that attempt to visually represent the nature (amplitude, tone, emotion) of sound production. There are four specific programmes for use with different age-groups and different verbo-auditory abilities of the individual subject: 6 months to 3 years; 3 to 7 years; 7 to 16 years; adults.

Using this method on a 5-year-old child, we noticed how receptive she was during the fitting sessions and how quickly she adapted to the various inputs. Her tolerance levels increased. Within two days, she passed from intense discomfort (she cried and pulled off the receiver at the first impression of sound) to tolerance of discomfort and to total acceptance of sound. She developed systematic pattern perception making almost immediate use of them. This led to the spontaneous creation on her part of games involving listening and association between visual, auditory and motor stimuli. In fact, even during the second session, the child suggested using a game that she had invented herself based on associations between perception of sound intensity (soft, normal, loud) and physical size (small, medium, large). The game involved interaction with the therapist and made use of castanets as the acoustic stimulus and graphic representations of a house as a visual stimulus. It is this sort of insight into complex perceptive processes on the part of the child that makes her an ideal candidate for application of the 'musical rhythm' method. For such a child, there are two to three sessions per week and the mother takes part in all sessions. Once a month, one session is video-recorded in order to monitor the progress of the child using video analysis described by Tait (1993).

Conclusions

Our experience in the rehabilitation of both adults and children (Bosco, Argirò & Ballantyne, 1995; Filipo et al, 1995) is that implantees must have a valid reference point, the implant centre; that is, a centre capable of coping with the multifaceted needs of each individual. The members of the team must have experience in the field of deafness. They must be able to communicate without bias both with the deaf person and with the family. Interaction between the various members of the team is also fundamental, including a united goal and respect for the relative roles of each. When working with children, liaisons between the centre, schools, family and subsidiary workers (when needed) are essential.

Furthermore, it is important to create a relationship, where possible, with the deaf community and with organisations of parents of deaf children in order to favour a realistic approach towards the advantages, limits and progress made in the field of cochlear implantation.

The rehabilitation process, even though based on well-defined procedures, must be flexible enough to adjust to the various needs of the individual patient and should also consider the social and cultural environment in which the patient interacts. The successes we have experienced have encouraged us to expand our programme further and to integrate the existing procedures with two new groups of cochlear implant candidates: children between the ages of 3 and 5 years and blind–deaf patients. The Deaf–Blind Project is to be started in cooperation with the UIC (Unione Italiana Ciechi) for the implantation of blind, postlingually deaf adults.

We hope that our contribution in this book has offered other rehabilitationists a different view of techniques and we look forward to the continued opportunity to learn new methods for the best implementation of rehabilitation protocols that take into account the specific needs of each individual cochlear implant wearer.

References

Bosco E (1991) La diagnosi funzionale del bambino ipoacusico. Aggiornamento delle schede operative. L'Educazione dei Sordi 1: 23–24.

Bosco E, Argirò MT, Ballantyne D (1995) Procedure for the rehabilitation of implant patients in relation to age and onset of deafness: questions, answers and results. Paper presented at the 3rd International Congress on Cochlear Implantation, Paris, 27–29 April.

Bosco E, Argirò MT, Filipo R (1993) Il processo riabilitativo nell'impianto cocleare in caso di sordità di vecchia data. In Proceedings of National Congress Italian Society of Audiology, Abano Terme, Italy, CRS: Milano, 13-16 October.

Bosco E, Argirò MT, Ballantyne D, Filipo R (1995) Selection protocols for cochlear implants in adults and children. In Proceedings of the Second Twinship Stockholm–Rome, Karolinska Institut, Stockholm, in press.

Bosco E, Argirò MT, Ballantyne D, Filipo R (1994) Relationship between psychological selection criteria and choice of rehabilitation protocol in Italian children using the Clarion device. Paper presented at the 2nd European Symposium on Paediatric Cochlear Implantation, Montpellier, France, 26–28 May.

Canestrari R (1990) L'Adoloescenza. In Canestrari R Psicologia generale e dello sviluppo. Bologna: Clueb, pp 577–605.

Clark GM, Blamey PJ, Brown AM, Busby PA, Dowell RC, Franz BK-H, Pyman, BC, Shepherd RK, Tong YC, Webb RL, Hirshorn MS, Kuzma J, Mecklenburg DJ, Money DK, Patrick JF, Seligman PM (1987) The University of Melbourne Nucleus multi-electrode cochlear implant. Advances in Otorhinolaryngology 38.

Collins AM, Lofts EF (1975) A spreading activation theory of semantic processing. Psychological Review 82: 407–28.

De Filippo CL, Scott BL (1978) A method for training and evaluating the reception of ongoing speech. Journal of the Acoustical Society of America 63: 1186–92.

Downs MP (1987) The deafness management quotient. Hearing and Speech News 1: 67–73.

Drezancic Z (1982a) Il ritmo musicale nella rieducazione del linguaggio. Strutture create per il metodo verbotonale. Turin: Omega.

Drezancic Z (1982b) Schede musicali: la voce parlata, il ritmo, l'intonazione. Turin: Omega.

Drezancic Z (1989) Il metodo creativo, stimolativo, riabilitativo della comunicazione orale e scritta con le strutture musicali di Zora Drezancic. Urbino: Quattroventi.

Fenn G, Smith BZD (1987) The assessment of lipreading ability: some practical considerations in the use of the tracking procedure. British Journal of Audiology 21: 253–58.

Filipo R, Argirò MT, Ballantyne D, Bosco E (1995) Experience with the Clarion device in children: surgical aspects, choice of strategy for stimulation and rehabilitation. Preliminary results. Advances in Otorhinolaryngology 50: 72–77.

Freud A (1968) L'Io e I meccanismi di difesa. Florence: Martinelli.

Hellman SA, Chute PM, Kretschmer RE (1991) The development of a children's implant profile. Annals of the Deaf 136(2): 77–81.

Owens E, Telleen CC (1981) Tracking as an aural rehabilitative process. Journal of the Academy of Rehabilitative Audiology 8: 79–84.

Robertson D, Irivine DRF (1989) Plasticity of frequency organization in auditory cortex in guinea pigs with partial unilateral deafness. Journal of Comparative Neurology 282: 256–71.

Rossi M. (1994). Indirizzi riabilitativi. Audiologia Italiana XI:360–376.

Ryals BM, Rubel EW, Lippe W (1991) Issues in neural plasticity as related to cochlear implants in children. American Journal of Otolaryngology 12: 22–27.

Tait M (1993) Video Analysis: Monitoring Progress in Young Cochlear Implant Users. Nottingham: Carnival Printers

Chapter 13
A Psycholinguistic Approach to the Rehabilitation of Cochlear Implant Children

HELMUT L. NEUMANN, RENATE MEIXNER

Introduction

Implantation in children requires ethical and thoughtful consideration. In children the surgery and its outcome may be the key to spoken language, unlike the situation for adults where the implant serves to provide a restoration of auditory communication. Its effects will impact on the entire future of a child.

When parents consult a hospital, they are searching for the most promising rehabilitative assistance available for their child. They are well aware of the need to make a decision that will be beneficial. Moreover, they are also aware that some individuals and interest groups are against implantation in children. An implant team concerned with the rehabilitation of children, therefore, must fulfil a number of specific responsibilities.

Responsibilities of an implant team

Parents are interested in knowing about the potential advantages obtained for their child immediately after the operation and what they can expect in the future. The team must be able to answer their questions comprehensively and provide some educational information and counselling. The team must explain that the hearing capacity of the child will not suddenly become normal after surgery. It must be clearly stated, and reconfirmed to the parents, that the child will develop auditory skills gradually as a result of support and motivation.

Educational situations must also be considered. Teachers at kindergartens and schools and the parents need to have a coordinated aim in promoting linguistic development in the child. All should be informed that the new sensory impressions will make new teaching methods and content essential. Questions about changes that might take place in the schools should be discussed in a supporting and trusting manner with the teachers. The teachers should understand, most importantly, that placing pressure on the child to make progress should be avoided. Children with cochlear implants need time to catch up with what hearing children have been learning for years.

The responsibility for the care of the child should be built up and maintained in a carefully woven network of support and after-care services. From the viewpoint of the psychologist and rehabilitationist, information and counselling about the postoperative stages are even more important than the success of the operation and the specific preliminary examinations.

In Aachen, an interdisciplinary team makes use of its psychological and linguistic knowledge to develop and implement pre- and postoperative assessments and parent counselling. As a consequence of the rehabilitative experience with deaf and hearing-impaired children, it promotes cooperation between schools and rehabilitation institutions.

Assessment

Although it is beyond the scope of this chapter, we would like to emphasise the need for psychological examinations and educational reviews during the preoperative phase. They can lead to an understanding of essential factors relevant to the feasibility and future prospects for implantation in a particular child. They may give rise to new talks with parents and shed valuable insights on implementing an auditory/verbal education. We acknowledge that there may be medical reasons disqualifying a child from a cochlear implant, but there are also psychological and/or rehabilitative reasons that might indicate whether or not an implant will be useful or disappointing, and whether reproaches are likely to follow (Meixner, 1992).

After a successful operation, some parents tend to overestimate the newly acquired capabilities of their child. They might wish to place their child in a kindergarten for normal-hearing children, or into a regular primary school. This means that counselling must emphatically explain to the parents that all children are different, and that progress will depend on the circumstances of each child. It is even worthwhile to focus on the importance of the speech processor fitting and that time is needed to provide the most useful programme to the child.

Lipreading and auditory education

In kindergartens and schools for hearing-impaired children who use hearing aids, learning takes place mainly through acoustic impressions and the children learn language through hearing. This is true even though they learn in less favourable conditions. Still, they learn in a natural way through natural auditory pathways. Even for these children, their speech is atypical, their vocabulary is essentially reduced in comparison with normal-hearing children and, for the most part, they speak with incorrect grammar. Importantly, though, they have a naturally developed relationship to spoken language.

Teachers for the special education of children describe those who are deaf in the following way. They are able to gain little or no auditory information even with the use of the best-fiting hearing aids. These children do not have a natural relationship to spoken language. They receive spoken language as a lipread message. Alich describes deafness as: 'The sensory feedback is interrupted. The deaf speaker cannot lipread himself. Therefore, the study of lipreading is very difficult. The signals used for lipreading are called 'kinemes'. They are not as efficient as the speech sounds (phonemes) or alphabetical letters. There are about 11 to 12 kinemes' (Alich, 1977). The relative number of kinemes compared with the wealth of alphabetical letters suggests that deaf children learn German or English as if it were a foreign language. They do not have a basis for a mother tongue. Taking into consideration that deaf individuals are able to grasp only what is directly spoken to them, and that they are not in a position to follow the conversation of others, it is easy to imagine that they must remember many features. An illustrative example is provided by Tigges (1977), who states that even for hearing children, it becomes evident how difficult lipreading can be for the English and German languages. He illustrates how Latin words, for example, can be visually grasped – an advantage for lipreading. In both English and German, the ending morphemes of the verbs are more complicated for the lipreader.

Latin:	eo	is	it	(no pronouns)
English:	I go	you go	he goes	(pronoun and ending)
German:	ich gehe	du gehst	er geht	(pronoun and three endings)
Perfect:	Latin:	ii		
	English:	I have gone		
	German:	ich bin gegangen		

Deaf children make much slower progress in kindergartens and schools than the hearing-impaired children simply because of the complexities of grasping language.

Auditory/verbal education and motor theory

Teachers must guide children with cochlear implants through their first experiences in mastering the world of sound, music and language. The children will learn to hear, step by step, what they could previously only grasp visually through lipreading. Gradually, they will realise that they are now always surrounded by language, that they spontaneously grasp much more language and that they are able to differentiate sounds and words through hearing. This does not mean that all cochlear implant children should be integrated immediately into classrooms where more linguistically competent children are learning.

It is our impression that children older than 5 years of age should not be placed in the same classrooms as hearing-impaired children of the same age immediately after receiving their speech processor. However, they also should not be put with children who are much younger. In Aachen, we handled this problem by scheduling several children who were in the same school to be implanted at the same time. When they received their speech processor, they were placed in a special classroom together until they could be more effectively streamed into the other classes where hearing-impaired children with hearing aids were being taught. This process of integrating the children and their education took place at the Aachen School for Deaf and Hearing Impaired and is described in more detail by Meixner (1992).

The lessons offered to these children and the auditory-verbal education programme used were based on the motor theory as described by Liberman (1963) and Braun (1969). 'Any residual hearing is enough to notice acoustic events. It takes adaptation to language; equivalent supporting information from other sensory systems and a background of linguistic knowledge and skill to discover that the acoustic events are about language' (Braun, 1969). Further to this, Fry states: 'We govern our articulation by reference to what we hear of our own speech. We do this by the acoustic cues that have evolved from speech reception to the monitoring of our own movements' (Fry, 1975). The importance of the motor theory is supported by the work of Novelli-Olmstead and Ling (Ling, 1984; Novelli-Olmsted & Ling, 1987). They found that children who repeated names of objects and pictures that had been read aloud to them made particularly remarkable progress in language learning compared with children who had not been given similar practice (Robertson & Flexer, 1993). It was characteristic of the auditory-verbal approach provided to the Aachen students that they first grasped language through a combined approach, i.e. reading and simultaneously hearing the teacher (or themselves) read aloud. This means that acoustic and visual information were combined.

In many instances, we even used a stronger multisensory approach that involved the listening–reading–speaking method of Ewing (Ewing & Ewing, 1964). Different teaching materials were necessary for this and needed to be designed specially for a hearing-impaired population.

Special materials

The education of hearing-impaired children in German schools involves learning reading skills as early as kindergarten (Loewe, 1994). This allowed us to have a relative amount of freedom in developing new materials at Cologne University that supported a multisensory approach to learning language (Jussen & Neumann, 1985; Jussen, Neumann & Holdau, 1994). Games designed to teach language to small children between 3 and 4 years of age included pictures and written cards that represent persons, objects and activities. The concepts and images were chosen according to psychological and linguistic criteria (Jussen, Neumann & Holdau, 1994). Moreover, they consider age-related interests of children at appropriate linguistic levels for particular training goals that are relevant to everyday life situations. To enhance perception, easily understood cards have also been designed that can be explained separately through writing or lipreading (see Figure 13.1).

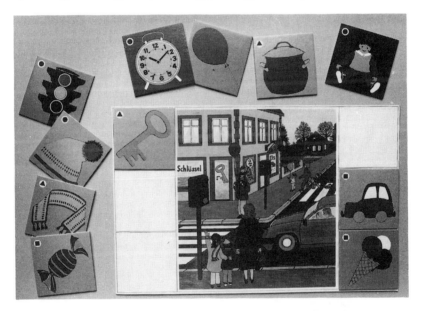

Figure 13.1: Materials designed to teach language to small children between 3 and 4 years of age using pictures that represent persons, objects and activities

Lipreading practice should contain clear mouth shapes, especially for younger children. It should contain as many kinemes as possible which, according to Alich (1977), are easy to grasp (labio-dental kineme, bilabial kineme, rounded-dental kineme, broad palatal kineme and broad velar kineme). When looking at text, children orientate themselves strongly on the different beginning letters of words, upward-sweeping letters (*d, l*) and downward-sweeping letters (*g, p*), and not necessarily on the length of a word. This means that even reading ma-terials can be specially adapted. Help for the auditory comprehension of spoken words is given by the prosodic features of language, by varying lengths of words and, in the German language, by the wide variety of vowels.

The speech of a child must always be regarded in the context of an action, i.e. something that really happened. That is why games for learning language contain pictures showing action and objects, both of which are known to the children. Thus, language learning supported by materials developed especially for hearing-impaired children can promote the perceptual capacity of children by the use of general pictures. It can induce them to recognise and name objects which they will eventually assign to individual representations.

For the next stage, a series of pictures that represent stories were developed. The picture-reading booklets depict everyday conversational situations that occur with the family, in kindergarten and at school (*Talk Situations in Everyday Life* [Jussen & Neumann, 1985]). The pictured pages contain comments and the conversation is written in balloons. The 4- to 6-year-old children can try to follow the text and listen to educators and parents as they read the stories aloud. A special feature of these books is that they not only tell a story, but also convey meaning and information about language. Again, acoustic and visual information are combined.

Hearing children learn at an early age to understand picture books because they have learned as their parents read to them aloud. In this regard, hearing-impaired children may not have the same advantages. They may need to be instructed to look at a series of pictures from left to right. They may need to be taught that a course of events in picture books can be presented as a sequence of pictures (see Figure 13.2). They

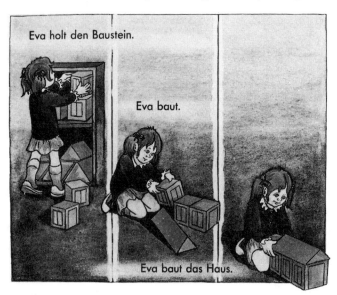

Figure 13.2: A sequence of pictures which show that one action follows another and that pictures can represent a series of events: Eva gets a building block; Eva is building; Eva builds the house

should also understand that the same person can be shown on different pages and in a variety of positions or that for one picture following another, the same person may have changed place, having moved from one room into another (Figures 13.3a and 13.3b).

Starting with two persons, the children may be shown that word

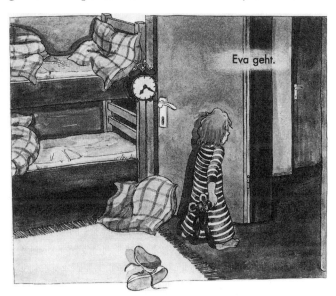

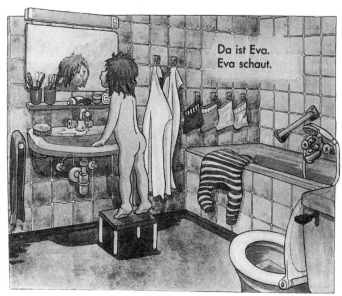

Figure 13.3: Pictures demonstrating that the same person can appear in a series of illustrations where the situation is completely different: (a) Eva is going (girl leaves her bedroom); (b) This is Eva. Eva is looking (girl looking at herself in a mirror in her bathroom)

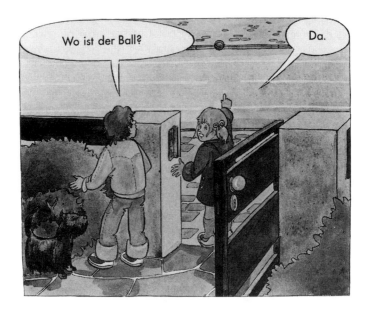

a

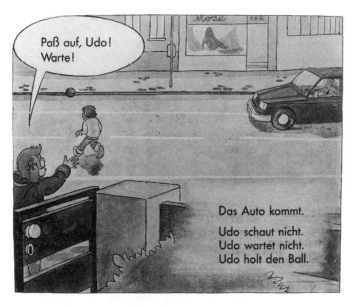

b

Figure 13.4 a-b: These illustrations have word balloons that show the relationship between simple verbal action: (a) Where is the ball? Over there; (b) Watch out, Udo! Wait! [The car is coming. Udo doesn't look. Udo doesn't wait. Udo is getting the ball].

balloons describe simple verbal actions that are related to one another. Thus, the first steps toward meaningful reading develop. The children ultimately learn to read and to understand accompanying text (Figures 13.4a–d). This is extremely important for implant-wearing children with reference to phonetic development. We consider these materials essential

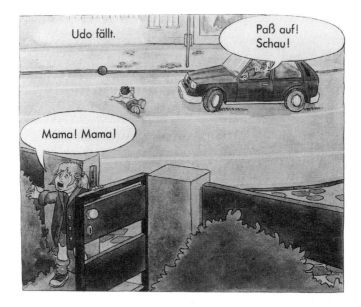

c

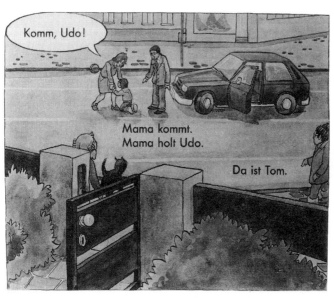

d

Figure 13.4 (cont.) (c) Mama! Watch out! Look! (d) Come on, Udo! [Mama comes. Mama gets Udo. There is Tom.]

because they give children an understanding of language in a multisensory way, so that they can grow into using spoken language by hearing and expressing themselves.

The materials described above not only promote early reading, they also enable a multisensory-orientated linguistic support especially for children with cochlear implants (Neumann, 1992). Picture-reading booklets provide this phenomenon because they represent the common conversations that take place in families, kindergartens and during school games with children of the same age.

Education and support in kindergartens

The value of a cochlear implant can only develop to its fullest when there are experts qualified to support and instruct the child postoperatively. The earlier children receive their implants, the more easily they can gain a natural perspective towards spoken language. Our experience lies with children who received their implants after the age of 3 years. In these cases, it was important for them to come into contact with hearing-impaired children. Most German schools have departments for deaf and for hearing-impaired children. In the kindergartens, there are parallel groups for deaf and hearing-impaired children, too. This is important for the careful observation of auditory development of children with hearing aids. Ultimately, only those who are unable to learn language via the auditory pathways, using the best hearing aid possible, and who, therefore, must rely on lipreading are united into classes. This careful division of kindergarten classes according to auditory capabilities makes it easy to take implant-wearing children out of their current group and bring them together with children who are hard of hearing. Hard of hearing, in educational terms, describes children who are in a position to grasp and learn language quite normally with the help of a hearing aid, but who require the aid of lipreading.

In Aachen, educators are in charge of the individual kindergarten groups. In addition, there are teachers for special education in every group. Working with two or three groups, their particular task is to promote speech and language. These teachers are also in charge of the special support given to cochlear implant children. They assure that the language level of each individual child is evaluated before the implant surgery. This is important because the child's pre-implant, existing knowledge of language must be taken into consideration when planning the post-implant educational programme.

Linguistic improvements for implant-wearing children who are integrated with hard-of-hearing children lead to the possibility of mainstreaming into classes with normal-hearing persons. Moreover, before deciding to move a child into a mainstream situation, it provides the opportunity to assess progress in relation to classmates and to normal-hearing children. The results of the evaluation assure the appropriateness and timing of mainstreaming.

Our experience has led us to favour a gradual transition into a mainstream situation for several reasons. First, we observed that children who had been mainstreamed immediately after implantation were not able to integrate socially with the other children easily and completely. As a result, they were not motivated or supported to improve their language skills. Second, the classrooms were large, in comparison with special education classes, and availability of personnel to help the children was limited. Third, the willingness to take implant-wearing children was not always present in the class. Finally, there is a risk that the cochlear implant children might be placed in the role of an outsider in spite of the sincere efforts of all those involved in integrating them into schools for normal-hearing children.

Support of students with cochlear implants

Linguistic support should always be action-orientated no matter what age the children. It should also be consistent with the curricular aims associated with developing competence in the areas of grammar and vocabulary. The opportunity to test this idea arose because of the unique situation in Aachen where three boys and one girl of the same age all received their implants at the same time. Once their speech processors had been fitted at the ENT Department of the Technological University in Aachen, they joined a special class at the David Hirsch School for Deaf and Hearing Impaired. The students were in the final class of primary school and were between 10 and 11 years old. They continued to be taught language by the same teacher who had instructed them before surgery. She knew the linguistic level of the students and incorporated the appropriate steps of the auditory-verbal approach into the newly formed class. It was important for students of that age to learn that the implant is really a support for the acquisition of language. A short while after the adjustment of the speech processor they discovered that they were able to decode their names auditorily and discriminate them from prosodic features.

Prior to receiving their implants, the students had monitored their speech movements via an 'inner feedback loop' (Meyer-Eppler, 1969). That is, they monitored sensations associated with the pressure changes and location sensations of speech organs. Soon they learned to their great astonishment how they could perceive hearing what they, themselves, had said. In the sense of the motor theory, the teacher gave them insight into the ability of mastering their own words in an auditory way. They advanced in reading, speaking and hearing. Step by step, they experienced the ability to participate in casual conversations, thus growing more and more confident with spoken language. Many grammatical rules which were previously difficult to store in memory could be self-monitored auditorily. The students learned that consistent rules governed language. They experienced this again and again in their daily lives. Their own speech became increasingly fluent and their voice pitch became lower.

For the students it was extremely impressive that the implant enabled them to remember verb conjugations more easily. The German language contains many more finite verb forms than the English language. These finite verb forms are difficult to grasp and differentiate through lipreading because the ending morphemes are formed subtly. This difference is illustrated in the following example:

English	German	English	German
I go	ich gehe	we go	wir gehen
you go	du gehst	you go	ihr geht
he/she goes	er/sie geht	they go	sie gehen

If the many German plural forms are compared with those existing in English, one is impressed by the difficulty deaf German students face in remembering the different forms:

English	German
ship/ships	Schiff/ Schiff*e*
car/cars	Auto/Auto*s*
garden/gardens	Garten/G*ä*rten
train/trains	Zug/Z*üge*
train/trains	Bahn/Bahn*en*
house/houses	Haus/H*ä*u*ser*
scooter/scooters	Roller/Roller
bag/bags	Tasche/Tasch*en*
picture/pictures	Bild/Bild*er*

The relief the implant brings must be like a liberation for deaf students. It is really an important change for them when they begin to realise that their self-confidence at grasping and differentiating speech is developing because of hearing.

Another problem for deaf German students is forming appropriate grammatical units. These are 'stress patterns' that carry important information. In spoken language, these stress units function to focus the attention of the listener. Of course, for deaf children, hearing and learning to produce stress patterns is very difficult. This is a particular problem in German because the stress unit changes depending on the tense of the verb and whether or not the verb is separable.

Examples of changing the stress unit from the beginning part of the sentence to the end are:

Example 1: (verb tense changes: present versus perfect). In this case, the object of the sentence is located between the predicate and the participle:

| I have a dog | Ich *habe* einen Hund |
| I have had a dog | Ich *habe* einen Hund *gehabt* |

Example 2: (separable verb). In this case, the object of the sentence lies between the stem and the prefix, a separable portion of the verb:

to lift	aufheben
I pick up the stone	Ich *hebe* den Stein *auf*

It is not surprising that deaf German-speaking children have difficulty in remembering to produce correct stress units. Basically, it is easy to give students an impressive demonstration of how their abilities will grow and precisely what kind of help they should receive from their implants. As they progress, they see their hopes confirmed and they are prepared to participate in the steps leading to mainstreaming. At the Aachen school, we were able to introduce these measures after one year. Our goal was to help the students reach a certain level through auditory-verbal education so that they could be integrated into classes for hearing-impaired students of their own age. We felt it more practical for them to be with peer-age students rather than younger ones. The latter case might have lead to depression and possibly the idea that they were unable to cope with linguistic tasks needed to communicate with similar aged students.

Steps towards integration

Transition of children with cochlear implants into classes for hearing-impaired students only seems justified if their linguistic level has been examined beforehand. After one and a half years of special auditory education for implant-wearing students, we thought that the time for a transition into the department for hearing-impaired children had come. We decided to test the students' abilities to express themselves freely as they described a series of pictures (Neumann, 1968). Our colleague, Gitta Grunert (1966) examined 265 spontaneous speech samples according to criteria developed by Grunert and also Kainz (Kainz, 1964; Grunert, 1966). The linguistic data gathered from the assessments of hearing-impaired children were compared with those obtained from normal-hearing children. She examined several aspects of the speech samples:

- the number of word categories being used;
- the percentage of nouns;
- the percentage of mistakes made in language forms;
- the share of incomplete sentences;
- the number of the parts of sentences;
- the beginning of the sentences;
- the form of presentation of the whole.

The analysis of the samples clearly indicated that the hearing-impaired children had a significant delay in learning to use different pronouns.

Grunert, therefore, extended the usual number of word categories to 16 and devised the following classification for her revised test:

nouns	other pronouns	prepositions
personal pronouns	numerals	conjunctions
reflexive pronouns	auxiliary verbs	inclusives
demonstrative pronouns	verb	interjections
possessive pronouns	adjectives	articles
relative pronouns	adverbs	the conjunction 'and'

Based on these examinations, she characterised seven stages of linguistic development for hearing-impaired children with ages as young as 2 years to the end of primary school (12 years). The results of our testing revealed that the students of the Aachen school were at a lower level than expected. In practical terms, this meant that for a transition to the classes for hearing impaired to take place, the children should have achieved the following results: (1) mastery of more than 10 word categories, (2) the percentage of nouns in spoken language should not exceed 25%, (3) errors in language forms should not exceed a ratio of 1:20, (4) incomplete sentences should not occur, (5) spoken language should be composed of sentences consisting of four or five parts, (6) the beginning of the sentences should consist of attributes or adverbs in 33% of the sample and, finally, (7) the spoken concepts had to be coherent, as well as relevant to the topic.

The findings from the examinations showed the following capacities: without any exception, all sentences constructed by the children started with the subject; no personal pronouns were used and only one possessive pronoun was identified in all of the samples. There were several positive characteristics including the finding that the sentences were structured at age-appropriate levels and that it seemed to be possible for the cochlear-implant wearers to make up for the language delay they experienced because of profound deafness. This was discovered by comparing their results with those of hearing-impaired students using hearing aids. It was also found that the percentage share of nouns was dependent on age. Finally, most of the language structures were meaningful (Neumann, 1994).

The results of the study demonstrated to us the need to work on the students' vocabulary. After the pronoun categories had been carefully reviewed, the children were encouraged to incorporate them into their speech. Moreover, we endeavoured to strengthen some of the weaknesses displayed in their use of word categories by requesting that they form verbs and adjectives from nouns. We also designed exercises that helped the children discover direction adverbs, which are frequently used in German. These included such words as (drehen) to value and (abdrehen) to devalue.

Even though children have received a cochlear implant, they still tend to use the same forms of sentence building they learned and practised before implantation. Sentences usually begin with the subject. Before changing into a class with hearing-impaired students, they need to move away from this habit. This is especially true for the German language where sentences usually begin with prepositions or attributes. Methods for teaching more flexible sentence building were carefully planned to ensure that it would not cause confusion. We used sentences following the pattern: *Wir verreisen eine Woche* changes to *Eine Woche verreisen wir*. In English, that would be: *We are travelling for one week* changes to *For one week we are travelling*. Sentences obeying the structure subject + predicate + accusative object were useful to demonstrate the flexibility of language and to motivate the children to talk with other hearing-impaired peers.

It is not our purpose to check the linguistic capacity of cochlear implant children in order to discover whether their approach to language is similar to that of normal-hearing students. The only important question is whether or not the children have reached a level of communication that allows them to interact with other children of a linguistically equivalent age. Basically, examinations with a similar structure may be useful when children receive an implant at an early age and when the intention is to mainstream them in kindergartens with hearing-impaired or, later, even normal-hearing children.

The linguistic method described by Clahsen (1986) appears to be particularly suitable in this context. It leads us to a better understanding of the linguistic level of kindergarten-age children. Progress must be recorded very carefully at these young ages. The most important points in the German language are: the parts of sentences which are spontaneously used, the order in which the ending of the verbs is acquired and applied, the development of the morphology of cases and the position of the verb in the sentence. This is in contrast with the observations made for the English language. Clahsen (1984) describes the five steps of speech and language development in early childhood which he considers to be significant. According to his examinations, young children turn to the use of verbs after they have outgrown the mere use of nouns. During the first stage, they employ finite forms of the third person singular and the first person plural. Of course, there are tendencies to over-generalise. It is only in the relatively later phases that structures concerning the position of the verb and the development of cases are within the bounds of possibility. Examinations for the acquisition of grammatical skills are frequently applied when evaluating children's language. They are useful in discovering language-related learning disabilities or handicaps. Our purpose is to use long-term observations in order to gain information about the linguistic level of young cochlear implant children regarding integration possibilities.

The future

Successful implantation is a reason for joy. The main task of all persons involved in the rehabilitation of children with cochlear implants is to make them aware that their lives now have a new dimension. Now they are not only able to respond when they are spoken to directly, but they find themselves in a world of sounds, noise and language. Step by step, they learn how easy it is for them to be in touch with the world because they can be addressed and can hear spoken language. They eventually, almost without noticing, begin to participate in conversations and in the exchange of thoughts and ideas. They gradually notice how much easier it is to grasp the real meaning of words and that they can repeat them. Their burden of remembering becomes noticeably relieved as they continue to listen to words and sentences in various contexts. They are able to recognise and to remember grammatically important features and forms.

Every hearing disability has a syndrome of characteristics. It not only harms linguistic development of children but it may also hamper the development of personal and social behaviour, as well as the growth of intellectual capacities based on learning through spoken language. Remediation through the use of a cochlear implant should, therefore, not be considered a cure for deafness. The support that is necessary for children must encompass the entire human being. That is what our examples in this chapter have aimed to demonstrate, as described in the work in kindergartens and schools and from the resulting steps towards integration. That is why this type of support, rehabilitation, requires so many professional groups and their interdisciplinary cooperation. Language is more than a pure means of communication. It is the means through which we gain an idea of the world. It is one of the keys to keeping up with the spirit of the times. Our efforts in working with implanted children should be to help them become members of our language community, which is a community of people using the same mother tongue leading them to adopt similar customary ways of thinking.

Acknowledgements

All translations of the quoted materials have been undertaken by the authors.

References

Alich G (1977) Sprachperzeption über das Absehen vom Munde. Sprache Stimme Gehör 1: 90–96.
Braun A (1969) Über das Verhältnis der Hörerziehung zum systematischen Sprachaufbau und der Sprachanbahnung. Neue Blätter für Taubstummenbildung 23: 24–30.

Clahsen H (1984) Linguistische Aspekte der Spontansprachdiagnostik im Frühbereich. Sprache Stimme Gehör 8: 38–43.

Clahsen H (1986) Die Profilanalyse. Berlin: Marhold.

Ewing A, Ewing I (1964) Teaching Deaf Children to Talk. Manchester: Manchester University Press.

Fry D (1975) The role and primacy of the auditory channel in speech and language development. In Ross M, Giolas TJ Availability Management of Hearing Impaired Children: Principles and Prerequisites for Intervention. Baltimore: University Park Press.

Grunert G (1966) Die Spontansprachentwicklung schwerhöriger Kinder im Vergleich zum normal hörenden Kind. Die Sonderschule 11(4): 194–203.

Jussen H, Neumann H (1985) Gesprächssituation im Alltag. Berlin: Marhold.

Jussen H, Neumann H, Holdau KR (1994) Kölner Sprachlernspiele. Aachen: Holdau.

Kainz F (1964) Sprachentwicklung im Kindes- und Jugendalter. München: Reinhardt.

Liberman A (1963) A motor theory of speech production. Proceedings of the Speech Communication Seminar, Stockholm.

Ling D (Ed) (1984) Early Intervention for Hearing-impaired Children: Oral Options. San Diego: College Hill Press.

Löwe A (1994) Unausgeschoepftes Potential. Leseprobleme hochgradig hoergeschaedigter Kinder muessen bereits in der Vorschulzeit angegangen werden. Sprache Stimme Gehoer 18: 162–67.

Meixner R (1992) Pädagogische Aufgabenteilung bei Schülern mit Cochlea-Implantaten. Hörgeschädigtenpädagogik 46: 91–99.

Meyer-Eppler W (1969) Grundlagen und Anwendungen der Informationstheorie. Berlin: Springer.

Neumann HL (1968) Sprachliche Einschläge in sogenannten sprachfreien Tests. Gesichtspunkte zur Untersuchung Taubstummer. Kettwig: Verlag Hörgeschädigte Kinder.

Neumann HL (1992) Aufgaben des Pädagogen als Mitglied einer multidisziplinären Arbeitsgruppe bei Schülern mit Cochlea Implantat. Sprache Stimme Gehör 16: 1–52.

Neumann HL (1994) Peadagogical and psychological tasks regarding children and teenagers being considered for cochlear implants. In Advances in Cochlear Implants. Proceedings of the 3rd International Cochlear Implant Conference, Innsbruck 1993. Wien: Manz.

Novelli-Olmstead T, Ling D (1987) Speech production and speech discrimination by hearing impaired children. Volta 86: 72–80.

Robertson L, Flexer C (1993) Reading development: a parent survey of children with hearing impairments who developed speech and language through the auditory-verbal method. Volta 95: 253–61.

Tigges J (1977) Charakteristika eines systematischen Sprachaufbaus bei Gehörlosen. Sprache Stimme Gehör 1: 59–64.

Chapter 14
Adolescents and the Cochlear Implant

CARMEN PUJOL, TERESA AMAT

Introduction

Cochlear implantation of adolescents is a challenging process for all those associated with the implantee. Factors that influence the selection and rehabilitation are broader in this population because of psycho-social circumstances that surround these young people. It is possible that clinics will limit their selection of teenagers for implantation because they present too many difficulties for the rehabilitation process. This chapter presents an optimistic viewpoint on the treatment of deaf adolescents who receive cochlear implants.

Considerations

We believe it is of great importance to have extensive contact with the adolescent before initiating treatment with the cochlear implant. This involves all areas of speech and language evaluation, as well as detailed understanding of the child's social and family background. We need to know about the young person's hopes and expectations and, above all, interests. Based on this information, a pre-implant programme can be devised. It should contain clear objectives for all of the involved professionals, keeping in mind that the ways to achieve the objectives can never be rigid. Rehabilitation objectives, especially for this population, should be flexible.

Postlingual adolescents

Emotional Support

An easy classification for adolescents is between those who have pre- and postlingual deafness. In the case of postlingual adolescents, where spoken language is usually preserved, we have not encountered any serious difficulties when implementing the rehabilitation process. Nevertheless, we bear in mind that adolescence is a difficult period of development (Corbella & Valls, 1993) and requires emotional support from the rehabilitation team, the teachers and the family.

It is clear that a certain amount of time must pass for the recognition of new perceptions to develop. The amount of time will vary from one individual to the next, and will depend on their expectations, abilities and the duration of their deafness. Although teenagers may be clear about their expectations, especially when they have an opportunity to hear descriptions of listening experiences from other implant users, they are slightly apprehensive until they experience the sensations for themselves. Once this happens, a period of over-optimism occurs at which time the teenager goes dizzily in pursuit of auditory information and attempts to process it all at the same time.

Training

We can take a more analytical approach to the suprasegmental aspects of language (intonation, stress, duration and articulation) and the components of speech (consonants and vowels), progressing quickly through the stages of detection, discrimination, identification, recognition and comprehension (Huarte, 1990) with postlingual teenagers. They achieve higher levels of performance more quickly and with less stress than those with prelingual deafness. In part, this is because there are many overlapping and interlinked elements which can be introduced rapidly into the rehabilitation sessions. The exercises utilise phonetic opposition (paired comparisons), telephone work, listening to different types of music, vocabulary building, and incomplete sentences to be completed by the listener (We buy medicine in a _____ [pharmacy]), word games (Hangman, I-Spy, Scattergrams), vignettes (short stories) and pictured sentences. These types of exercises are usually well accepted and successful from the onset of the rehabilitation programme. They are, after all, pleasant and create enthusiasm in the teenagers because they experience success. It is possible to move quickly into exercises that focus more specifically on recognition.

Prelingual teenagers

There are many subtle differences within the group of teenagers who have had their deafness from birth or before establishing spoken language, although they also have common characteristics. Some important distinctions need to be recognised. Although, in principle, the subjects' expectations might be very clear, their age leads to a natural impatience to see results. The rehabilitator needs to be reminded that adolescence is a delicate phase, where impulsivity and impatience need to be controlled. At the same time, motivation needs to be maintained in the teenagers. This can present a very difficult balance which is challenging for the rehabilitationist to maintain.

Another consideration is that, in one way or another, these children have worked harder throughout their lives than any hearing person of the same age. They have done this without achieving the same educational levels or the same results. They are tired of special programmes, of support teachers, of speech therapists, of diction exercises, of various types of training. They are simply tired of making so much extra effort. The cochlear implant is a new adventure. This is a key point of which we, as rehabilitationists, must take advantage. The cochlear implant is a new stimulus. It is one that, for the first time, provides auditory feedback. Using this idea as a base, we should make the sessions agreeable and directly involve the adolescent from the start. The sessions should not be another task or just more work. That is why it is so important to find out not only what they know, but also what their experiences and interests are. This understanding serves as the basis from which we develop individual programmes. It is also the source for providing support and motivation (Martincz Torralba, 1992).

Training

Once we know the individual, we select a central theme from which any element for training might radiate. It should lead us to global communication because the child is interested in succeeding and sharing information. It is obviously necessary to work on audition, but language is communication.

The proposals for working with an individual are varied, although we always follow general patterns that can be modified according to the individual's environment. For example, the circumstances in which the children find themselves in background noise are different for those who live in the city and those who live in the country. The sound of tractor engines, the chirping of crickets or the crowing of cockerels will not be frequent sounds in a noisy city full of ambulance sirens, lorries or the screeching of car brakes.

We begin rehabilitation with the detection of sound and with changes in its intensity and frequency. Thus, the presence or absence of sound (sound/silence) will be the first parameter taught. The practice for this is expanded through the use of what we term a *listening set* consisting of expected or announced closed-set sounds. The next step is gradually to introduce unexpected sounds which are to be detected while the teenager is carrying out some other task. In this case, the subject is not alerted to the presence of a sound and whatever auditory reaction cccurs is carefully recorded by the clinician.

The localisation of sound is another of the exercises proposed. These follow when we have maximally structured the auditory environment. This means that the teenager is able to distinguish the presence of environmental noises, the presence of voices and changes in inflection. The next step is to work on associating sounds at different distances; that is, the concepts of nearness and remoteness. Some sounds come gradually closer (an aircraft, a siren) while others become more distant (the sound of a church bell with its echo that slowly fades). At first, we employ aids, especially visual aids, but these are gradually withdrawn as the subject progresses.

Inflection (see Figure 14.1) and pronunciation are areas in which everyday phrases prove very useful. Everyday phrases have a double purpose: on the one hand, the teenager uses very common, repetitive phrases; phrases that appear constantly in the environment. On the other hand their use in the context of developing better speech production also provides opportunities for identification and, later, recognition. The repetition of the commonly spoken phrases provides a platform for practising changes in intonation and stress patterns associated with affirmative and negative sentences, questions and exclamatory sentences.

Reading Exercises

Reading is a gratifying exercise that we propose for our adolescents. They follow a text while the reading rhythm is varied. For this exercise, the individual has a text to follow while the therapist reads aloud. The teenager cannot see the reader's lips and must follow the text by listening. We vary the prosodic characteristics throughout the text (reading

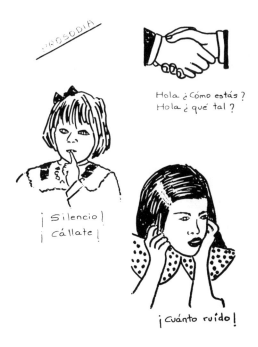

Figure 14.1: Illustrated common phrases emphasising prosodic differences

quickly, slowly, moderately quickly) and the subject signals which word in the text has been reached. This is known as paragraph tracking (Mecklenberg, Dowell & Jenisen, 1991).

To summarise the approach for prelingual teenagers, the following represent useful activities: distinguishing between the absence/presence of sound; use of words that sound like what they represent (onomatopoeia, see Figure 14.2); identifying duration characteristics; detecting expected and unexpected sounds; discriminating environmental noise; identifying both the presence of voices and different voices, repeating auditory speech signals without visual cues and localising near and remote sounds (Gajik, 1985). It should be noted that we work on localisation with those who use both a cochlear implant and a contra-lateral hearing aid. We encourage the use of a hearing aid in the non-implanted ear as a bridge between deafness (what they have known before the implant) and the objectives of useful spoken language (utilising the cochlear implant). The level of the exercises, whether concerned with rhythm, words, actions or phrases, will depend on the level of previous language development in the individual. Further, they will be linked to the teenager's knowledge, experiences and interests (Marchesi, 1987).

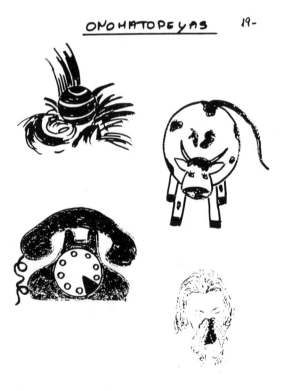

Figure 14.2: Words that sound like the images they represent (onomatopoeia) such as: rrrrrrr... = ring/telephone; achooo...= sneeze; mooo...= cow; splash...= ball landing in water

Use of sign language

We have encountered adolescents whose only means of communicating is through sign language. They usually have a low communication level. This has led us to develop a language programme similar to one we might use to teach a young deaf child to speak. However, it takes into consideration the experience an adolescent has with receptive, signed languages as well as the audition provided throught the implant. The exercises can be used in a positive way to ensure that the adolescent does not feel he/she is being treated like a baby. To avoid giving the adolescent this impression, the materials should be adapted to his/her chronological age rather than linguistic age. This is a different approach than is usually recommended for younger children.

We make one proviso: we know that profoundly deaf persons who only communicate with sign language are not ideal candidates for a cochlear implant. This is because their auditory environment is usually poor and their oral productions are usually scarce and limited. However, although we know from the start that we will be faced with a difficult challenge, philosophically we do not believe that this reason alone should condemn them to a life of silence espicially for someone who really wants to hear. The selection process for cochlear implant candidacy for such teenagers, however, must be very critical. The person must want to hear and be part of the hearing world. This means he/she must have a need to communicate with hearing friends and family. During the pre-implant counselling, we emphasise the effort involved in learning to hear. There can be no misunderstanding about this. Rehabilitationists, also, need to adjust their own expectations. The signing children will start at a lower baseline of performance. Their results will be different from those obtained from oral children. Rehabilitation will focus on the acquisition of concepts as well as training the subject to speak intelligibly. These elements will take up a large part of the time and training.

Developing a rehabilitation programme that emphasises language

We shall take, for example, sports (see Figure 14.3) or travelling (see Figure 14.4) as our themes. These are interesting to adolescents. We select certain concepts related to the theme. If these do not exist, they must be introduced. For example, let us assume that the concept of *table* is not a familiar one. First, we show the teenager a series of pictures illustrating different table designs. Next, we introduce table designs that have not been shown and mix them with other pictured objects. This shows the teenager's ability to generalise the concept. Finally, we teach the word 'table'. Once conceptualised, we work on articulation, using a variety of exercises to achieve correct production.

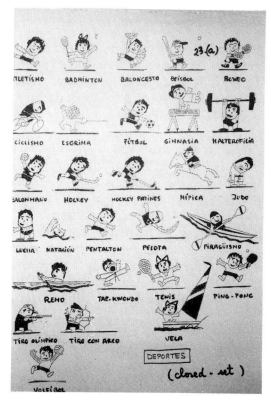

Figure 14.3: Words and images representing different sports activities

We believe that a person needs the concept of the word before working on the auditory perception of the word. We continue using the same methods to teach discrimination (with and without lipreading), words of different lengths and different phonetic features, i.e. pass-port (two syllables) and des-ti-na-tion (four syllables). We begin with highly contrasted words and gradually introduce similar sounding words along with changing the pitch and other speech features. The same theme allows us to work on onomatopoeia (motorcycles, ships, trains and so forth).

Again, building from concept to word, the technique allows us to designate and discriminate between words in closed sets (forced choice), such as: transport/travel, clothes/travel, items/cities/countries or in open sets (free choice). We can introduce adjectives in games using antonyms: fast/slow, cold/hot, comfortable/uncomfortable, open/closed. Without a verb there is no sentence, so actions and verb conjugations also merit our attention. The subject of travel allows us to introduce: seeing, admiring, knowing, discovering, strolling, buying, writing, noting, drawing, eating, drinking, resting, photographing, filming, asking and many more action words (Vergara et al., 1993). In this way,

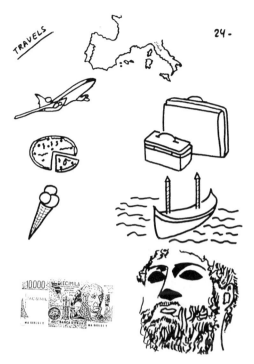

Figure 14.4: Pictures associated with travel

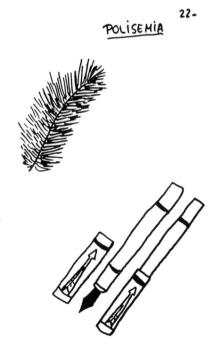

Figure 14.5: Words that have polysemious meaning (e.g. quill, pen)

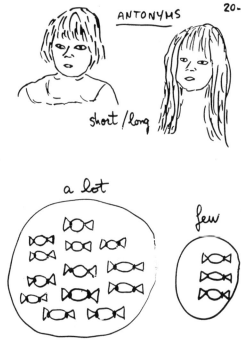

Figure 14.6: Words that have opposite meanings (antonyms)

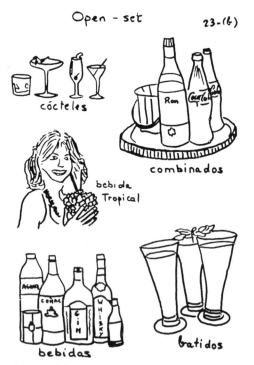

Figure 14.7: Cued or modified open-set words, such as things to drink

we arrive at sentences. The first stage is to discriminate them with the purpose of later asking the teenagers to create them own. Step by step, we let our adolescents acquire the abilities necessary to perceive speech and to become involved in the complex framework of language. An interesting topic, for instance, is the understanding of time and space; responding to questions of where, when and how, and so forth. The process is more than an exercise, it is one which involves discovering the world through spoken language. We have found that our subjects enjoy this approach to rehabilitation because it sharpens their imaginations and broadens their vocabulary.

Vocabulary building is useful. We encourage looking up new words and expanding indexes or lists (with visual aids in the majority of cases). Table 14.1 provides some examples of vocabulary-building topics (see also Figures 14.5, 14.6 and 14.7).

Table 14.1: Vocabulary-building topics

- Two-word expressions (suspension bridge)
- Three-word expressions (ace of spades)
- Derivatives (act, actor, actress)
- Words with more than one meaning (craft)
- Antonyms (a little/a lot)
- Collective nouns (group, team, flock)
- Letter soups
- Semantic fields (medical vocabulary, the vocabulary of the weather)
- Classifications (types of shoe, types of drinks)
- Association of ideas
- Set expressions
- Popular sayings
- Colloquial language (juvenile slang)
- Words or phrases with two meanings or metaphorical meanings
- Riddles, etc.

We have provided concepts and verbs but we are still at a rudimentary stage of comprehension. We often find that young deaf people who have assimilated a concept and who know of an action may still have a problem putting the two together to form a coherent sentence. They also have problems differentiating between the subject and the object. What normally occurs is that they conceptualise them as two isolated elements and are unaware of how to join them to produce a final meaningful notion.

We are not suggesting the need to develop an extensive vocabulary on the PARADIGMATIC level (vertical): Example: 'The *boy* eats bread' (or dog or bird)

This might seem to be the case in our example. The goal is to instill in those given cochlear implants the ability to control words (see Figure 14.8). That makes it possible for real communication to take place because they learn to dominate (or have power over) syntactical relationships. Choosing from the range of possibilities offered by a common noun could be likened to an isolated perpendicular line. It leads up and down, but not laterally. We offer verticality. In grammar, this verticality is composed of eight parts. We see the horizontal aspect or 'the linear nature of language', as described by Saussure (1971). Being able to relate these parts on the syntactic level implies being at the level of formal speech. We do not introduce these parts all at once. The first step is to categorise the words as noun, verb or article; however, if we introduce any part first, it would be the verb. With these three elements, there exists a functional, simple sentence. The next step is comprehension. Here, we ask simple questions based on a traditional grammatical model: What is it? Who is it? What is he doing? (Herren, 1982). Strangely enough, answers given to the last question (about a picture of a child swimming) have included: (a) child, (b) water and (c) swimming pool. All of these are common nouns, but do not even comply with the features of a given framework as they do not belong to the same semantic categories.

Our final objective is to reach the deep structures of language, but this is not always possible. We are aware of the difficulties this presents on the linguistic level and in the understanding of the transformations that the rules of language can generate. It is possible, from a treatment point of view, to become too involved in the language therapy. The rehabilitationists must keep in mind that our subjects are idealistic and impatient adolescents whose three basic objectives are to hear, to understand and to have fun (Recasens, 1988; Guillermo & Palacios, 1989; Estienne-De Jong, 1991).

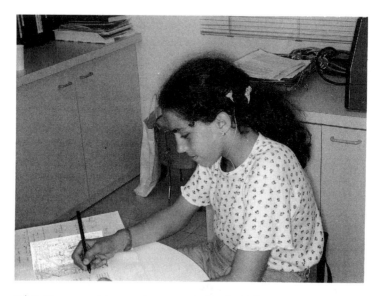

Figure 14.8: Teenage girl at work on vocabulary building exercises

Our aim is to create situations and to share in activities that facilitate access to language. In this way, the subject grasps and organises the language forms spontaneously (Aimard & Abadie, 1992). Audition is one of the props of training. There are exercises in our repertoire that are designed for independent work and others designed for use at home or with friends. In the first case, recognising, discriminating and identifying environmental sounds are very useful. The exercises do not have to be boring, which is how many teenagers see any type of assignment. We make a serious effort to provide an enjoyable task. In this case, they might be related to sounds in the room, the telephone, footsteps or the clicking of high heels, the sound of paper being crumpled, a pen falling to the floor, and other current and relevant sounds. These are everyday noises that hearing people often do not even notice. Other sounds may be more artificial, such as sound-location Lotto or cassette recordings. We can make these sounds even more relevant; for instance, going to the bar for a drink gives us the sound of glasses clinking together, the noise of the coffee machine, the sound of coins when we go to pay and so forth.

Individual exercises might include listening to the sound of one's own voice when reading aloud. This can be gratifying as well as useful in learning to regulate and use intonation correctly. Following the lyrics along with the rhythm of music in a karaoke bar can also be extremely appealing and something new. At home, there are endless sounds to discover and identify, and discriminating the voices of relatives and friends (their different timbres and tones) can be a fascinating adventure.

Music appreciation

Music warrants a chapter of its own both in terms of the type of instrument and the type of music. At first, very different, highly contrasted types of music should be employed (jazz, pop, classical). More subtle differences can then be introduced gradually (Cooper, 1991).

Unfortunately, there are few materials available on the market that meet our specific needs, especially because these needs vary for each child. The therapist involved with adolescents requires creativity, imagination and patience to discover the right choices for each person. There are, nevertheless, certain topics prevalent at this age. A simple list includes: certain sports, social events, current events, studies in school, outside interests and music. It is possible to develop or create materials from these. There are sporting materials; albums with pieces of different material that provide opportunity for distinguishing names and textures; fashion magazines; newspapers which give us the opportunity to comment on the most spectacular events of the day; travel brochures; dossiers on jobs and much more.

Voice quality

Voice quality is another area about which most deaf adolescents are concerned. To complicate matters, this is a time when teenage boys experience voice breaks. Both boys and girls need work on modulation and intensity control. The programmes provided by the commercially available Phonetic Visualizer (Kay Elemetrics Corp) are very useful for voice therapy. The children find them enjoyable and realise characteristics of their speech that would, otherwise, be difficult to teach. The programmes provide speech models which the children can imitate. They can monitor their own progress as they more closely approach the programmed model. Computer programs provide exercises for work on verb tenses, sentence structure, temporality and sequencing. Teenagers are computer literate.

Video cameras also provide interactive games that encourage improved language skills, in particular, diction and lipreading. The camera records youngsters holding a spontaneous conversation on a given theme (where they gives opinions, without a script). The subjects later watch themselves on the screen and try to transcribe the conversation (by lipreading what they said). Errors of diction frequently crop up which can then be corrected immediately.

Our centre offers individual therapy for adolescents outside the school system. Ideally, contact is maintained with the educational facility through interaction with the teachers who provide the academic training. The communication is mutually beneficial because we learn what the children are studying in school. This helps us to keep our session materials more relevant to the child. The teachers learn from us what to expect from the cochlear implant. Because we are an outside clinic, we can bring children together from different school programmes. Group therapy with two or three of these adolescents, who have similar characteristics and levels of performance, stimulates them with spontaneous competitiveness. This results in more attentiveness even to the point where they discriminate new sounds and show rapid increases in performance.

Telephone training

With the postlingual group, we usually achieve high levels of interactive conversation. Prelingual teenagers receive training that allows them to hold simple, short conversations which are useful in their daily lives. There are different aspects to telephone training for the two groups. The first problem to overcome is to ensure that the fear which may be associated with speaking and hearing over the telephone is reduced. They need to be encouraged to attempt to use the telephone and assured that whatever they achieve will be accepted as a success. The steps progress from very simple closed-set tasks and proceed slowly: initially, differences between a male and female voice, closed-set (well rehearsed) names and then simple sentences with these same names (I'm Mary, Where is Mary? Call Peter). Other closed-set topics are: yes/no, days of the week, places (at the cinema, to the theatre, have dinner) and transportation (by train, by car). Numbers are covered in detail: in isolation, time, telephone numbers and numbers in sentences (at three o'clock). The next stage emphasises a set of useful sentences (information, greetings, farewells). We specially design the sentences together with each teenager, as the sentences should be important. Examples of information sentences might be: I'll arrive on time. I'll be late. I won't come with you, I feel ill. Don't wait for me. Sentences used for greetings might be: How do you do? Hello. Who is speaking? Sentences which mean goodbye might be: See you later. OK. Bye-bye. See you on Sunday. An advanced exercise is to mix sentences and to understand what the important details might be. For instance, a series of sentences might be:

(a)	Hello	(listen to voice)
(b)	Who is speaking?	(listen for a name)
(c)	Message	(listen for day, time, place)
(d)	Goodbye	(listen for farewell)

The telephone, an important tool for social exchange, ceases to be a problem for most postlingual teenagers (Brimacombe et al., 1989). It also becomes useful for some prelingual children and even becomes a practical tool for some. To date, very few prelingual teenagers can hold a telephone conversation. However, they do attempt to speak and give short messages, as well as learn to discriminate familiar sentences, especially in a closed set.

Summary

The majority of adolescent implantees have shown positive emotional changes and important social reactions. We can highlight the following factors which may be useful when counselling parents of teenagers and the children themselves. The concern about the cable which, for aesthetic reasons, initially worries both parents and the teenagers becomes a minimal or non-existent problem. Sport, especially football for boys, does not create special problems. This is an important issue because sports and the wearing of a cochlear implant may seem incompatible at first. Our experience is that the children simply stop thinking of the implant as something alien. They incorporate it into their everyday activities, viewing it as a necessary and irreplaceable tool in the same way that people needing visual assistance adapt to their eyeglasses.

All of the teenagers in our programme have experienced improvements in their voices and their diction. We view this as an aid to their becoming more integrated with their peers and friends. It gives them a sense of confidence in the world of hearing people. It also has an impact on their independence and willingness to make decisions. They realise that without the implant they would experience more difficulties in everyday life. Specific examples from our population relate to successes in school. They are more independent in areas of transport such as getting their driving licences or travelling unaccompanied in the city. Again, they are more independent of their parents, going out with friends, going to parties, the cinema, concerts or on holiday with friends. Their self-confidence increases and they dare to ask more questions and even go shopping where they will face the challenge of communicating with normal-hearing people.

Conclusion

The biggest challenge with adolescent cochlear implant patients is not whether they will utilise auditory sensations effectively, but whether they will identify themselves as hearing individuals. This is a time when both self-image and peer pressure have a significant impact. It means that rehabilitationists are more than speech and hearing therapists: they are partners in working with young adults to enhance self-confidence and independence. Our experience has been rewarding. We encourage other cochlear implanters to include this population in their patient selection.

References

Aimard P, Abadie C (1992) Intervención precoz en los transtornos del lenguaje del nino. Barcelona: Mason, pp 108–32.

Brimacombe JA, Beiter AL, Barker MJ, Mikami KA, O'Meilia RM, Shallop JK (1989) Speech recognition abilities over the telephone for Nucleus 22-channel cochlear implant recipients. In Fraysse B, Cochard N (Eds) Cochlear Implant: Acquisitions and Controversies. Toulouse: Paragraphic, pp 345–52.

Cooper H (1991) Training and rehabilitation for cochlear implant users. In Cooper H (Ed) Cochlear Implants. London: Whurr, pp 219–38.

Corbella J, Valls C (1993) Davant una edat difícil-Psicologia de l'adolescent. Barcelona: Columna, No. 6.

Estienne-De Jong F (1991. De la créativité a l'écoute et la discrimination. In Estienne-De Jong Plaisir et langage. Brussels: Editions Universitaires, pp 59–79.

Gajik K (1985) Habla y audición. Método verbo-tonal. Valencia: Nou llibres.

Guillermo M, Palacios A (1989) El taller de las palabras. Madrid: Seco-Olea.

Herren H (1982) Estudio sobre la educación de los niños y adolescentes sordos. Barcelona: Médica y Técnica, pp 117–20.

Huarte A (1990) Manual de rehabilitación del implante coclear. Pamplona: Servicio de Publicaciones de la Universidad de Navarra.

Marchesi A (1987). El desarrollo cognitivo y lingüístico de los niños sordos. Psicología, 204–7.

Martinez Torralba I (1992) El desafío de la integración. Barcelona: Milán, pp 23–29.

Mecklenburg DJ, Dowell RC, Jenisen G (1991) Rehabilitation Manual. Sydney, Australia: Cochlear Pty Ltd.

Recasens M (1988) Actividades de estructura de las palabras y vocabulario. In Recasens M Como jugar con el lenguaje. Barcelona: CEAC, pp 81–130.

Saussure F (1971) Curso de lingüística general. Buenos Aires: Losada.

Vergara KC, Oller DK, Eilers R, Balkany T (1993) Curricula objectives for educators of children with cochlear implants. In Fraysse B, Deguine O (Eds) Cochlear Implants: New Perspectives. Basel: Karger, pp 216-19.

Appendix A: Resource materials in Spanish for speech therapists

Kent LR, Basil C, Del Rio MªJ (1989) Programa para la adquisición de las primeras etapas del lenguaje. Madrid: Siglo XXI de España Editores.

Lafon J-C (1987) Los niños con deficiencia auditiva. Barcelona: Mason.

Pita Gherardi E, Arribas J (1986) Estructuras básicas de la comunicación oral. Madrid: CEPE.

Silvestre N, Martínez I (1987) L'educació del deficient sensorial. Barcelona: Fundació Caixa de Pensions.

Wood D (1983) El desarrollo lingüístico y cognitivo en los deficientes auditivos. Madrid: Infancia y Aprendizaje no. 3.

Chapter 15
Therapeutic Concepts for Training Cochlear Implant Patients Who Have Good Preoperative Language Skills

GEORGE A. TAVARTKILADZE, ELSA V. MIRONOVA, RAISA A. BOROV-
LEVA, INNA A. BELYANTSEVA, GREGORY I. FROLENKOV

Introduction

Speech perception performance of cochlear implant users depends on a variety of factors. Some of them, such as the duration of rehabilitation period, the period of deafness prior to operation, pre- or postlingual deafness onset and age of the patient at the moment of implantation, have been well recognised (Dowell, Mecklenburg & Clark, 1986; Deguine et al., 1993; Gantz et al., 1993a, 1993b). Nevertheless the great diversity in postoperative, hearing-only results has been reported even within the groups of patients specially selected according to the above-mentioned factors (Dawson et al., 1992; Dorman, 1993; Lehnhardt & Aschendorff, 1993). Thus, we are still very far from a good prognosis of the postoperative scores of a particular individual on the different speech recognition tests (Dawson et al., 1992; Dorman, 1993). To some extent, postoperative results could be related to the preoperative spoken language skills but there are only scarce data on this subject (Geers & Moog, 1994). We take the opportunity, here, to describe our experience with the rehabilitation of patients using the Nucleus Mini System 22. The focus is directed particularly on the subjects who had good spoken language skills before implantation. Such a group of patients offers the opportunity to utilise the general principles of re-habilitation without the significant influences usually facing the thera-pist of duration and age at onset of deafness, and whether the patient has enough language to use a variety of training materials. Further, these patients frequently show good open-set speech recognition scores so that evaluation materials relating to different linguistic levels (sentences, words, quasi-words, meaningless phoneme complexes, phonemes) can be developed. Such tests were found to be particularly helpful in testing the performance of our cochlear implant patients.

Multidisciplinary team

Our cochlear implant rehabilitation team consists of five professionals, all involved in the programme on a part-time basis. There is the coordinator who is an otolaryngologist and a physiologist responsible for overseeing the progress of each patient. The team manager is a biophysicist who is responsible for administering the pre- and postoperative audiological assessments and counselling, technical support of the cochlear implant equipment and programming of speech processors. A physician–physiologist performs routine speech processor programming and any necessary psychophysiological tests. This individual is also involved in pre- and postoperative counselling, as well as in some preoperative testing. Individual rehabilitation programmes are designed by a speech therapist/special educator who also administers all necessary performance measures, is involved in patient selection and participates in pre- and postoperative counselling. A teacher of the deaf completes our team. She is responsible for carrying out the training at each rehabilitation session. All the specialists meet to discuss results and to plan strategies to be implemented in further rehabilitation sessions for each patient.

We also have specialists who help with preoperative evaluations. There is the surgeon who is responsible for the coordination of all activities concerning surgery and the entire clinical stay. Another surgeon-audiologist performs promontory stimulation tests. Finally, a physician-audiologist performs routine preoperative audiological assessments.

Counselling: pre- and postoperative

During preoperative psycho-educational counselling, a cochlear implant candidate and the normal-hearing relatives are interviewed about what they know and expect of cochlear implantation. Usually the information they have needs to be corrected and expanded. We ask whether the family is certain of their decision to proceed with the operation and if they are aware of all the possible outcomes. It is also important to determine the possibility for the patient to make regular visits to the centre for training and testing, whether the family is capable of carrying out home training and who, exactly, will do it and whether the candidate is prepared for the long-term, postoperative rehabilitation. We also investigate the speech production skills of the candidates and their speech perception abilities with the use of lipreading with and without hearing aid(s).

Our experience has revealed that there are certain areas in preoperative counselling which require special attention. It should be made clear to the adult implant candidate and to families of children that there is a wide range of speech perception results obtained among the cochlear implant users. It should be emphasised that it is not possible to predict exactly how a particular candidate will benefit from the implant, either in the short or long term. Families and patients must be aware that usually a long rehabilitation process is necessary in order to achieve the best possible results. Finally, a proper psychological environment should be available for the cochlear implant user to enhance the opportunity to experience success. Such factors as maximum exposure to listening opportunities, clear speech on the part of the speaker (not necessarily the implant user) and a general atmosphere of oral communication are essential.

Sometimes a discrepancy may be found between the expectations of potential candidates and the clinician. Clinicians usually expect that implantees (both adults and adolescents), regardless of the degree of progress in speech perception using only audition, will easily be aware when a speaker is addressing them face to face. This is a minimal expectation and such levels of performance are reported for the majority of cochlear implant users (Anon., 1994). On the other hand, some of our candidates expect to understand speech without lipreading, understand speakers on the television or the radio and freely use the telephone shortly after implantation.

Postoperative counselling includes a description of some typical steps in the cochlear implant user's performance, arrangements to have a conversation with the best, previously implanted patients and a detailed description of home tasks and the individualised rehabilitation programme. At postoperative consultations, the implantee and relatives report on any observed changes in auditory sensations and reactions to various non-speech and speech sounds. The patients are questioned about any sources of discomfort during implant use. If problems exist, the electrode levels are re-checked. Indications for necessary programme adjustments are degradation in speech discrimination, an increased need for repetitions, complaints about unpleasant sensations caused by loud sounds or reports that all sounds are too quiet.

Patient overview

All our patients were implanted with the Nucleus Mini System 22 cochlear implant and all are native Russian speakers. The first patient was implanted in 1991. Originally, the rehabilitation programme for Russian-speaking cochlear implant patients was developed on the basis of our experience with postlingually deafened adults. Later it was expanded, using the main principles of the programme, for application to any subject who is characterised by a relatively high educational level compared with others of a corresponding age, relatively normal grammatical patterns and well-developed oral speech production that has a normal speaking rate. This approach has resulted in a rapid growth in speech recognition skills for all such patients, including a congenitally deaf child and a deaf–blind subject.

Training

Both speech and non-speech auditory signals are presented to the cochlear implant users to establish the recognition of these sounds and to accentuate the differences between these two major types of signal inputs. This already occurs during the first days after the initial fitting of the speech processor. This general introduction is followed by the use of individually selected speech materials.

Guidelines

The foundations for all the therapeutic materials that have been developed in our clinic are based on several guidelines. First, only meaningful speech materials are selected for training. This means Russian words, word combinations (phrases), sentences and paragraphs or texts. The materials are limited to everyday vocabulary at the first stages of rehabilitation and become progressively more complex at following stages. Second, training sessions are usually conducted with only auditory input and a shield to eliminate the possibility of using lipreading (i.e. a mesh screen held in front of the face of the therapist while speaking). Combined hearing and lipreading is used only for instructions and sometimes for the correction of the patient's answers.

Third, each training exercise is designed on the basis of some speech material or conceptual framework which is familiar and meaningful to the patient. Exercise phrases and sentences are built around a particular kernel or keyword. For example, a teacher might choose the word 'fish' and suggest for the training passages different word combinations with this word: goldfish, tasty fish, fish plant, fish swims, flying fish, fish soup, fishermen, fish with mushroom sauce and so forth. Of course, the patient is instructed to recognise the word combinations containing this word. Another example is the recognition of items out of known sequence (days of the week, numbers, set of colours and others).

Fourth, a factor of vital importance for the success of rehabilitation is to select and design training tasks that are appropriate for each individual. At each training session, the correctness of all patients' answers are recorded. After the session, the overall percentage of correct answers is calculated. We try to keep this percentage between 60% and 80% for each patient's session by selecting appropriate speech materials. This value was found to be sufficiently high to encourage the patients and sufficiently low to produce fast performance improvement.

Fifth, after training sessions, cochlear implant patients are instructed by the therapist as to which exercises should be repeated during home training. Some exercises are repeated over the phone with the most advanced adults and teenagers.

Sixth, it is also helpful to introduce some self-training exercises. For example, a teacher could instruct the patient with the following: 'Please ask several people in the street how to find some place (known to you), or what time it is now, or something else where you could predict the answer to some extent. Try to hear and recognise all the words of the answers given by different people.'

Additional considerations for children

For the cochlear implant children, in addition to the specific hearing training, the rehabilitation programme should include special procedures aimed at enriching the development of linguistic and speech production abilities, as well as the reading capabilities, mathematical symbolisation and many other skills. Although older cochlear implantees can be trained with a unisensory approach, both auditory and visual inputs should be utilised for children.

The rehabilitationist instructs the parents of the cochlear implant child on how to perform home training. The parents acquire the training techniques while following the teacher's examples during training at the centre. The tasks are selected taking into consideration the child's individual abilities, along with appropriate aims of a particular rehabilitation stage. It is also essential to take account of the abilities of the parents. It is not reasonable to expect that all parents have comparable training abilities.

Performance measures

The first evaluation materials we used were the screening tests (word length identification, sentence length identification, second formant discrimination, open-set common sentence perception) recommended by the rehabilitation manual for the Nucleus device (Mecklenburg, Dowell & Jenisen, 1991) and adjusted to the Russian language. Although these are still useful during the very early stages of rehabilitation, we have found it necessary to develop a complete test battery more appropriate for our advanced patients. Many of the principles behind the development of these test materials may be applied broadly for other languages.

Open-set Word Recognition

This skill is tested with 50 sets of specially selected Russian words; each list has 50 items. Some decades ago, these word lists were designed for testing the clarity of speech transmission over various telephone lines (Pokrovskij, 1962). Eventually the word lists were found to be helpful in testing speech perception performance through different sensory inputs with or without assistive devices (Mironova, 1977).

There were four underlying principles used to develop this test. First, the words reflected the syllable-stress pattern used in normal Russian language. Stress position within a word is quite essential and meaningful in the Russian language. The term 'syllable-stress pattern' designates the number of syllables in the word with the exact position of stress on a particular syllable. Second, the proportion of different categories of words (nouns, verbs, adjectives, etc.) represented in these lists was similar to that in the normal Russian language. Third, the order of the words in the lists was arranged so that no contextual relationship between any two sequential words occurred. Finally, all the words are unique so that no two words occur more than once in all 50 sets. Each list generally contains a similar number of occurrences of different phonemes. An interesting aspect of this test is that it is similar to the commonly used MTS test (Erber & Alencewicz, 1976) because scores can be calculated for both the number of correctly perceived syllable-stress patterns and whole words. However, this test is open set in contrast with the MTS which is a closed-set task. The chance for a patient to learn the test materials is eliminated because of the large number of lists.

Open-set Recognition of Quasi-words

Quasi-words are commonly known as nonsense words or word-like sound complexes. The test consists of eight sets of 50 specially created items (Mironova, 1978). Quasi-words were derived from phonetically balanced Russian word sets (Leongard, 1965). These sets were designed to evaluate the speech intelligibility of deaf, school-aged children. The child read the words into a tape recorder and the normal-hearing listener wrote the perceived word. To refer this to an English-speaking population, it could be considered similar to the McGarr Test (McGarr, 1983).

Deriving from these sets, quasi-words preserve syllable-stress patterns of original sets, but the meaningful relationship between the syllables is changed so that they do not represent real words. The manner in which the quasi-words were created required that each original word be divided into its syllable units and then recombined. As a result, five groups of syllables were obtained: the stressed vowel, the first pretonic (the syllable preceding a stressed syllable), the second pretonic (two syllables before the stressed syllable), the first post-tonic (the first syllable following the stressed syllable) and the second post-tonic. Monosyllable quasi-words were selected from the group of stressed-vowel syllables. Then pretonic and post-tonic syllables were attached to the stressed-vowel syllables exchanging the syllables exactly within the above-mentioned groups of syllables. A total of six different quasi-word, syllable-stress structures occur. Thus, the set of quasi-words preserved all syllable-rhythmic, as well as, phonetic relationships peculiar to the original word set.

Open-set Recognition of Meaningless Phoneme Complexes (MPC)

This test was derived from the standard materials recommended for the assessment of the quality of speech transmission channels (Anon., 1971). Sets of recommended phonetically balanced phoneme complexes (31 items) were used. Single phoneme recognition scores are estimated as a percentage of corresponding answers containing this particular phoneme irrespective of the correctness of the phoneme position in the answer (see Anon., 1971).

Open-set Sentences Recognition

Originally, this test was developed for the assessment of lipreading skills of deafened adults (Mironova, 1980). Later, it proved to be suitable for the testing of children and teenagers who have good spoken language skills regardless of the sensory input type: lipreading alone, hearing alone or hearing combined with lipreading. In total six sets of 24 sentences are used. All lists are balanced so that they are equally difficult to each other list for perception either in hearing-only conditions or in lipreading-only conditions. Mean percentage of correctly perceived sentences (regardless of some small errors that do not change the exact sense of the sentence) are calculated.

Some typical results of open-set speech material recognition by audition only

The results were gathered in a very specific manner. Each item of all speech material tests was presented at least twice by the live voice of the same female speaker. Following the patient's request, an item presentation could be repeated. Patients' responses to all presentations were recorded. The overall percentage of correct responses was calculated separately for both the first presentation alone (first trial result) and for the correct responses to at least one of the presentations (maximal score).

The growth rate for word recognition tended to be higher in subjects with a shorter period of deafness prior to implantation, which is well correlated with previously reported data (Dowell, Mecklenburg

& Clark, 1986). Syllable-stress pattern recognition was always found to be better than word recognition regardless of the type of material used: natural words or quasi-words (see Figure 15.1). Improvement in word recognition over time was shown to be preceded by syllable-stress pattern recognition improvement in all our patients. As one could predict in advance, the recognition of senseless information (MPC and quasi-words) always yielded the poorest results in our test battery. Surprisingly, in the majority of subjects the recognition of MPC was better than that of quasi-words, probably due to shorter duration of test items. The recognition of the single phonemes was always between syllable-stress pattern recognition and nonsense material recognition (Figure 15.1).

Cochlear implantees usually perceive natural words better than meaningless information but the diversity of results is greater (Figure 15.1). We are not sure of the reason for this greater variability of word recognition results but it could be related to the individual differences in language skills. Recognition of sentences is always better than word recognition, apparently due to the addition of contextual help.

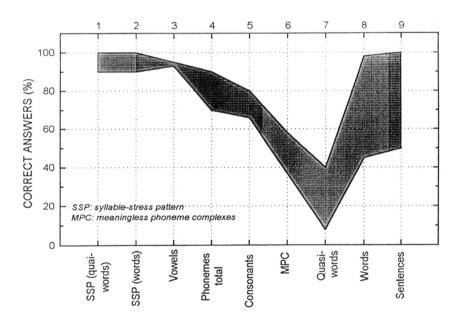

Figure 15.1: Recognition scores of speech materials of different linguistic levels (indicated at the bottom) in a group of cochlear implant patients who achieved no less than 40% word perception (open-set, audition only.) Shaded area corresponds to the range between maximal and minimal results in this group. Subjects perceived test materials in open-set hearing-only conditions (see description in text)

Experience with a well-educated congenitally deaf child

The progress in perceptual skills of congenitally deaf children after cochlear implantation is usually much slower than that of postlingually deafened subjects (Dawson et al., 1992; Gantz et al., 1994). These children generally are able to obtain high levels of open-set speech understanding only after several years of continuous rehabilitation work (Gantz et al., 1994). Of course such long-term speech therapy needs special programmes. Nevertheless, for some of these children, under appropriate conditions (early diagnosis of deafness, early onset of hearing aid use, intensive and appropriate speech therapy), it is possible to achieve high levels of spoken language skills before implantation, within the first 3–5 years of life. We have only one such child who was successfully implanted at age 9 years. It was quite easy to use the therapeutic principles described above for the rehabilitation of this child after cochlear implantation. Surprisingly, the dynamics of her speech recognition results were no worse than those of the best-performing, postlingually deafened subjects. Six months after receiving her speech processor, recognition scores were in the ranges shown in Figure 15.1. These results are probably related to the intense speech therapy she received during the preoperative period.

Experience with a deaf–blind adult patient

It was necessary to adapt our therapeutic techniques only slightly for use with a deaf–blind patient. We applied standard test materials and found that several lists could not be used because some of the sentences were related specifically to people who could see, i.e. what did you see at the movies? What colour is...? Therefore, the lists were adapted to eliminate such sentences. The first training sessions used both sound and finger spelling for the deaf. In a way, this is similar to the principle we reported earlier where both lipreading and sound are used. In this case, it means that we used the finger spelling for instructions only and slowly excluded its use.

Rehabilitation of deaf–blind cochlear implant patients is of particular interest because of their extraordinary abilities to concentrate attention on hearing sensations. Relatively small amounts of data have been published on the performance of deaf–blind cochlear implant users (Ramsden et al., 1993). Although the deaf–blind patient in our centre obtained good open-set speech recognition scores and was capable of free conversation with unfamiliar speakers, her performance did not differ qualitatively from the performance of our best cochlear implant users without blindness.

Natural rehabilitation outside the clinic

Most of the rehabilitation outside the clinic takes place at home with specially designed home exercises. The most exciting progress was observed, however, when some of our patients started to share their time with a normal-hearing boyfriend or girlfriend. These patients learned to utilise the information provided through the cochlear implant more rapidly than those who continued their friendships more or less exclusively with hearing-impaired people or with parents.

Summary

The rehabilitation of postlingually deafened adults who receive cochlear implants presents a convenient model to develop training and evaluation materials. We have described some of the guidelines applied in our clinic for this population. One interesting aspect is that once developed for a rather high-performing group of patients, the materials could be generalised and individualised for both a prelingually deaf child and a deaf–blind adult. We have also found that counselling is an essential element of the rehabilitation process, as is motivation. The responsibility of each cochlear implant team is to assure accessibility, continuity of service and interest in the individual patient as a unique person who has the potential to interact through aural–oral communication.

Acknowledgements

We would like to express our gratitude to the invaluable contributions given to help establish our programme by Professor Ernst Lehnhardt (Hannover University) and Drs Monika Lehnhardt and Ernst von Wallenberg (Cochlear AG). We would like to address our special thanks to Dr Dianne Allum-Mecklenburg for the continuous encouragement and support of our work. We also wish to acknowledge gratefully the editorial help of Sophja Kamenetskaya.

References

Anon. (1971) Speech Transmission over Radio Communication: Requirements for Speech Intelligibility and Methods of Articulation Measurements. Moscow: State Standard of the USSR, GOST 16600–71.

Anon. (1994) Cochlear Implants: Issues & Answers. Sydney, Australia: Cochlear Pty Ltd.

Dawson PW, Blamey PJ, Rowland LC, Dettman SJ, Clark GM, Busby PA, Brown AM, Dowell RC, Rickards FW (1992) Cochlear implants in children, adolescents and prelinguistically deafened adults: speech perception. Journal of Speech and Hearing Research 35: 401-17.

Deguine O, Fraysse B, Uziel A, Cochard N, Reuillard-Artieres F, Piron JP, Mondain M (1993) Predictive factors in cochlear implant surgery. Advances in Otorhinolaryngology 48: 142–45.

Dorman MF (1993) Speech perception by adults. In Tyler RS (Ed) Cochlear Implants: Audiological Foundations. London: Whurr Publishers, pp 145-90.

Dowell RC, Mecklenburg DJ, Clark GM (1986) Speech recognition for 40 patients receiving multi-channel cochlear implants. Acta Otolaryngologica 12: 1054-59.

Erber N, Alencewicz C (1976) Audiologic evaluation of deaf children. Journal of Speech and Hearing Disorders 41: 256–67.

Gantz BJ, Woodworth GG, Knutson JF, Abbas PJ, Tyler RS (1993a) Multivariate predictors of success with cochlear implants. Advances in Otorhinolaryngology 48: 153–67.

Gantz BJ, Woodworth GG, Knutson JF, Abbas PJ, Tyler RS (1993b) Multivariate predictors of audiological success with multichannel cochlear implants. Annals of Otology–Rhinology–Laryngology 102: 909-16.

Gantz BJ, Tyler RS, Woodworth GG, Tye-Murray N, Fryauf-Bertschy MA (1994) Results of multichannel cochlear implants in congenital and acquired prelingual deafness in children: five-year follow-up. American Journal of Otology 15(Suppl. 2): 1–7.

Geers A, Moog J (1994) Spoken language results: vocabulary, syntax and communication. Volta 96(5) (monograph): 131–48.

Lehnhardt E, Aschendorff A (1993) Prognostic factors in 187 adults provided with the Nucleus cochlear mini-system 22. Advances in Otorhinolaryngology 48: 146–52.

Leongard EI (1965) Speech intelligibility determination in deaf children of school age (in Russian). News Acad Pedal Sc (Russia) 140: 3–75.

McGarr NS (1983) The intelligibility of deaf speech to experienced and inexperienced listeners. Journal of Speech and Hearing 26: 451-58.

Mecklenburg DJ, Dowell RC, Jenisen G (1991) Rehabilitation Manual. Sydney, Australia: Cochlear Pty Ltd.

Mironova EV (1977) On the oral speech perception by the postlingually deafened subjects (in Russian). Defectology N2: 72–83.

Mironova EV (1978) Visual, tactile-visual and hearing perception of rhythmic and phonemic structure of quasi-words by deafened adults (in Russian). In Geilman IF (Ed) Sovershenstvovanije sredstv obshenija gluhih I slaboslishashih v uslovijah sluhorechevoj reabilitacii. Leningrad: Rehabilitation Center for the Society of the Deaf, pp 27–31.

Mironova EV (1980) Evaluation of Lipreading Skills with Standardized Speech Material (in Russian). Moscow: Pedagogika.

Pokrovskij NB (1962) Calculations and Measurements of Speech Discrimination (in Russian). Moscow: Svjazizdad.

Ramsden RT, Boyd P, Giles E, Aplin Y, Das V (1993) Cochlear implantation in the deaf blind. Advances in Otorhinolaryngology 48: 177–81.

Chapter 16
Maximising Overall Communication Abilities for Cochlear Implant and Hearing Aid Users

BRIGITTE EISENWORT, WOLFGANG BAUMGARTNER,
ULRIKE WILLINGER, WOLFGANG GSTÖTTNER

Take care of the sense
and the sounds will take care of themselves
(Lewis Carroll)

Introduction

Little guidance on rehabilitation strategies exists in the literature although rehabilitation of cochlear implant users is generally considered to be an important aspect of most of the cochlear implant programmes. To date, there are few definitive conclusions that can be made about the effects of intensive aural rehabilitation programmes (Tucci, Lambert & Ruth, 1990; Gagne et al., 1991).

Cochlear implant users form a special group within the population of those with hearing impairment. Their performance varies from the ability to recognise some environmental sounds, differentiate voices, use auditory cues as a support to lipreading up to comprehension of speech in the auditory-only modality. They are a special group because of the kind of signal they receive and the fact that they experience an abrupt change from a 'world of silence' to a 'world of sound'. In addition to these special characteristics, cochlear implant users have similar problems and needs comparable to hard-of-hearing individuals fitted with conventional hearing aids. Both groups must learn to make maximum use of their auditory, visual and communication ability to cope successfully in everyday communication situations.

Our group started in 1978 with the implantation of deaf and severely hard-of-hearing adults. We started to collect rehabilitation materials systematically and to develop and describe exercises. It has been our goal to develop and describe a large variety of exercises for the improvement of auditory abilities, speechreading and communication skills.

During the early 1980s, we concentrated on auditory training exercises (Burian, Eisenwort & Pfeifer, 1986). In discussions with our patients, speech pathologists, deaf teachers and many others, we have learned to understand that the ultimate goal of an intensive rehabilitation programme should be the improvement of communication ability in everyday life rather than speech perception in the auditory-only modality. As a consequence, intensive work on the development of communication exercises started. Recently, we have modified many of these exercises (Eisenwort, Burian & Viehhauser, 1990) and have also added new ones. We have also focused on developing training units for the improvement of speechreading ability (Eisenwort, Viehhauser & Bigenzahn, 1992). Currently, the Vienna Rehabilitation Program comprises 112 exercises (37 speechreading, 36 communication training and 39 auditory training [33 exercises without background noise and 6 with background noise]). They are divided into auditory training, speechreading training and communication training and a summary is listed in Table 16.1 found at the end of this chapter.

Auditory Training

The conceptualisation of the programme followed a progression from exercises at a basic level to those that encourage and support everyday interactions. The basic level includes training with respect to sounds: the frequency, intensity and duration of stimuli, as well as length of pauses. These discriminations are clearly determined by a patient's individual hearing ability. Environmental sounds are selected which can be discriminated easily by the patient. Duration of stimuli and length of pauses also are adapted to the patient's individual needs. Speech elements are part of the basic training. In this case, the presentation of speech stimuli is very slow, clearly articulated and with marked stress and intonation. Presentation is in a natural manner, but extremely clearly articulated.

The everyday level also contains exercises for both sounds and speech. For sounds, normal frequency, intensity, duration of stimuli and pauses are used. Environmental sounds are presented in the same way as they occur in everyday life. The speech training uses an average conversational style. Presentation of stimuli is fluent with stress and intonation presented as it occurs in everyday speech.

Speechreading Training

Our speechreading training programme consists of 22 individual exercises and 15 group exercises. It is composed of both synthetic and analytic exercises and also includes role playing and transfer of skills to everyday situations. The individual exercises are designed for patients who are absolute beginners. The prerequisite for attending the group rehabilitation and exercises is based on a speech tracking rate of 10 words per minute. Candidates who have lower scores need individual training. Patients and therapists discuss their success and problems in speechreading.

All adult patients who will receive a cochlear implant should be able to speechread everyday communication. For poor speechreaders, we offer speechreading training preoperatively.

Communication Training

The communication training consists of 36 group exercises designed to help cochlear implant users improve their communication ability in interactive activities. It is only presented as a group activity. The average group size is six. The age of the participants can range between 17 and 70 years. The groups should be organised so that they are composed of individuals with comparable age, linguistic and communicative competence and especially speechreading ability. Motivation is very important for participation in this group activity and so is the willingness to speak about individual problems.

Rehabilitation management

The Vienna Cochlear Implant Team

Our team consists of two ENT doctors, two speech therapists, two psychologists and one technical engineer all of whom care for patients in the age range between 2 and 71 years.

The medical doctors are responsible for clinical examinations and organise all preoperative tests. They explain the results of all tests to the patients and decide, in agreement with the team, whether a cochlear implant can be helpful to the potential patient or not. They determine the surgery date, organise hospitalisation and implant the chosen device. They carry out postoperative wound care and are present at the first fitting. Sometimes they also attend a rehabilitation session to see which benefits are achieved and to motivate a patient.

Speech therapists perform audiometric tests and evaluate receptive (auditory and audiovisual) abilities, speech production and language skills. Preoperatively, they offer speechreading training and auditory training with conventional hearing aids. They are involved in the selection of the appropriate device. Postoperatively, they attend the first fitting sessions and are responsible for rehabilitation.

Psychologists perform the psychological evaluation of candidates and offer counselling sessions. Psychological evaluation of adults comprises administration of an intelligence test (e.g. HAWIE [Wechsler, 1986]), a personality profile (e.g. Freiburger Persönlichkeitsinventar [Fahrenberg, Selg & Hampel, 1973]) and special questionnaires such as the Denver Scale of Communication Function (an expectation questionnaire) and an interview with the patient and family. Counselling sessions are offered pre- and postoperatively. In our department, objective measurements are done by a neuropsychologist who is specialised in objective audiometry.

Engineers perform the preoperative subjective electrostimulation test with the ENT doctors using the MED-EL Electroaudiometer, and also work with the neuropsychologist performing the objective auditory brainstem and electrostimulation tests.

Rehabilitation Management in the Preoperative Period

This offers the possibility to run each programme either separately or as individual training units for the different topics. During the preoperative period, ENT doctors and psychologists offer counselling (Eisenwort, Brauneis & Burian, 1985). Speech therapists offer speechreading training and auditory training with conventional hearing aids.

An example of how we might modify this programme to meet the needs of a particular patient is illustrated by the case of a postlingually deafened cochlear implant candidate with little residual hearing (500–1000 Hz: 85 to 95 dB). He is amplified with two conventional hearing aids and is a poor speechreader with a speech tracking rate of 10 words per minute. The individual training programme might consist of speechreading exercises 1 to 22 (see Table 16.1). In parallel, one could begin with exercise 8 from the auditory training programme to help this patient use suprasegmental cues as an aid to speechreading. If there is an ongoing group activity, this patient could join during his preoperative period.

Rehabilitation Management in the Postoperative Period

During the postoperative period, the focus is on the auditory training programme. Earlier, when we first designed this programme, particular attention was given to the hierarchical structure contained in the first 14 exercises (Eisenwort, 1985). We realised, however, that many patients are not motivated to spend a great deal of time counting and classifying tones and sounds. They want to perceive and comprehend speech. Therefore, we usually combine exercises 1 to 5 with the early exercises for speech discrimination. As a result of recent technical developments in cochlear implants, patients learn to comprehend speech earlier. This means that later exercises become more important.

Patients can attend counselling sessions with the psychologist or ENT doctors, if they wish. When communication training in a group is offered, two therapists (a psychologist and a speech therapist) are responsible. We have recently realised that speech tracking techniques are very useful for the improvement of everyday communication. The original speech tracking technique of DeFilippo and Scott (1978) was the first method we offered. Later, we understood that hearing-impaired individuals need to learn to take an active part in communication and for this we now prefer the USCF-Tracking Procedure (Owens & Raggio, 1987).

Again, let us consider the postlingually deafened patient who now has a cochlear implant, excellent psychoacoustic skills, but suffers from psychological problems caused by his hearing loss. An individual programme for him could consist of five training units in which exercises 1 to 21 are performed and 10 training units focusing on word and sentence comprehension. Psychological counselling and participation in communication training with the aim of overcoming the crisis caused by his hearing loss would be an important support for this patient.

Duration of programme

Between 1980 and 1990, many patients who lived in other countries or distant parts of Austria received cochlear implants at our clinic. It was necessary for them to stay in a hotel near the clinic during the pre- and postoperative rehabilitation period. When an intensive preoperative training programme was necessary, we offered are for two weeks, twice daily, one hour of speechreading training or auditory training with conventional hearing aids. Postoperatively, patients living far away had to stay for four weeks in Vienna for speech processor adjustment and rehabilitation.

Today, there are other cochlear implant centres in Austria. Therefore, most of our patients are local, from Vienna and Lower Austria. This means we can offer preoperative and postoperative rehabilitation once or twice weekly over longer periods of time. This also offers us the opportunity to maintain our patient profiles of rehabilitation for a long time.

Summary

In our experience, nearly all cochlear implant patients profit from intensive rehabilitation if they are treated from a holistic point of view. This is because managing everyday communication successfully is more important for their life quality than speech perception in the auditory-only modality in a clinical setting. Thus, we have developed the comprehensive rehabilitation programme as presented in this chapter.

References

Burian K, Eisenwort B, Pfeifer C (1986) Hörtraining: Ein Trainingsprogramm für Kochlearimplantatträger und Hörgeräteträger. Stuttgart: Thieme.

De Filippo CL, Scott BL (1978) A method for training and evaluating the reception of ongoing speech. Journal of the Acoustical Society of America 63: 1186–92.

Eisenwort B (1985) Rehabilitation of the post-implant patient. In Schindler RA, Merzenich MM (Eds) Cochlear Implants. New York: Raven, pp 517–20.

Eisenwort B, Brauneis K, Burian K (1985) Rehabilitation of the cochlear implant patient. In Gray RF (Ed) Cochlear Implants. San Diego, CA: College Hill Press, pp 194–210.

Eisenwort B, Burian K, Viehhauser G (1990) Kommunikationstraining: Förderung der Kommunikation bei hochgradig hörbehinderten Erwachsenen. Stuttgart: Thieme.

Eisenwort B, Viehhauser G, Bigenzahn W (1992) Ablesetraining. Heidelberg: Julius Groos.

Fahrenberg J, Selg H, Hampel R (1973) Freiburger Persönlichkeitsinventar. Göttingen: Hogrefe.

Gagne JP, Parnes LS, LaRocque M, Hassan R, Vidas S (1991) Effectiveness of an intensive speech perception training program for adult cochlear implant recipients. Annals of Otology, Rhinology and Laryngology 100: 700–7.

Owens E, Raggio M (1987) The UCSF tracking procedure for evaluation and training of speech reception by hearing impaired adults. Journal of Speech Disorders 52: 120–28.

Tucci DL, Lambert PR, Ruth RA (1990) Trends in rehabilitation after cochlear implantation. Archives of Otolaryngology, Head and Neck Surgery 116: 571–74.

Wechsler D (1986) Hamburg Wechsler Intelligenztest für Erwachsene. Bern: Huber.

Table 16.1: Comprehensive list of exercises for auditory, speechreading and communication training

Level no.	Auditory training	Speechreading training: individual	Communication training: group
	Aim: Selective attention to tones and sounds (detection and discrimination)		
1	Detection of tones	Patient learns to recognise which factors may have a negative influence on speechreading ability	Patients meet each other
2	Countable tones and other sounds (maximum 10) where frequency, intensity, off-time (silence) and stimulus duration are varied	Strategies to compensate for the influence of these factors are introduced	Possibility to speak about their problems and expectations
3	Discrimination of temporal features: long/short durations are proportionally varied	Presentation of an overview of the speechreading programme	Relaxation training: the ability to relax is an important prerequisite for the acquisition of successful communication strategies
4	Discrimination of loudness: loud/soft contrasts are gradually reduced for different frequencies and sound durations	Speechreading of the visual aspects of the rhythmic structure of speech	Relaxation training
5	Discrimination of frequency: high/low pitch contrasts are gradually reduced at different intensities and for different sound durations	Speechreading of the vowel /a/	Relaxation training

Table 16.1: (contd)

6	Discrimination of environmental sounds: (a) gross (clock ticking/door slamming); (b) fine (clock ticking/telephone ringing), recorded or live	Differentiation between /e/ and /I/	Relaxation training
7	Discrimination of voices: recorded or live	Differentiation between /o/ and /u/. This completes speechreading training of vowels	Relaxation training

Aim: Suprasegmental features

8	Syllable number: (a) monosyllables; (b) polysyllables	Speechreading of diphthongs /au/, /ai/ and /oy/	Relaxation training
9	Sentence duration: build sentences of only monosyllabic words	Speechreading of diphthongs /au/, /ai/ and /oy/ (continued)	Focus on hearing tactics from two perspectives: listener and speaker
10	Word length: paired comparison: (a) compounds and their parts (Fenster/Fensterbrett); (b) words selected according to their length (Tag/Marille)	Speechreading of diphthongs /au/, /ai/ and /oy/ (continued)	Focus on hearing tactics from two perspectives: listener and speaker
11	Phrase and sentence length	The patient has a sheet with written word shapes but with missing vowels. The therapist produces a word and the patient should recognise the vowels and fill them in on the page	Focus on hearing tactics from two perspectives: listener and speaker
12	Different word stress in sentences: (Das FLEISSIGE Mädchen lernt/ Das Fleißige MÄDCHEN lernt)	Focuses on speechreading bilabial consonants /m/, /b/ and /p/	Focus on hearing tactics from two perspectives: listener and speaker

13	Discrimination of stress patterns in polysyllabic words. Minimum of three-syllable words	Recognition of labiodental consonants /f/ and /v/	Speech tracking
14	Sentences: questions/statement discrimination (pairs of sentences) or identification (single sentences)	Speechreading alveolar consonants /n/, /d/ and /t/	Speech tracking
	Aim: Suprasegmentals and/or segmentals		
15	Syllable number and/or word accent and/or many vowels and consonants	Speechreading sibilants /s/ and /ʃ/	Speech tracking is trained
16	Words differing in several features with vowel emphasis: syllable number and/or word accent – many vowels	The liquid /r/	Strategies for group discussion are developed
17	Words differing in many vowels	Speechreading velar consonants /k/, /g/ and /x/	Focus on improvement of the ability to combine information on the phonological level
18	Minimal pairs: vowel change (Tante/Tinte)	Similar to E11, E18 consists of recognising and filling in consonants	Focus on improvement of the ability to combine information on the phonological level
19	Words differing in several features with consonant emphasis: syllable number and/or word accent – many consonants	Patient learns to analyse words	Focus on improvement of the ability to combine information on the semantic level
20	Words differing in many consonants	Focus on flexibility training	Focus on improvement of the ability to combine information on the semantic level

Table 16.1: (contd)

21	Minimal pairs: consonant change (Mappe/Matte)	Patients are taught to analyse sentences	Focus on improvement of the ability to combine information on the syntactic level
	Aim: Auditory comprehension: exercises for the acquisition of word comprehension		
22	Familiar versus unfamiliar words: identify familiar word in group	Completion of the individual exercises	Focus on improvement of the ability to combine information on text level
23	Unfamiliar versus familiar words: identify unfamiliar word in group	**Begins group exercises;** patients meet each other	Focus on improvement of the ability to combine information on text level
24	Sentences with the structure noun–verb–object: fill in the missing part	Strategies are taught that are helpful for the speechreader	Focus on improvement of the ability to combine information on text level
25	Closed-set word identification supported with pictures	Patients learn to know their individual mouth shapes	Reception of body language as a support to reception of oral language
26	Modified open-set identification for categories of words (fruit, food, etc.)	Focus on word comprehension	Reception of body language as a support to reception of oral language
27	Identification of polysyllabic number word	Focus on word comprehension	Reception of body language as a support to reception of oral language
	Aim: Auditory comprehension: exercises for the acquisition of sentence comprehension		
28	Recognition of simple, everyday sentences	Reception of body language	Reception of body language as a support to reception of orel language

#			
29	Identification of sentences supported by composite pictures	Reception of body language	Reception of body language as a support to reception of oral language
30	Recognition of common phrases and more complex everyday sentences	Reception of body language	Role playing
31	Identification of familiar versus unfamiliar sentence: emphasis is on the familiar sentence	Focuses on sentence comprehension	Role playing
	Aim: Auditory comprehension: exercises for the acquisition of text comprehension		
32	Picture-story and text comprehension	Patients speechread texts	Role playing
33	Text comprehension	Patients speechread texts	Role playing
	Auditory comprehension with background noise		
34	Exercises 28 to 33 are repeated with background noise. The therapist should speak at a level approximately between 60 and 70 dB SPL. At first, the patient should listen to soft background noise. Gradually, the intensity of the background noise should be increased until it is equal to the voice of the therapist	Role playing	Role playing
35		Role playing	Role playing
36		Role playing and complete the group exercises. This supports a transfer from the training programme to everyday life interactions	Finally in E36, patients reflect on their improvement and the problems they still have
37		Patients reflect on their improvement and the problems they still have	

Chapter 17
Rehabilitation in Adult Cochlear Implant Patients

ANGELIKA STRAUSS-SCHIER, UTE ROST

Introduction

The majority of nearly 400 adult patients provided with a cochlear implant at the Medizinische Hochschule in Hannover (MHH) since 1984 have late onset of deafness and, therefore, are postlinguistic. Our experience has shown that a short, intensive hearing rehabilitation phase is one important factor influencing the success in effectively using a cochlear implant for this group. It is necessary for the implant centre to provide long-term, direct therapy in only a few cases. Individuals who require extended training are usually supported by speech therapists in their local regions. We therefore work with the patients intensively after they are first fitted with the speech processor and then periodically monitor their performance and offer reinforcing rehabilitation exercise periods. We are also a ready resource available for providing information. Further, because our clinic is always active with cochlear implant patients, we easily accommodate those who wish to drop in for support, programming checks or friendly conversation.

After the first fitting for the speech processor, we offer a basic, progressive rehabilitation programme in which exercises gradually increase in difficulty. This prepares the patients for daily communication. They learn to interact through audition more effectively with a cochlear implant, how to maintain the device, to apply lipreading skills in association with hearing and/or to achieve open-set speech recognition. The rehabilitation programme is designed for the individual requirements of a patient. After the basic rehabilitation, we do not stop seeing our patients. They return to our clinic at regular intervals and we offer an extensive after-care programme outside the hospital because learning with a cochlear implant is an ongoing process for a recipient's entire life.

Programme structure

The Basic Rehabilitation

Every patient receives basic hearing training in the clinic after the cochlear implant operation (see Table 17.1). It starts 4–6 weeks postoperatively once the wound and mastoid region is completely healed. The programme lasts at least two weeks. It consists of the speech processor programming and daily hearing training with a speech therapist. The hearing training is carried out twice a day for one hour. For additional rehabilitation, the patient has the possibility to use some audiovisual devices for self-training such as video, tape recorders and touch screen (Willenbockel & Lambusch, 1986). The patient is also seen during this time for frequent programme checks to fine tune the speech processor. At the end of the basic rehabilitation, we administer a series of tests to evaluate speech perception performance, and we discuss further rehabilitation possibilities and needs with the patients.

Table 17.1: Basic rehabilitation hierarchy

1. Environmental sounds
   - (a) Detect sounds in the surroundings
     - (i) Horn honking
     - (ii) Knock on the door
   - (b) Discrimination of musical instrument sounds
   - (c) Suprasegmental speech
     - (i) High-pitched/low-pitched
     - (ii) Long/short
2. Discrimination
   - (a) Syllable patterns in words and sentences
     - (i) Stress
     - (ii) Intonation
     - (iii) Segmental speech
   - (b) Words with different syllable pattern, stress and vowels
     - (i) Sounds with all three features
     - (ii) Sounds with only two features
     - (iii) Sounds with only vowel differences
   - (c) Words with different syllable pattern, stress and consonants
     - (i) Sounds with all three features
     - (ii) Sounds with only two features
     - (iii) Sounds with only consonant differences
3. Identification
   - (a) Sounds
     - (i) Vowels
     - (ii) Consonants
   - (b) Words
     - (i) Closed set
     - (ii) Numbers
   - (c) Semantic field
     - (i) Sentences
     - (ii) Closed set
4. Speech tracking
5. Telephone training
   - (a) Discrimination: Yes–No tactic
   - (b) Identification
     - (i) Closed-set sentences
     - (ii) Open-set speech recognition

Clinical Check-ups

The patients return at regular intervals to our clinic. The time frame is first after three months, then after six months and continuing at yearly intervals. It is during the return visits that we check the program of the speech processor, measure performance on speech perception tests and offer additional exercises in hearing. An otologic examination is also made by the physician during these visits.

Local Rehabilitation

There are some cochlear implant patients who either wish for or need further rehabilitation after finishing the basic training at the MHH. These patients are offered the possibility to obtain auditory training from a speech therapist in their local region. About 30% of the patients use this opportunity for ongoing training. The hearing training usually takes place once a week and lasts between 10 and 20 sessions. Of course, if required, further sessions may follow. To help our patients find speech therapists in their vicinity, we provide them with a list of names and addresses of those practising in their neighborhood or near their place of residence. Our patients also receive therapy materials with ideas that are specifically designed for the particular patient concerned. They also receive a rehabilitation report to give to the speech therapist. Further, we answer any questions they might have through telephone conversations.

This referral process is the usual way in which many patients find a local speech therapist. Unfortunately, this is not always the case. Sadly, at the moment, there do not seem to be enough speech therapists who can carry out hearing training for cochlear implant patients. There may be long waiting lists of patients wanting therapy or patients may have to travel long distances to reach available therapists.

The spreading of information about cochlear implants to speech therapists, and sharing auditory training techniques for cochlear implant users is, therefore, still a very important part of the clinic's patient follow-up. Along with the opportunity to go to a speech therapist, there also exists the possibility to continue the hearing training with a family member, with friends or with others in the family circle. Further, if there is interest, we offer the family members or the friends of our patients the chance to come to the hospital and observe our auditory training programme.

Patients' Associations

All cochlear implant patients have the opportunity to organise themselves into a cochlear implant society. Such organisations provide broad support for the patients and their families. Most of the patients visit one of the 15 local self-help groups in Germany that organise meetings for information dissemination, speech therapy and some hearing training or lipreading training. These societies also offer social activities and the opportunity to share experiences.

Training for non-resident foreign patients

Though cochlear implant operations have become a routine procedure in many countries, our hospital also receives foreign children and adults who could not be provided with a cochlear implant in their own home region. We have also treated patients who simply preferred to come to Hannover. Most of the foreign children are from Arab countries and need to be trained in their native language. In terms of their rehabilitation programme, this means that the advice to parents concerning home training and instructions for learning in school are the most important factors (Bertram, 1996).

We try, however, to support language acquisition and hearing discrimination skills by giving the children examples in their native language. This, of course, depends on the therapist's foreign-language abilities. This language competence also applies to the case of non-resident foreign adults. If therapist and patient cannot find a common language, it is important to have an interpreter. The interpreter can be a family member, a close friend or any acquaintance willing to offer assistance.

Working through an interpreter requires sufficient amounts of time, a great deal of good will and abundant patience. Because the interpreter assumes the role of the therapist, not only is it necessary to translate the German material of the therapy session, it is also necessary to find the equivalent phonetic word material for discrimination and identification in the native language. The examples worked out during the sessions serve as the basis for the ensuing home training.

Supervision helps the interpreter to learn to pronounce, speak and present the native language spoken in a way that is suitable for the cochlear implant patient. This point should be clarified before planning the rehabilitation phase with the patient. Careful choice of a person who is genuinely willing to take part in this extensive work as an interpreter and therapist is essential for the care of foreign-language patients.

The vowel–consonant test, the number identification test with live voice and the speech tracking test are given at the end of the basic rehabilitation. The results, however, can only be interpreted in terms of intra-individual development and are not comparable to the results of other German-speaking patients. This is because the number of syllables per word, which relates to the speech tracking rate and the respective stress patterns, are different in every language. All our foreign patients receive adapted basic rehabilitation as well as individual support. They return to our clinic twice in the first year and then annually for fitting, testing and counselling.

Hearing training in groups

Hearing training additional to our basic rehabilitation programme is sometimes offered at weekends for 10 cochlear implant patients per course, at most. Relatives may accompany them. The hearing training takes place in Hannover and is located in various public institutions. Most recently sessions have been held in the new 'Wilhelm Hirte' Cochlear Implant Center. The sessions require rooms with good acoustic conditions and lighting, as well as a pleasant environment. Such an arrangement offers optimal conditions for improving listening in a relaxed atmosphere.

These meetings are very important for long-term deafened patients who still need further encouragement in hearing with their cochlear implant as well as for patients who want to improve their listening skills after the basic rehabilitation programme. We have named this hearing training 'Having fun with listening'. The name implies, on the one hand, that patients want to have fun when working on the discrimination tasks and, on the other hand, that they also want to be able to communicate successfully with other cochlear implant users and normal-hearing people too.

There are two alternative ways to carry out the hearing training: (1) the therapist speaks while the patient discriminates or (2) one patient speaks to another and the listener answers or repeats in the course of the ongoing hearing exercise or hearing game. The cochlear implant patients in the group always receive written material to be completed through hearing discrimination. They are seated in a circle round a table so that the hearing exercise can be combined with lipreading. It is up to the individual patient to determine his/her own level of difficulty. The patient may do all exercises by hearing only or combine hearing with lipreading.

In addition to hearing training, these sessions offer other important aspects for every cochlear implant patient. Coming together and talking to other cochlear implant patients is psychologically beneficial and thus may help the patient to identify more with the cochlear implant and accept the condition of being hearing impaired.

The participants also learn to develop communication skills such as the acquisition of good pronunciation, a slower and clearer manner of talking, a more careful choice of words, use of another word instead of the one not understood by the other listener, etc. Depending on the patients' confidence in their own hearing, a highpoint of the training programme could be provided by an excursion organised by the patients themselves. For instance, they may choose an evening to visit a cultural event or go to a local fair.

The hearing training is open to all users of cochlear implants, regardless of the type of device, the original implant clinic or the level of hearing. Obviously, most patients have been provided with a cochlear implant in Hannover. We know these patients personally and are aware of their hearing abilities as they are currently and as they were at the beginning of basic rehabilitation. Similar courses offered by therapists elsewhere in Germany would be most welcome. These could contribute new ideas and bring forth other aspects of the therapy.

Contents of rehabilitation

The basic hearing training at the MHH is built up in hierarchical order and involves the following aspects: detection of environmental sounds; discrimination of vowels and consonants; identification of words, numbers and sentences; comprehension of speech and telephone training.

The structure and the time frame of the hearing training always depends on the patients' abilities. Their preoperative experience with lipreading, hearing aids and hearing tactics as well as their duration of deafness will influence the kind and the degree of difficulty for the discrimination and identification tasks. The hearing exercises can be done with hearing plus lipreading and with hearing alone. The rehabilitationist chooses the degree of difficulty for each training phase and guides the well-motivated patient to individual success.

Detection and Discrimination of Environmental Sounds

Patients must accustom themselves to the new hearing and the quality of incoming new sounds after the first processor setting. For some of the patients, this is pleasant from the first day, but many need experience in the basic ability of detecting sounds. The therapist provides some examples of how the patient can explore surrounding noises such as car engine sounds, horns honking, water running, knocks at the door and so forth. The patients are also encouraged to experiment by themselves and report back to the speech therapist. After a short introduction to the functions of the speech processor and the rehabilitation training to the new hearing, the patient learns to discriminate specific sound parameters such as number, length, pitch and intensity. There is also the opportunity to discriminate between various musical instruments.

Discrimination of Suprasegmental Speech

Before the patient can understand speech, the therapist usually draws attention to general aspects of speech. The patient learns to identify syllable patterns in words and sentences and to discriminate different stress and intonation. This helps the patient identify independent speech segments as meaningful units.

Word Discrimination

The patient learns to discriminate pairs of words which have differing syllable patterns, stress patterns and vowels. Progressively, pairs of words with more similar features are presented as exercise materials. The first task, which is the easiest, is when the paired words vary in all three features of syllable duration, stress and vowels. Next, the paired words differ only in stress pattern and their vowel content and, finally, words differ only in their medial vowel. After this step using vowels, word discrimination exercises begin again using the same progressive steps, but with consonants.

Identification of Vowels

Coinciding with the word discrimination training, the patient specifically learns to discriminate vowels. These are offered in a consonant–vowel–consonant context in nonsense words: biit, beet, baat, boot, buut, bit, bet, bat, bot, but. In addition to the live-voice nonsense words, the patient has the possibility to practise identification skills through the use of audiovisual devices (see Figure 17.1).

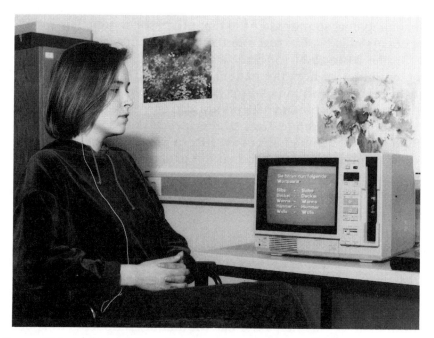

Figure 17.1: Adult practising self-training through the use of video

Identification of Consonants

Consonants are also presented in nonsense words in a vowel–consonant–vowel context, such as: ama, aba, apa, and so forth, until all of the consonants are represented. We have developed some special exercises for guiding the patient to the best methods for using hearing combined with lipreading. The consonants are grouped by the place of articulation (labial, dental, velar). The patient is asked to discriminate the manner when seeing the same picture of the lips. A special exercise for hearing alone is to group the consonants by manner (fricative, nasal, plosive) and ask the patient to discriminate the place of articulation.

Identification of Numbers

The comprehension of numbers starts with polysyllabic numbers, then bisyllabic numbers and, finally, monosyllabic numbers. Once the patient can identify the various numbers, the numbers are embedded in common, everyday sentences that represent relevant situations such as repeating telephone numbers, birth dates, time, prices and measures.

Identification of Words

The patient first learns to discriminate words in a closed set, i.e. by choosing from a known group of words. The patients is presented with a list of a maximum of 10 words with a known theme; for example, fruit. One word is spoken at a time and the patient repeats what has been heard. If the patient is able to do this, the therapist offers another word from the same semantic field but one which is not written down. If the patient continues to understand the unknown words, she is told only the topic of the word field and is asked to identify the words.

Identification of Sentences

As in the previous exercises, the patient begins with sentences in a closed set. The sentences are read in order, one after the other, by the therapist and, eventually, then mixed so that the patient must discriminate the spoken sentences. Next, the therapist exchanges some words or parts of the sentence. If the patient is able to identify unknown parts, he/she is given only the topic as a guide to identifying the sentences and must identify the whole sentence correctly.

Speech Tracking

Speech tracking is a method for training word-in-context comprehension. The therapist reads phrase by phrase from an ongoing text and the cochlear implant patient repeats back each spoken word. If the listener cannot understand a word, the therapist repeats a word, provides an alternative word (synonym) or paraphrases the sentence until the patient is able to repeat the sentence correctly (Mecklenburg, Dowell & Clark, 1986). The cochlear implant patient sits one metre directly in front of the therapist while listening to the story. The first condition is hearing combined with lipreading and then, if the cochlear implant patient is able to perform this task, the sentences are given without the opportunity to use lipreading (hearing alone). The initial materials for speech tracking are commonly known fables with a length of approximately 100–200 words. Adult fiction novels with normal adult reading levels are used for more advanced training (De Filippo & Scott, 1978).

Telephone Training

Telephone training concludes the basic hearing training in the clinic. The ability to communicate by telephone is very important for a cochlear implant patient. It is rated top of all the patient's goals in hearing and communication with regard to using the implant system. The therapist offers some strategies relative to the specific hearing abilities of the individual patient. A very easy way to communicate over the telephone is with the Yes-and-No tactic (Castle, 1980). The cochlear implant patient asks the listener some questions and the listener answers with yes or no. The next step is the comprehension of everyday sentences in a closed set. The cochlear implant patient is asked to discriminate the known sentences and repeat them correctly. The same technique used for sentence identification (as above) is applied for telephone training; that is, words or parts of sentences are interchanged. Once the patient is able to repeat the different sentences, only known topics such as sport, weather, hobbies and so on are discussed over the telephone. If the patient is able to understand specific subjects over the phone, open-set speech recognition is practised where the therapist speaks freely as in normal conversation.

Method-Framework

The framework for hearing training is a guide for the therapist that suggests steps in how to train a patient to acquire useful hearing through a cochlear implant. It is not an absolutely structured programme, but allows for flexible application of the therapeutic techniques. The choice of exercises must be based on the individual abilities of each patient. The framework includes general learning strategies where exercises progress from easy to difficult and from analytic to synthetic.

For all exercises that relate to speech perception, the patient receives a set of words or sentences that can be reviewed. The therapist reads the sentences or words aloud as the patient follows the written text. Next, the therapist presents the reviewed sentences or words in random order and the patient is asked to repeat what was said. Patients should always be asked to make the effort to repeat the word with the goal that they listen to their own voice and further develop sound–meaning associations. All these exercises have two levels of difficulty: hearing with lipreading and hearing only. If the patient is able to do most of a particular task correctly, the therapist progresses to the next step. If the patient is unable to achieve a satisfactory level, the therapist uses the same sentences or words for further practice, as well as adding similar types of sentences and other words to the exercise. This means that there should always be more than one list of words or sentences available for each session.

Summary

Most of our patients, as mentioned earlier, are postlingually deafened adults with an average duration of deafness between 7 and 8 years. This means they progress through the early stages of training (environmental sounds, suprasegmental speech) very rapidly. The major part of rehabilitation is spent on word and sentence understanding for daily communication. Generally, exercises are practised in the condition of hearing alone, if possible. In this group of postlingually deafened adults, lipreading and hearing are used when the patient demonstrates that hearing alone is too difficult. This strategy may also be used as a preparation for hearing-only tasks.

For the long-term deafened adults with more than 20 years of deafness, it is important to integrate hearing and lipreading. The majority of exercises concentrate on this combined approach. Not all of our patients are able to achieve open-set speech recognition, but they all obtain better speech communication skills. Experience has shown us that the patients in this group usually achieve some level of open-set speech understanding but only after several years of experience with their cochlear implant. Analysis of the development of the communication rate, measured by the speech tracking technique over a period of 10 years (Strauß-Schier et al., 1995), has proven that the majority of cochlear implant patients have shown positive development both in hearing combined with lipreading and in hearing-alone conditions. Even the remainder have shown improvement in hearing with lipreading. Therefore, they need encouragement to continue improving their listening skills. Often, it is necessary to provide this group with more counselling support and to develop an innovative means of motivating them. Because of the large number of patients we have seen, we fully expect most of them, eventually, to understand simple conversations with familiar speakers. This means that we are able to counsel the patients about the need for both patience and persistence.

Telephone training needs to be given to all cochlear implant patients regardless of their level of hearing skills. The ability for cochlear implant users to reach a satisfactory communication level over the telephone is variable. This means that even those who do not have open-set speech recognition skills need to experience some success in using the telephone for communication. For this reason, there are different exercises which vary in difficulty between simple yes–no tasks, closed-set sentences and open-set recognition. We believe that in today's modern society telephone communication is an integral part of every adult's life and, therefore, exercises for telephone training provide excellent motivation. It is very important that patients experience success and, therefore, the exercises should be carefully selected.

It is not only the hearing training exercises alone that help to aid cochlear implant patients achieve better auditory communication skills, it is also counselling support. Further, we should always remember that comprehension and communication take place whenever the therapist and the patient interact. This means that when instructions are given, when hearing tactics are discussed or when questions that are posed by the patient are answered, patients are gaining listening experience and are learning to associate sounds they hear with words that have meaning. The implication is that the therapist should only communicate with the patient when the speech processor is turned on so that every exchange is an auditory one and provides the opportunity for useful listening.

Conclusion

When our clinic handled fewer patients, our aspirations for the provision of rehabilitation included much greater direct contact with the patients. However, this became less manageable after about 200 patients. We learned that an efficient programme containing intensive training immediately following the initial fitting of the speech processor, with periodic visits to the clinic, is effective. We have utilised the techniques reported in this chapter for several years now, and have found that they provide a supportive therapeutic programme in which patients obtain positive experiences with their new hearing. Further, we know that they will have continuing access to support services. Without really planning for the need, these external services developed because of the sheer number of post-rehabilitation cochlear implant users who wanted them. It has taken more than 10 years for these services to be firmly in place throughout Germany. Today, we are confident that our patients, after basic rehabilitation, will have access to an environment where cochlear implant use is encouraged through support groups, hearing-training groups and continued follow-up visits to our clinic.

References

Bertram B (1996) An integrated rehabilitation concept for cochlear implant children. In Allum DJ (Ed) Cochlear Implant Rehabilitation in Children and Adults. London: Whurr, pp 52–64.

Castle D (1980) Telephone Training for the Deaf (course materials). Rochester, NY: National Institute for the Deaf, Rochester Institute of Technology.

De Filippo CL, Scott BL (1978) A method for training and evaluating reception of ongoing speech. Journal of the Acoustic Society of America 63: 1186–92.

Mecklenburg DJ, Dowell RC, Clark GM (1986) Speech tracking – Verfahrensweise und aergebnisse. In Lehnhardt E, Hirshorn MS (Eds) Cochlear Implant: Eine Hilfe für beidseitig Taube. Berlin: Springer, pp 153–59.

Strauβ-Schier A, Battmer R-D, Rost U, Allum-Mecklenburg DJ, Lenarz T (1995) Speech tracking in adults. Annals of Otology, Rhinology and Laryngology 104 (9, Part 2, Suppl 166).

Willenbockel C, Lambusch M (1986) Audiovisuelles Selbsttraining. In Lehnhardt E, Hirshorn MS (Eds) Cochlear Implant: Eine Hilfe für beidseitig Taube. Berlin: Springer, pp 92–93.

Chapter 18
Clinical Application of the Landscape Montage Technique for Counselling Cochlear Implant Recipients and Families

MASAE SHIROMA, SOTARO FUNASAKA, KUMIKO YUKAWA, SHUKUKO KAWANAMI

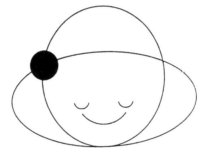

Introduction

The greatest handicap of an acquired hearing loss is frequently the behavioural problems that it produces in the individual; thus, a rehabilitation programme for cochlear implant recipients should include provisions for psychological counselling. We have chosen to employ the Landscape Montage Technique (LMT), an art-psychotherapeutic method. We use the method for two purposes: to assess changes in attitude before and after implantation and for counselling not only for the patients but also for their families.

Attitudes towards deafness

Deafness sometimes equates with isolation, especially for individuals whose onset was sudden; for example, as a result of head trauma or meningitis. The aftermath of such incidents may leave confusion, depression or anxiety for the future, not only for the afflicted person but also for the family. There are various responses to the problem of sudden deafness. In our experience, many of the cochlear implant recipients resented the period of time that they were without hearing. Some of them preferred to ignore the hearing handicap by not wearing hearing aids or learning and/or using sign language in public. Others confessed that they even thought about committing suicide rather than living under the tremendous pressure of newly acquired deafness. Deafened children present with a more complicated set of problems because counselling must be directed toward the child's parents as well as the child. Inappropriate attitudes on the part of the parents influence not only the child's ideas towards the hearing impairment but also may affect the maximum use of the cochlear implant prosthesis. Parents need guidance to accept the child's handicap and release themselves from a sense of guilt. For instance, mothers (parents) whose children's hearing loss is of sudden onset due, for example, to meningitis may feel that they are responsible for their child's deafness. A clinician should be empathetic toward the parents because they are confused about not knowing the best way to communicate and cope with the needs of their own children. Another problem for parents is overly high expectations. Some parents view the cochlear implant as a panacea whereby the deafness will be completely healed, or they may believe that the cochlear implant will relieve them of the need to return to the hospital or hearing institutes. No matter how much a clinician may stress the importance of strong family support and responsibility for the success of the implant, one may meet some parents who expect an overnight miracle. The teenage group is another population that needs special attention. The mental stress due to the deafness, low self-esteem, insecure self-identity and self-body image may cause special psychological problems.

Degree of satisfaction for cochlear implant recipients

Not all cochlear implant recipients are satisfied with their cochlear prosthesis. Collaborating with the national cochlear implant patient-support group in Japan, ACITA (Association of Cochlear Implant Communicators through Audition), we were able to conduct a survey of 122 adult cochlear implant recipients (see Appendix for questionnaire). The purpose of the investigation was to understand the degree of satisfaction expressed by recipients using an implanted prosthesis, as well as the behavioural and psychological changes found over time with the prosthesis.

According to 118 of 122 recipients who responded to the questionnaire, 59% were satisfied with the implant, 25% were dissatisfied and 16% avoided answering the question either positively or negatively. The reasons for dissatisfaction were that it was very difficult to communicate on the phone freely, the sound was unnatural, the speech processor picked up too much noise, using the implant was tiring, the cosmetics of the implant system were not stylish, and so on. On the other hand, the majority of the recipients responded that they would have difficulty answering the question of what would happen if they could not use the prosthesis for some reason. The responses suggested how much the recipients value the use of the cochlear prosthesis in daily life. We found that 85% of the recipients thought that it was useful, 10% felt that it was of little use and the rest (5%) made no comment.

Those who were satisfied with the prosthesis numbered only 11.9%, but 60.1% of the population felt that the prosthesis was very useful and 73.3% felt that they would be very distressed if they could not use the device. Thus, we learned that the expectations and the goal of hearing through a cochlear implant can be quite different within the same individuals. Some answered that they were quite happy with only a result of 50% on auditory perceptual tests whereas others felt that the cochlear implant was useless because they could not talk over the phone freely. We found that even users who answered that they were dissatisfied or mostly dissatisfied seemed to recognise the usefulness of the cochlear prosthesis. From our survey, we found that the top five items suggesting changes in attitude were related to communication (see Table 18.1). Our interpretation of the results suggests that the stability of the communication mode, either non-verbal or verbal, is highly related to the stability of behaviour and mind. The LMT is helpful in understanding mental stability and in demonstrating behavioural or psychological changes that occur between pre- and post-cochlear implant surgery. Further, to better understand the patients' goals and expectations we have used the interpretation of the LMT for our patients since 1992.

Table 18.1: Behavioural and psychological changes due to cochlear implantation ($n = 112$)

	Improved (%)	Same (%)	Decreased (%)	No answer (%)
Family conversation	59	31	4	6
Conversation with others	58	32	7	3
Concern about surroundings	54	29	7	10
Initiation of conversation	54	36	4	6
Laughter	49	41	5	5
Watching TV and video	41	44	11	4
Going out	39	54	5	2
Reading	29	59	10	2
Attendance at meetings	27	53	14	6
Shopping	27	66	4	3
Expanding to new hobbies	26	62	6	6
Helping at home	26	66	4	4

Description of Landscape Montage Technique

The Landscape Montage Technique is a non-linguistic (non-verbal) therapeutic method that can be applied to individuals who have poor verbal skill. LMT is an 'art therapy' which implies the use of drawing, painting, finger-painting and plastic art, such as clay modelling or pottery. As a mode of psychotherapy, it may also incorporate dance, play, literature and other means to demonstrate the imagination functions which, in turn, may elicit a self-healing tendency through images. Cognition, feeling, thought, desire and experiences are directly connected to art therapy as a basic indicator regardless of the means of expression selected, whether it be language, music or art. The former two require language and time characteristics whereas art relies on a visual, non-verbal space for expression. By means of pictorial projection, art therapy encourages symbolic communication, both non-verbal and also verbal, if the client verbalises the work. In any case, the purpose of using art therapy is to understand and elicit an individual's internal feelings and thoughts. The projected feelings may eventually lead to personal healing. Naumberg (1966) states, 'Art therapy recognizes that the unconscious as expressed in a patient's fantasies, daydreams and fears can be projected more immediately in pictures than in words. Art therapy should be differentiated from the art work of patients in a treatment setting who utilize art for recreational or artistic purposes.'

We selected LMT, as opposed to many other art therapeutic methods, for counselling the cochlear implant recipients for several reasons. First, it is a non-verbal psychotherapeutic approach that can be used in the course of an interview when a verbal reaction cannot be attained. It is sometimes easier for one to express feelings and thoughts by drawing than by verbal articulation. In a different sense, it may be useful for some hard-of-hearing individuals who cannot articulate clearly. Second, as the method does not require linguistic ability, the technique can be used not only for adults but also for children whose language competence is limited. Third, it is easily applied longitudinally in a diagnostic sense; the process involves the study and examination of changes in consecutive drawings. It is, again, very useful for children who require long-term observation to determine effective use of the cochlear implant. Fourth, landscape drawing is considered to be future orientated, and to require positive attitudes by the painter. Finally, it is less time consuming than other methods; most clients are able to accomplish the work within a 50-minute session, including the interview. It can be administered pre- and post-operatively along with several other psychological assessment tools.

Development of the Landscape Montage Technique

The Landscape Montage Technique (LMT) was invented by a Japanese psychiatrist, Hisao Nakai, in 1969 (Yamanaka, 1984). He was enlightened by Naumberg's 'Dynamically Oriented Art' (Kalff, 1966) especially from the standpoint of 'participant observation' as a non-verbal approach to the client. LMT is considered to be a derived form of an art-therapeutic technique involving clients drawing a landscape by composing 10 items and/or additional elements into a picture. The basic 10 items are river(s), mountains(s), field(s) or meadow(s), house(s), tree(s), person(s), flower(s) and/or grass, animal(s) or living creature(s), rock(s) and/or sand.

There are several distinctive characteristics of LMT (Kaito, 1994). It is defined as a 'projective technique' yet is a structural, pictorial technique. The client transfers his/her own three-dimensional image of the landscape onto a two-dimensional space. As the word 'montage' implies, it is a process of making one pictorial composition from many items closely superimposed onto each other. It should be noted, however, that the objectivity of it as an assessment test in terms of measurement is low, as there is a risk of misinterpretation of the results even though the characteristics of degrees of freedom as a test are high. Experience is required on the part of the clinician.

The original purpose of applying LMT was to observe and elicit the characteristics of so-called 'psychological space characteristics: classifying H- and P-types' in the mind of schizophrenic patients who had just overcome (or were just about to overcome) a critical period as expressed through their drawings (Yamanaka, 1984; Kaito, 1994). Today, the method has been widely used among Japanese psychologists, psychiatrists, psychotherapists and those in special education not only as a therapeutic method but also as a means of assessment to understand human behaviour, personalities and individuals' psychological state, in general.

Materials

A plain sheet of paper a little larger than letter size (297 x 210 cm) is used in our clinic. The size does not have to be specific, although it is difficult to complete the picture if the paper is too large. A broad-nibbed pen or felt pen is needed. The advantage of a felt pen is that it is possible to see the form of the lines even from the back of the paper (the ink penetrates the paper) after the client has coloured the picture. For this reason, a pencil should not be used as an alternative. Finally, 12–24 coloured crayons should be available.

Procedure

The procedure and interpretation described below are adapted from the work of Yamanaka (1984) and Kaito (1994).

Instruction to the client

The client is asked to produce a landscape picture by drawing 10 items, with or without additional items. Every item can be drawn either once or in multiples. For example, the client can draw a house or several houses, or even draw as many rivers as she wants. The client should be gently encouraged to draw because many hesitate to begin. Bear in mind that the activity can be frustrating when one feels discouraged in being unable to express visually what one has in one's mind. Remind the client that you are not looking for skill but a drawing done in any manner. Skip a particular item if there is resistance. For the individual who cannot understand the verbal instructions, use an alternative communication mode such as sign language.

Drawing the frame

It is important that the clinician draw a frame on the paper in front of the client. The function of the concrete visible 'frame' is to limit and restrain the patient's non-verbal expressions. In a sense, the frame is a protection. At the same time, it assures and releases the client from making an early decision about the drawing. The frame phenomenon, according to the study of Osanai et al. (1989), has an indivisible threefold function: (1) articulation of the world into two different frames of reference, as well as articulation of the world into self and non-self, (2) evocation of self-existence and (3) actualisation of world (others) self-relation.

Beginning to draw

Hand the pen to the client and gently prompt the client to start after you have drawn the frame. As the patient draws the landscape, watch over it as a painting partner. This is referred to as 'therapeutic alliance' and implies a working together rather than one person doing something to, or for, another.

Items to draw

The 10 items are grouped into three: (1) large items (distant view or spectacular view) such as the river, the mountain, the field and the road, (2) middle items (middle-distance view) such as the house, the tree and the people and (3) small items such as the flowers or plants, the animal and the rock. Additional items may be put into the landscape evolving from the client's spontaneous imagination.

Drawing the large items

The clinician can start with a phrase such as, 'First, the river. Would you draw a river or rivers for me?' Starting the drawing with the river is the main point of this technique. It divides the available space. The clinician can observe the client's work quietly so as not to increase the tension. Clients may draw a river as a rapid stream, as meandering, wide in the middle, completely narrow, and so on. In order not to impose any pressure, the manner of prompting is important. 'All right. We have the river there, it may be nice if we have mountains, too.' One may draw a mountain, another may put in a range of mountains; sharp or dull, large or small, in the middle or the corner. Next comes the field. The rice field is a familiar scene for Japanese. It may not be applicable to some countries so, alternatively, it could be a cornfield, wheatfield, or some sort of agricultural field or meadow. When one draws rivers, mountains and roads on paper, they collectively form a landscape. The point to observe in the drawing of large items is the partition or proportion of the use of space.

Drawing the medium items

When guiding the client, the clinician should change the manner of giving an instruction, by tone of voice or altering phrases, sometimes, in order to make the client feel as if you are creating the landscape together and not ordering the task. The sense of mutuality is important even though the clinician ought not to make any comments while actual drawing is taking place. Lead the client with a phrase such as, 'Let's put a house or houses somewhere'. Afterwards, have the client draw tree(s) and person(s). For some clients, the task of drawing a human figure seems to be a burdensome one, and they refuse to do so. Skip the item and continue with the next one.

Drawing the small items

Many clients appear to be relieved after being asked to draw a psycho-logically burdensome item like a human figure(s). However, clients who refuse to draw a person may still draw an animal. These clients may think that animals are trustworthy, whereas people are not. Rock (or sand) is the last item of the 10. The item is not conspicuous and almost all clients who have rejected drawing other items put these in the picture. Moreover, it is possible to gather deep insights from the way patients draw rocks.

Drawing additional elements

The instruction for the additional elements is, 'That is all I have to say. If there is anything else you want to put in the picture, please feel free to add it. I will wait until you finish the picture.' The majority of clients draw the sun and clouds in the sky. Some add a bridge over the river and put fish in the river, windows and doors in the house, and so forth. The main point is that these extra items should be left to the patient's spontaneous discretion.

Colouring

After finishing the rough sketch, colouring comes next. Hand the crayons to the client asking that the drawing be coloured freely; there is no order in colouring. Partial colouring and/or rejection of colouring are, of course, accepted.

Exploring the casual interactions of the landscape

Once the art work is obviously completed, the clinician can put the materials back into their boxes and ask some questions about the picture in a casual manner. The clinician should wait expectantly for the client to tell a story about it and may ask questions such as 'Can you tell me about the season?', 'What about the time of day?', 'What direction does the river flow in?', 'How old is that person?', 'Is it a man or a woman?', 'What is he doing', and so on. A word of caution: in terms of interpretation of the client's work, the inexperienced clinician may risk losing some of art therapy's valuable treasures at either end of the spectrum by either over-reliance or under-reliance on the verbal description of the art work by the client. In such circumstances, erroneous interpretations can frequently be made, often confirmed by the interpreter's frame of reference. Much of this sort of 'mind reading' may be avoided by sensitive questioning of the artist.

Interpretation

In spite of the fact that LMT has been used widely and studied academically in Japan, especially in comparative study with other art therapy methods or other objective psychological tests, the interpretation is not standardised. No matter how brilliant the standard of the interpretation might be, the risk exists of losing the liveliness of the work of the client by applying a standardised interpretation. However, a basic interpretation is introduced below, based on the work of Yamanaka (1984) and Kaito (1994), as mentioned earlier. Studying sand-play technique (Kawai, 1969) and Jung's psychology will also be helpful to the interested clinician. Needless to say, the clinician's observations during the drawing process and interaction with the client are also very important for the interpretation. Bear in mind that each painting should be interpreted in relation to two or more paintings by the same individual over a certain period of time and not relative to other people.

For the pictorial characteristics, one observes the drawing's organisation, use of space, balance of form, colour, line, focus or direction, and motions. We can assume some processes in the image function to exteriorise (externalise) what is represented in the client's mind. The first is the primary imaging process which divides the 'primitive image' into sensory images and the second is the secondary imaging process, which associates the sensory images with each other to build up a context. To review the clinical application of the LMT as it applies to cochlear implant recipients, the reader is referred to several cases which have already been described by Yukawa et al. (1994). In their paper, results of the LMT were contrasted with those obtained from psychological measures. Paintings of those who showed an improvement from the psychological standpoint were characterised by several features: (1) the space is filled, (2) colours become softer and lighter, (3) the picture is well balanced, (4) it is wider in perspective rather than focusing on a frontal view. Figures 18.1 and 18.2 are paintings done by a 10-year-old boy, pre- and two months post-implantation. Our clinical psychologist interpreted the second picture to mean that the boy was showing signs of stress and strain even though he seemed to show interest in the outside world. The audiologist needed to change the method of training so as not to pressure the child to discriminate speech and to be more flexible in order to enjoy new sounds. LMT was also administered to his parents as part of counselling in order to have them effectively involved with the rehabilitation programme.

Interpreting Individual Characteristics.

Although the impact of visual expression is always observed in its totality, it is necessary, for discussion purposes, to examine individual characteristics separately, keeping in mind that there is always a high risk of arbitrary interpretation.

Distribution of space

Starting from the symbolisation of the space characteristics, the space to the left on the drawing represent one's mind or inner world, and to the right represents the outer world. Space at the upper left projects one's mentality, spirituality and religious mind, whereas space at lower left projects impulse and origin. Upper-right space projects the social and function, and lower-right space projects the family and emotion.

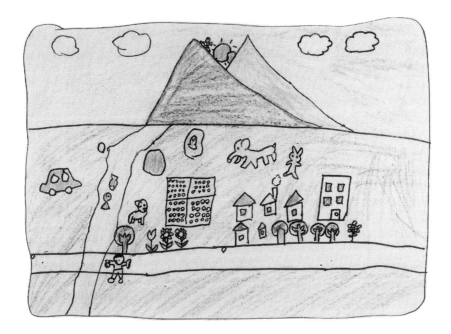

Figure 18.1: Pre-implantation – self-comment: A sunny spring afternoon. Animals are playing together, fish are in the river and ponds

Distorted use of space such as every item being drawn in one corner or separated far apart from one another with no relevance are not normal for adults. This test may not be applicable for children under 6 because they have not developed the use of space and connection of each item in a process of structuring a landscape.

Colour

When the whole colour is vivid or dark, it may indicate aggressiveness and troubles, while softer and lighter colours indicate psychological stability. Refusal to colour, colourlessness or partial colouring (less than half of the picture) can be observed in schizophrenia.

Frame

Drawing on or out of the frame implies that the individual has difficulty adapting to reality. When lines of the rough sketch do not meet the frame, this can be interpreted as pathological.

River

The river and its force represents the stream of unconscious. The volume of water may indicate the fullness of psychological energy of the unconscious; the force of the current indicates uncontrolled vigour. For the direction of the flow, current streams from right to left indicate that the stream of consciousness aims at the internal world, while current flowing from left to right is interpreted as energy approaching the outside world. From the viewpoint of space characteristics, the river fixes the direction and the depth of space in the picture. Observe its position, the direction of the current, width and depth, where/if it straightens, the way it spreads or narrows, the way it separates, whether it shows reversed current and so on. Be careful to observe whether there are objects such as rocks or islands placed in the river which obstruct the flow or something that makes it easier to cross the river, such as a bridge. A meandering river indicates obstacles or distorted energy. It is desirable to have a mildly winding river rather than a sharply turning one.

Mountain

This represents the distance between reality and the ideal, indicating problems the client feels need to be solved. It indicates the present condition and how the client feels about future prospects. It determines

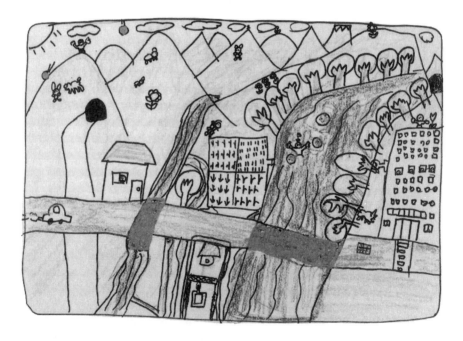

Figure 18.2: Post-implantation – self-comment: One evening in spring. A man is about to drown. Interpretation by the clinical psychologist: The first impression is of confusion, as if these two pictures have been drawn by a different person. Looking at the pictures drawn later, the boy seemed to be under a lot of pressure even though he gained in energy and interest to interact with the outside world. Finally, because the flow of the energy may change over time, this person needs to be followed up

the proportion of sky and earth, and the gross space is set by where and how the mountain is positioned. Points to observe are the slope of the mountain, a range of mountains, their placement, colour and so on. When a mountain is painted as sharper and independent, bigger and darker compared with the previous picture, it can be interpreted as an increase of problems for the client. When it is drawn peacefully and smoothly, it is understood as the settling of the matter that was bothering the client.

Field

This sometimes indicates the season and time that the client leans towards psychologically such as 'the good old days', 'prime time', 'bright future'. It also indicates how the client views her task, responsibility, study and so on, because the concept of the field is connected to labour. Interestingly enough, those who quit school or work have a tendency to draw a lot of people in a large field. It may indicate psychological compensation for their own idleness, but it sometimes indicates the will to work at a given task. An individual who draws the field precisely, even down to the ears of the rice plants, might have suffered from an obsession. Points to observe are its width, spatial placement, coordination, season, etc. Distortions in the spatial sense tend to be exposed when one draws this item. A colourless field can be pathological.

Road

The road represents the stream of consciousness in living, and it indicates future direction. The road of an individual who looks to the future will be wide and straight, while that of one whose direction is uncertain is narrow and distorted. Many direct types of roads can be expected such as those that become wider and open towards the front, are straight, diverge into two or more roads and so on. The observation point is to see its direction; whether it is parallel to the river or blocked by the river; paved or unpaved and so on. It is also important to check whether the item is reversed with regard to the river at the point of colouring, as mentioned earlier: this is a sign of schizophrenia. The road can also be related to the mountain and the field. The distortion of space becomes obvious after drawing the four largest items: river, mountain, field and road.

House

This indicates the home and family relationships. The whole house indicates the body, and the roof indicates the mind, thinking and psychological stability. Its windows show the viewpoint towards the outside world, and the entrance door reflects interaction with other people. The ideal house will be placed on the right-hand side of the paper with a door open to the right. The base of the house should be stable (set on the ground), and several houses are preferable to one house.

Tree

This indicates the unconscious self-image and balance of mind.

Person

This indicates the self, as well as interpersonal relationships. The last three items (house, tree, person) are used quite often as part of the projective-drawing method called the H-T-P technique (Buck, 1948). They can be used individually or together. Koch (1952) introduced tree drawing as 'The Baum Test' in Europe and established drawing as a personality assessment test categorised under the projective technique, and its interpretation was based on Jung's depth psychology. Regarding drawing a person as a projection method in the clinical study of psychopathology, a paper on 'Personality projection in the drawing of the human figure' was reported by Mochover (1949).

Animal

The psychological energy of the client may be determined from the size of the animal drawn, and further interpretations can be made by considering other attributes of the animals. For example, animals such as 'kittens, dogs, koala' are to be petted, 'snakes and pigs' to be hated', 'dragons, crocodiles and sharks' indicate aggressiveness, 'gazelles and sheep' show quietness, and so on.

Rock and/or sand

These little items indicate the obstacles and burdens of life. The attributes of the items are frigidity, invariability or constancy. Some may be gem stones and some monuments. They can be colourless.

Additional elements

You can expect to observe that the majority of clients will draw the sun and/or clouds in the sky as additional elements in LMT. Ijyuin (1989) has reported focusing on the space seen as the sky, viewing it as the 'psychic field'. He attempted to make clients draw what is represented in the universe beyond the sky on a different sheet of paper after accomplishing the LMT. He observed in the drawings of schizophrenics, who often show dysfunction of the imaging process, the inability to paint blank spaces, the inability to relate to LMT and incapability of making 'vertical relationships'. The sky gives us an idea about the season, the weather and the time of day. It may be acceptable for an aged person to draw a landscape of dark autumn, but you would be worried if you saw a similar painting in the work of a child.

Conclusion

The cochlear implant has brought important benefits to the hard-of-hearing population and, indeed, many recipients have changed tremendously. As they improve their communication skill through the use of the cochlear implant prosthesis, self-esteem is seen to develop and personal relationships with others to improve; it might even be said that the implant has given them the 'strength to live'. However, there are still some recipients who are not satisfied with the outcome. These recipients and their families require more counselling than those who are content with the result regardless of the auditory perceptual ability obtained through the prosthesis.

Art therapy in various forms has been conducted by many professionals throughout the world and for many purposes. It may be because the word 'therapy' connotes sickness, disorder or pathology, that some may feel uncomfortable applying it to cochlear implant recipients who show no strange behavioural characteristics or psychiatric symptoms. However, expression through art actually stimulates fantasy, creativity and spontaneous, unconscious imagery that refocuses an individual's mind and thoughts.

As you read this chapter, we hope you have been encouraged to apply some kind of non-verbal art therapy to your cochlear implant recipients and their family members with the help of a psychologist or an art therapist. We are aware of the cultural differences in interpreting landscape because each country has its own manners and customs. We are simply hoping to convey the message that the client has the possibility of expressing herself through drawing as a tangible and comprehensible projection of an inner image. Although LMT is considered a projection method, which is analytical from the psychological point of view, one can use the method as a means of communication as well. There is sometimes an over-reliance on verbalisation for expressing our feelings and emotions. We find art therapy's unique power to be its ability to promote communication through images that then require only a small, further step for verbal exchange to take place. Even though we do not directly use LMT as a means of psychological therapy for the cochlear implant recipient, we believe it is a useful guide not only for hearing counselling but also to facilitate communication. In terms of expectations, even if we have only one recipient who is not happy with the pros-thesis, we believe it is our medical staff's responsibility and humane duty to meet that patient's needs as far as possible and help her to accept the limitations in what the prosthesis can do. We believe that counselling through LMT is a useful method to be employed in the rehabilitation process for cochlear implant users in our clinic.

References

Buck JH (1948) The H-T-P Technique – a quantitative scoring manual. Journal of Clinical Psychology Suppl. 5: 1–120.

Ijyuin S (1989) Sky/earth expressions and psychic fields in the Extended Landscape Montage technique. Japanese Bulletin of Art Therapy 20: 29–43.

Kaito A (1994) Landscape Montage Technique – Basic Principles and Practice. Tokyo: Seishin Shobo.

Kalff D (1966) Sandspiel – Seine therapeutische Wirkung auf die Psyche. Zurich: Rascher Verlag.

Kawai H (1969) Introduction to Sand-Play Technique. Tokyo: Seishin Shobo.

Koch C (1952) The Tree Test – The Tree-Drawing Test as an aid in psychodiagnosis. Berne: Hans Huber.

Mochover K (1949) Personality Projection in the Drawing of the Human Figure. Illinois: Charles C. Thomas.

Naumburg M (1966) Dynamically Oriented Art Therapy: Its Principles and Practice. New York: Grune & Stratton.

Osanai M, Sasaki T, Haraoka Y, Ono M, Tsukamoto R, Muraki A (1989) The effect of using a frame in the therapeutic situation – the original meaning of the frame and its practical application. Japanese Bulletin of Art Therapy 20: 7–13.

Yamanaka Y (Ed) (1984) Landscape Montage Technique – The Writings of Hisao Nakai. Tokyo: Iwasaki Gakujyutsu.

Yukawa K, Kawanami S, Shiroma, M, Funasaka, S (1994) Assessment of the 22-chan-nel cochlear implant patient. In Hochmair-Desoyer IJ, Hochmair ES (Eds) Advances in Cochlear Implants. Vienna: Manz, pp 616–20.

Appendix: Questionnaire for cochlear implant recipients (Association of Cochlear Implant Communicators through Audition)

1. Background

Name:_____ Date of birth: ____(yr)____(mo)____(da)
Age:____(yrs) ____(mo) Onset of deafness: Age ____(yrs) ____(mo)
Onset of hearing loss: Age___(yrs) ___(mo)
Occupation: Pre-implantation_____Post-implantation_____
Family members:_____

2. An encounter with the cochlear implant
  • How did you get to know about the cochlear implant?
     ____Newsletter ____TV ____Magazines ____Hospitals ____Friends ____Other
  • How long did it take for you to have the surgery after the first meeting? ____Days

- How long has it been since you received the implantation? Yrs___Months___
- Do you feel that the informed consent before the surgery was appropriate?
  ___very appropriate ___appropriate ___inappropriate ___misleading
- Compare the surgical result with your pre-surgical expectation.
  ___same ___almost the same ___neither ___different ___very different
- Describe the anxiety and fear you had before the implantation, if any:

_____

_____

3. Behavioural changes after the implantation

- Are there any behavioural or psychological changes observed in your life?
  ___became very active and/or positive about everything ___became a little more
  active and/or positive ___haven't changed ___became a little inactive and/or
  passive/negative ___became very inactive and/or passive about everything
- Are there any changes observed regarding the following activities?

Family conversation	___Increased	___Same	___Decreased
Conversation with others	___Increased	___Same	___Decreased
Concern about surroundings	___Increased	___Same	___Decreased
Initiation of conversation	___Increased	___Same	___Decreased
Laughter	___Increased	___Same	___Decreased
Watching TV & video	___Increased	___Same	___Decreased
Going out	___Increased	___Same	___Decreased
Reading	___Increased	___Same	___Decreased
Attendance at meetings	___Increased	___Same	___Decreased
Shopping	___Increased	___Same	___Decreased
Expanding to new hobbies	___Increased	___Same	___Decreased
Helping at home	___Increased	___Same	___Decreased

4. Degree of satisfaction

- How do you value your cochlear implant in general?
  ___very useful ___useful ___neither ___mostly useless ___useless
- What would happen if you, for some reason, lost access to use of the implant?
  ___very distressed ___distressed ___neither ___a little distressed ___don't care
- Are you satisfied with your cochlear implant?
  ___very satisfied ___satisfied ___neither ___dissatisfied ___very dissatisfied
- If dissatisfied, what are the reasons?
  ___very noisy ___very tiresome ___can't use the telephone ___hard to
  understand television ___can't understand music ___sounds are unnatural
  ___easily breaks down ___gives me a headache ___increased tinnitus
  ___makes me dizzy ___cosmetic reasons Other: _____

5. Sounds through the cochlear implant

- How long did it take to get used to the sound through the cochlear implant?
  ___Yrs ___Months
- How much can you understand in one-to-one speech in quiet surroundings?
  ___ understand with implant only ___understand with lipreading ___understanding is a little hard even with lipreading ___impossible to understand
- How much can you understand speech in the presence of several speakers?
  ___ understand with implant only ___ understand with lipreading

____ understanding is a little hard even with lipreading ____impossible to understand____able to understand with accessory kit such as external micro phone
- How much can you understand speech in noisy environments like the office?
  ____understand with implant only ____understand with lipreading
  ____understanding is a little hard even with lipreading ____impossible to understand
  ____able to understand with accessory kits such as FM or audio input selector
- How much can you understand speech outside the building?
  ____understand with implant only ____understand with lipreading ____understanding is a little hard even with lipreading ____impossible to understand
  ____able to understand with accessory kits such as FM or external microphone
- How much can you understand of speech such as lecture or plays?
  ____understand with implant only ____understand with lipreading
  ____ understanding is a little hard even with lipreading ____impossible to understand
  ____able to understand if used with FM or induction loop

6. Requests for others
- In order to help you to understand speech, what would you request in terms of a speaker's manner?
  ____speak slowly ____speak clearly ____speak face to face ____avoid noisy environment
  Other: _____
- What are the improper manners of speakers whom you hardly understand? (e.g. speaking with chewing gum in the mouth):
  _____
- What can families and friends do to help you improve your communication skill?
  ____patience ____more conversation ____learn sign language ____help with training Other: _____
- What can the clinic do to help you to improve your communication skill?
  ____patience ____lower charge ____more meetings ____skilful training
  Other: _____

7. Self-reliance
- What sort of effort do you make to use the cochlear implant more efficiently? (e.g. carefully monitoring the speech processor and microphone)
  _____

  _____

  (e.g. ask others to repeat when you can't understand)
  _____

  _____

8. What should the design of the cochlear implant be in future?
  _____

  _____

Listen carefully, talk cheerfully, and join in the circle for better communication!
Japanese Patient Support Group: ACITA
President: Mr. Yasuo Ogi
Address: 6-8-21 Kurihara
Zama, Kanagawa 228 Japan
Tel. & Fax.: 0462-55-0628

Chapter 19
Differences between Adult and Child Rehabilitation Approaches: Auditory/Oral versus Signing/Speaking

GÖRAN BREDBERG, EWA MARTONY

Introduction

The rehabilitation of hearing-impaired individuals is the responsibility in Sweden of Swedish society. In principle, this means that a cochlear implant is provided without cost to a hard-of-hearing or deaf person. The direct treatment, including surgical implantation and speech processor programming, is performed under the direction of Departments of Audiology at the universities in the larger cities. Services for hard-of-hearing individuals are also provided in smaller cities at hearing centres within Departments of Otolaryngology. The county councils are responsible for medical care, the communities for the schools for normal-hearing children and the state for schools for the deaf.

When the new method of treatment for deafness with cochlear implants became available in the 1970s, it was received with some caution. One reason for this was because there was a feeling of fear that this new, expensive technique could endanger the existing rehabilitation programmes, as well as remove financial resources allocated for teaching hearing-handicapped individuals. For example, the use of cochlear implants might affect the resources which were given for the early teaching of Swedish sign language to deaf children. Even for the postlingually deaf adult, rehabilitation with signing and signs to support speech were regarded as important. In Sweden, sign language is accepted as a language and, since 1981, every deaf person has the legal right to be educated in sign language. They also have the right to request signed interpretation, when desired. To the deaf population, the acknowledgment of sign language and the right to their own language is very important. Today, the deaf community is strong and influential comprising citizens who have a clear identity of being deaf individuals with a common language. At the University of Stockholm there is a full professorship in sign language. The implications of the important role of sign language in the education and socialisation of deaf individuals influences the type of rehabilitation provided to those who receive cochlear implants at our clinic.

Acceptance of cochlear implantation as a treatment for deafness

The method of cochlear implantation was regarded as expensive and results were questioned in 1984 when the technique was first introduced in Sweden. Also, resistance was initially shown by organisations representing the deaf (SDR), the hard of hearing (HRF) and deaf, hearing- and speech-handicapped children (DHB). However, with the development of multichannel, multi-electrode implant systems and more advanced coding strategies, the performance results of patients improved and some of the initial hesitation faded. Now these groups are supportive of cochlear implants in postlingually deaf adults. A critical attitude, however, persists against implanting children, especially those with congenital deafness, although a recent development from the Swedish Association for the Hard of Hearing (HRF) is encouraging. At the HRF Congress in May 1995, they expressed their attitude in an official statement that their association does not want to interfere in the decision that parents might take regarding implantation for their children. There remain two problems: the cost of the implant and the development of a suitable training methodology. This is especially true in the current atmosphere of a shrinking economy in relation to the medical care system.

Since 1984, our clinic has performed more than 100 operations (nearly 70% of the total number in the country). The majority of the patients have been adults, where the overall proportion of adults to children in Sweden is 5:1 and 6:1 in our clinic. This is changing. Presently at the Söder Hospital nearly 20 operations are done per year of which about 50% are on children.

The pre-implant phase: adults

Training with hearing aids always precedes candidacy for cochlear implantation whether it be for an adult or child.

Rehabilitation with Hearing Aids

The programme begins with the diagnosis and initiation of rehabilitation with amplification. An important part of the pre-implant rehabilitation is the contact with the specialist teacher who analyses the situation of the patient and teaches the handling of the hearing aid along with various listening strategies. The rehabilitation is provided at different levels of difficulty and in different stages depending on the severity of the hearing loss. The first step, in all cases, is to assure that the patient has well-fitting hearing aids. We also provide assistive devices such as amplifiers for TV, magnetic loop systems, optic signals for the door and telephone, and so forth.

When the hearing loss cannot be easily remediated with the application of hearing aids, contact is made with the social worker for analysis of the social and working situation. A three-week intensive rehabilitation course may be given at the Department of Audiology. If the hearing loss is more severe and is a hindrance in work or education, a more extensive rehabilitation programme may be undertaken and provided through a state rehabilitation center (AMI) with special occupational courses for hearing-handicapped individuals.

The patients are thoroughly informed about their hearing loss from medical, psychological and social viewpoints. Together with other patients who have similar impairment, they have the possibility to discuss their situation and share experiences. A psychologist also takes part in these discussions. In addition, different types of communication training – speech, voice and relaxation therapy, as well as telephone training – are made available to the patients.

These steps have served a very important role in terms of helping the patients to better accept their hearing loss. It follows that the hearing aid rehabilitation works to enhance a person's self-confidence and coping skills. The more pronounced the hearing loss, the more intense is the contribution of rehabilitation.

Preoperative Assessment and Counselling

Each patient who is a candidate for cochlear implantation goes through careful assessment and testing (see Tables 19.1 and 19.2). In the preoperative investigation and preparation of the patient, a very important element is to establish appropriate expectations with the patient; in particular, they should not be too high. It is much better for the person to be pleasantly surprised than the opposite! All our potential patients meet an active cochlear implant user. We are careful not to expose the potential candidate to 'star' patients. Postoperatively, then, most implantees receive better hearing than they had expected. Still, there are a few who are disappointed. Our experience has shown us that, in these cases, it is essential to provide continuous, strong support and further rehabilitation efforts. This is especially true because we have seen long-term effects of implantation where improvement was a very slow process.

Table 19.1: Preoperative assessment

Adult patients:

- First medical appointment. Information and discussion
- Establish status of hearing
- Optimal hearing aid fitting
- Psychosocial assessment and counselling
- First CI team discussion
- Estimating degree of tinnitus
- ENG/ABR
- Promontory stimulation
- Discussion with implantee
- Auditive and audiovisual testing
- Recording of voice
- Discussion with psychologist (when needed)
- Second medical appointment
- CT/MRI
- Second CI team discussion
- A recommendation of suitability is made
- Patient makes the final decision
- Date of surgery

Table 19.2: Preoperative test programme

Adult patients:

- Audiogram
- Hearing-aid Sound-field test
- Spondee Same/Different test
- Four-choice Spondee test
- Twelve-choice Spondee test
- Three Digit test
- Spondee test (open)
- Monosyllable test (open)
- Everyday sentences
- Speech tracking

Post-implant rehabilitation: adults

Initially when working with the single-channel implants, the greatest emphasis was placed on auditory training. Today, technically advanced multichannel implants that use more effective coding strategies allow the patient to obtain good results with less training. All patients go through a similar initial fitting programme over six days (three days each week for two consecutive weeks). Relatives are encouraged to accompany the patient for support during the fitting sessions.

The initial fitting period is divided into morning and afternoon sessions. The first day consists of a medical appointment, mapping (programming) and 'switch on' (initial fitting of the speech processor). The first afternoon and the second day are scheduled for therapy sessions. Day 3 ends with a technical check-up of the device, programming of the speech processor and a therapy session. The second week proceeds with further programming checks of the speech processor and therapy sessions spread out over the next three days. If there is strong disappointment, referral is made to a counsellor or a psychologist. For most patients, further training takes place at home mainly by using the implant, and device check-ups are scheduled at the clinic after six months. The check-up is then repeated yearly. In patients showing slow progress or other complicating factors, much more intense rehabilitation training may be needed. Continuous support from a counsellor or a psychologist is also important. This may be the case in long-term deafness, in partial or total ossification or in cases where other complications may occur such as facial nerve stimulation. In the latter cases, reprogramming, lowering or removing all stimulation on certain electrodes may be necessary. At the regular yearly check-up there is a postoperative test programme for evaluating perceptual abilities while using the cochlear implant (see Table 19.3).

Table 19.3: Postoperative test programme

Adult patients:

- Consonant and Vowel Confusion test
- Twelve-choice Spondee test
- Three Digit test
- Spondee test (open)
- Monosyllable test (open)
- Everyday sentences
- Speech tracking

This test programme is first presented at the time of 'switch on', after 6 and 12 months and thereafter at yearly intervals

The pre-implant phase: children

The experience with adults has led us to develop a systematic method of cochlear implant rehabilitation. Recently, we have turned our attention to children and the challenge to develop a rehabilitation programme is great because of the educational circumstances of deaf children in Sweden. The pre-implant phase is the most developed and consists of counselling, hearing aid training and assessments.

Counselling

Rehabilitation of hearing-handicapped and deaf children is done with a holistic approach. It is not only the hearing loss of the child which receives focus but the whole situation of the child in the family and in the social environment. The entire family is influenced by the discovery that the child has a hearing loss or is deaf. The physician gives the information about the diagnosis when both parents are present. Another appointment is often necessary after one to two weeks for further discussion about diagnosis, prognosis, possibilities for treatment, surgery, cochlear implantation, use of hearing aids and so on. Ongoing counselling is necessary because relevant questions often do not arise when the difficult message is given for the first time

The hearing parents are offered consultation with a psychologist or a social worker, often with both, before the educational rehabilitation of the child begins. This gives them the opportunity to talk about worries and about the sorrow or anger over the fact that their own child has been affected. Perhaps repressed, hidden feelings that are perceived by the parents to be forbidden (i.e. such as the sorrow over the fact that their child is not the perfect child they have dreamt of) need to have a free environment for expression. The parents have to learn a new kind of communication with the child. During counselling, all these feelings are allowed to be expressed openly. The parents have the possibility to continue the contact with the psychologist or the social worker as long as this is needed.

Most parents, of course, want their child to be as 'normal' or as ordinary as possible despite the hearing loss or deafness. The hope that the child will somehow learn to talk, even though deaf, is strong in the beginning. Parents may feel that their wish to restore the lost or missing hearing can now, to some extent, be fulfilled with a cochlear implant. There is an apparent risk that parents have too high and unrealistic expectations. It is important to allow the family enough time and opportunity to handle and work through the crisis so that they can approach acceptance of the hearing loss before the important decision is made for their child to undergo the cochlear implant operation.

During the preoperative evaluation, great emphasis is placed on information. That is why it is done by audiologically trained physicians, as well as psychologists, social workers and other members of the implant team. Information from parents of operated children, as well as meetings with these families, is mandatory. Those parents who decide to have their children operated on not only have their own mind to make up but may also meet suspicion and a negative attitude from parents who do not choose to have their child operated on. The latter parents may also be subjected to doubts regarding their own choice: maybe the child could have developed better with a cochlear implant? Thoughts about how the child might later accuse them of a choice poorly made may also arise. Not to let the operation be done is as active a decision as to go ahead. The negative attitude from patient organisations is also a factor which may make the decision more difficult.

Hearing Aid Training

The most common wish of the parents is to begin a hearing aid trial to learn whether or not it will provide a useful degree of hearing. They usually seek contact with a specialist teacher as soon as possible. Often the parents feel awkward and estranged around their own child after receiving the diagnosis. They need counselling assistance in order to initiate a communication process in a new and different way. It is usually the parents who decide on the timing for hearing aid rehabilitation. They also choose among the possible actions that can be taken in favour of communication training. Without parental cooperation, it is quite meaningless to initiate measures which the rehabilitation team regards as acutely necessary. If a cochlear implant is considered, the situation is even more problematic. Perhaps unconsciously, the training in using hearing aids and/or learning sign language may not be taken seriously by the parents. Because families may believe that it is the implant that will help the child in the best way, there is a great responsibility that lies with the implant team. They must clearly, fully and in a manner which will be easily comprehended by the parents, provide information about the consequences of the choice to provide a cochlear implant.

Post-implant rehabilitation in children: parallel language learning

Because cochlear implantation in small children has been performed for only a couple of years in Sweden, we are still working to develop a complete rehabilitation programme. It is based on parallel language learning. This means that there must be bilingualism where both signed and spoken languages are respected. During cochlear implant rehabilitation, there is an understanding of the use of sign language; however, there is an emphasis on the aural/oral possibilities provided through the cochlear implant. The therapist works to associate sound and signal. It is also possible to utilise the reading mode to make associations between sound and meaning because written language is always the second language for the deaf child.

The concept of bilingualism in rehabilitation means that oral language is not neglected. Every opportunity is made to encourage natural sound perception and speech production. Detection and identification of sounds for children whose first language is signing is made easier by explaining sound sources and what the sound means through association with signed symbols. At the same time, spontaneous opportunities to introduce meaningful sound are always integrated, which means that the children need to wear a well-functioning speech processor as much as possible, and as soon as possible after the initial fitting. Children are stimulated in a positive way so that they discover the benefits of the implant little by little.

Speech production can be encouraged for signing children through the use of software programs such as the computerised Speech Viewer (French IBM program adapted to Swedish). It can help stimulate the child to use voice, making sounds together with the teacher or the speech therapist, sometimes also together with another child. Depending on the child's ability to make speech-like utterances, it is also a useful tool to work on specific speech sounds. But, in a group of children where signing is the main language, even when the current (or active) language is speech, someone must always be prepared to take advantage of the possibilities offered through auditory stimulation.

In groups of two or three children, it may be possible to perform short language lessons using signing which is then interpreted into speech. It is important to awaken the child's curiosity, and to instill an interest in trying to understand and pronounce words. Many specialist teachers in Sweden are convinced that it is easier for a signing child to be interested in learning speech when it is interpreted and explained in sign language.

The challenge of developing a rehabilitation programme for signing children is for it to be compatible with the orientation of bilingualism. Indeed, cochlear implants have their limitations, but different situations demand different communication modes. The child with a cochlear implant needs to be offered the opportunity to take advantage of communication in both languages. One does not necessarily restrict the other. This is why we consider the development of parallel language learning to be a critical element in the care of deaf children who use their cochlear implant in settings with restricted, or limited, auditory input.

Educational circumstances for deaf children

The Specialist Teacher at Home and in Nursery School

Swedish specialist teachers working with hearing-impaired and deaf preschool children are trained as nursery school teachers with further training focusing on the consequences of hearing impairment and deafness. In the compulsory school for the deaf and for hearing-handicapped children, the teachers have a similar training.

Usually, a specialist teacher has already begun laying the foundations for rehabilitation before the child receives its implant. Information has been given to the parents about the role of the specialist teacher and about the need to reinforce all communication attempts made by the child regardless of whether they are in the form of speech or gesture. The most important aspect is to establish contact and initiate some kind of mutual communication between the parent and the child. The teacher and the parents plan a preliminary rehabilitation programme. Before and after the operation, the staff at the nursery school are also provided with clear goals for their work.

Swedish mothers often work outside the home. This means that most young children, including hearing-impaired and deaf children, stay in some kind of childcare centre during the day. It may be either an ordinary nursery school or a special nursery school, depending on the degree of hearing loss of the child and/or the community in which the family resides. The regular nursery school is either run privately or by the community. Children attending an ordinary nursery school receive a visit from the itinerant specialist teacher who instructs the parents. The staff of the nursery school is also instructed in ways to give the child the best possible support in its development even in an ordinary nursery school.

Interactive play between the teacher and the child is adjusted to the developmental level of the child. Together they choose the toys, pictures and books which will fit the current training. An excellent aid is the video camera which is very useful in recording the interactive communication in detail. The tape is replayed to the parents or the staff and the teacher can demonstrate the often indistinct responses of the child's communication attempts. Children are also encouraged to watch the videos and, of course, they always take great delight in seeing themselves on TV. Sounds, speech production, body language, gestures and signs are all recorded. This type of information is very useful for future training and gives feedback also to the cochlear implant team.

The Special Nursery School

The alternative to an ordinary nursery school is the special nursery school where the community council is responsible for the child's care and the county council for the rehabilitation. The specialist teacher is responsible for the special needs of the child. Between them, they assure that the child's needs are met each day.

The mixed group, with both deaf and hearing-handicapped children, automatically makes the common language of the group sign language. This is because it is the only language that can be used for deaf children who do not benefit from hearing aids. Indeed, for deaf children who do not use any technical aids this is a very positive solution. Sign language has a very high incidence of usage in Sweden and the children's sign language develops quickly and continuously. Those children who have usable residual hearing and are in such a group, whether by use of a hearing aid or a cochlear implant will, however, receive far too little stimulation to develop sound perception and speech production.

The current attitude is a belief that hearing-impaired children who develop good sign language skills will automatically be exposed to spoken language in the society outside the nursery school. It implies that little direct training in auditory perception and speech production takes place because children with residual hearing should naturally develop their own speech production skills. Clearly, this is a misconception resulting from inadequate knowledge about the possibilities that exist for hearing-handicapped children to acquire spoken language on their own.

If a child with a cochlear implant is part of such a group it may be doubtful whether there will be enough sound and speech stimulation. When parents have made the decision to choose a cochlear implant for their child, it is the responsibility of the rehabilitation team to give advice and instructions about what and how the parents and staff who are working with the child on a daily basis can do. One of the staff at the preschool must be chosen to be the main responsible person who does the daily training with the child. This person should take advantage of all natural sounds and encourage all the child's communication efforts. According to the Swedish view of rehabilitating children, the training must be carried out in a playful way.

The Compulsory School System for Hearing-impaired and Deaf Children

Currently, children using sign language as their first language attend the state-owned special schools for the deaf where they receive their education in their own language. Unfortunately, the most recent planning does not include the decision to use speech as part of teaching in regular classes. Classes where speech is used are voluntary. Speech is not a goal for deaf children in Sweden. On the other hand, children with relatively well-developed speech attend special classes for the hearing-impaired in public schools. These children are also offered sign-language classes in order to achieve bilingualism. Many hearing-impaired pupils are mainstreamed and have little knowledge of or contact with sign language. Several of these children receive support from itinerant teachers.

Discussions continue about ways to create a suitable education for children with cochlear implants. It is hoped that in the near future we will find a solution which will fit the needs of these children in the best possible way. This is our present dilemma. Our work to find a Swedish model for educating children with cochlear implants has only just begun.

Preliminary training programme for children

It is not always possible to tell after the first months with an implant whether a child will obtain good or minimal gains from the implant. As we consider the development of our rehabilitation programme, three facts are strongly embedded in our philosophy. First, sign language, or at least signing as a support to speech, is fundamental to the child's communication ability. Second, all training must be done in a playful way because the child is first of all a child! The teacher may use all her imaginative capacity to find stimulating activities. (It is interesting to note that some Swedish associations for the deaf and hearing impaired stress the idea that auditory training 'steals away' a child's right to childhood.) Third, and finally, whatever happens in the future, it is necessary to offer a child who has a cochlear implant the opportunities to achieve bilingualism, which means spoken language as well as signing.

The future

It is apparent that the situation in Sweden is different from that in most other countries because of the strong position of sign language. Postlingual adults have been able to integrate signing for support of auditory input into their lives. Deaf children have a different situation because they generally receive early training in sign language. It is interesting that studies of such children have shown that their cognitive, social and emotional development, as well as linguistic communication, have improved to a much higher level when comparing signing school-aged children in the late 1980s with contemporaries of the 1960s who were brought up in a strong oral tradition (Heiling, 1993, 1995). A consequence of this is that it is not defensible to neglect training in sign language until the individually implanted child can demonstrate equally good communication through listening and lipreading. Consideration must be given to the findings of linguistic research that clearly indicate that simultaneous learning of several languages is not a hindrance to language skills (McLaughlin, 1984). We need to define training programmes that stimulate the development of both languages. The new paediatric training method must have communication as its foundation but integrate training in sound perception and speech and articulation development. It must be based on bilingualism. We cannot continue only to stimulate the development of sign language in children who have received a cochlear implant. The parents also need knowledge about the possibilities and the limitations related to their child being competent in two languages. With the support of both the parents and the staff at the school, the child should integrate the use of the implant into daily life as soon as possible.

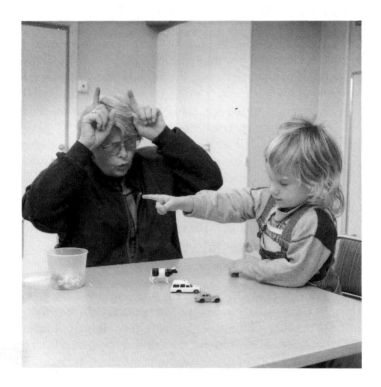

Figure 19.1: Training situation using both Swedish sign language and spoken language

A prerequisite for a good result after cochlear implant fitting is that not only the conditions of the child be evaluated but also both the parents and the team in the home community be thoroughly informed and, preferably, specially trained. Swedish rehabilitation has, by tradition, an extensive parent education programme that should be expanded to include knowledge about cochlear implants for parents of children with a prospective or recent implants. This will contribute to the defusing of the mystery about the new technique. The implant should not be allowed to become an 'escape' from the consequences that the child, in some sense, remains deaf or severely hearing impaired. In many situations it might, indeed, be necessary to rely on sign language. In the parent education, it is important to emphasise that despite the fact that the child will obtain some hearing through the use of the implant system there may still be problems in acquiring speech, and also that this process may take considerable time.

Experience with children shows that progress still continues even after three to five years of implant use; it is not necessarily immediate. Extensive further education is needed for specialist teachers, especially for those who work in nursery schools and in the lower and middle

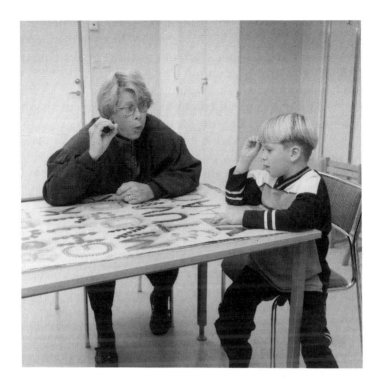

Figure 19.2: Blingualism offers the opportunity for signed and spoken language to complement each other for the rehabilitation of children with cochlear implants

grades of compulsory school. The other members of the rehabilitation team – psychologists, social workers and hearing aid assistants, speech pathologists and engineers – also need further training as a basis for their contacts with parents, children and members of the patient organisations. To achieve this, the first part-time university course began at the Stockholm Institute of Education in the spring of 1995. Participants in the course were mainly specialist teachers. An important and comprehensive part of the course is acoustics and articulation phonetics which gives a basis for the teachers to plan and perform stimulating listening, voice and articulation training. As mentioned earlier, such knowledge is no longer taught in the special training of specialist teachers. This training is not only needed for work with children using a cochlear implant but also for children with conventional hearing aids. With knowledge of phonetics, it is also possible to encourage the use of special training programs that are available via personal computers. Such programs are stimulating training tools which children enjoy.

Today's teams working with hearing-handicapped and deaf children may feel uneasiness and uncertainty about how to work with children using a cochlear implant. The Swedish model of rehabilitation is built on the concept that communication is the foundation for training. This we do not want to abandon, even though cochlear implants introduce a new dimension for providing useful sound to hearing-handicapped and deaf children who cannot benefit from well-fitting hearing aids. It is inconceivable to change to a method which is built exclusively on articulation and listening because functioning speech communication cannot be guaranteed for each individual child. In children with acquired deafness, however, we have already seen that many are regaining their spoken language skills within one or two years after implant surgery and device fitting. In congenitally deaf children using newer coding strategies some remarkable results are being reported (Archbold, Meyer et al, 1995 Lutman & Marshall, 1995; Waltzman, Cohen & Shapiro, 1995) although the full extent of the results is not yet known.

Conclusion

The use of cochlear implants in Sweden has brought up many issues. The goal of rehabilitation is to guide and support the development of communication skills and if there is access to meaningful auditory information such as that obtained through modern cochlear implant systems, the emphasis is on communication that utilises spoken language. We are on the threshold of developing such a functioning method for communication training irrespective of whether the primary language is signing or spoken language. This method will fit within the Swedish model used for treatment and care of hearing-handicapped adults and children.

References

Archbold S, Lutman ME, Marshall, DH (1995) Categories of auditory perception: a scale for documenting progress in young cochlear implant users. Annals of Otology, Rhinology and Laryngology 104 (9, Part 2, Suppl. 166): 312–14.

Heiling K (1993) Döva barns utveckling i ett tidsperspektiv. Kunskapsnivå och sociala processer (a thesis). Studia Psychologica et Paedagogica Series 153: 1–253.

Heiling K (1995) The Development of Deaf Children: Academic Achievement Levels and Social Processes. International studies on sign language and communication of the deaf. Stockholm: Hamling Signum Press.

McLaughlin B (1984) Second Language Acquisition in Childhood. New Jersey: Erlbaum.

Meyer V, Bertram B, Lenarz T (1995) Performance comparisons in congenitally deaf children with different ages of implantation. In Uziel AS, Mondain M (Eds) Cochlear implants in children. Advances in Otorhinolaryngology 50: 129–33.

Waltzman S, Cohen N, Shapiro W (1995) Effects of cochlear implantation on the young deaf child. In Uziel AS, Mondain M (Eds) Cochlear implants in children. Advances in Otorhinolaryngology 50: 125–28.

Chapter 20
Differences in Postoperative Management for Postlingual and Prelingual Adults and Children using Cochlear Implants

CLAUDE FUGAIN, MICHEL OUAYOUN, LUCILE MONNERON, CLAUDE-HENRI CHOUARD

Introduction

We have been providing cochlear implants with the aim of rehabilitating profound deafness since 1976 (Chouard & McLeod, 1973, 1976). Our rehabilitation programme has necessarily changed during these last 20 years in parallel with the devices used. Early experiences led us to adopt a very conservative attitude concerning expected results; however, present day cochlear implants offer broader applications. On one hand, we have changed our evaluation methods (Pialoux, Chouard & McLeod, 1976; Chouard et al., 1983) and counselling during the preoperative phase. On the other hand, postoperatively we have adopted more demanding, although shorter, management for most of our patients. The presurgical phase should serve not only as a selection process but also as the foundation upon which postoperative management is based. Pre- and postoperative management are interrelated for all patients. From the first encounters, we sensitise patients to the process involved in receiving a cochlear implant and, at the same time, we assess their current auditory capabilities and inform them about postoperative rehabilitation.

Our extensive experience, both in the number of years and the number of patients (more than 260), enables us to provide a well-informed description of the various devices we use, the expected performance gained through each, and their potentials and limitations. We

297

also are able to advise about realistic expectations for patients once implanted, especially in light of comparisons with careful audiological, electrophysiological, radiological, intellectual and psychosocial preoperative assessment.

The two major categories of patients seen in our department are those with postlingual deafness (adults, teenagers and children) and children suffering from prelingual deafness, whether congenital or neonatal. We also see those with perilingual deafness who we include in the second group. We have two different types of management for these two major types of patients.

Management of patients suffering from postlingual deafness

The first step for this group is to provide information. This occurs throughout the selection process and offers information about the various types of devices available in our clinic, their use and the reasons for choosing a particular device. The surgical procedure is explained along with the methods involved in postoperative management. Prior to surgery, all candidates for implantation meet one or several already-implanted patients who answer questions and provide reassurance regarding the capacity to understand speech and the opportunity to participate in the situations of daily living when using a cochlear implant. These presurgical encounters are essential because they render cochlear implants slightly commonplace for the future patient and demystify the device while providing reassurance. The strong solidarity between implanted patients facilitates these encounters which most often spontaneously continue during the postoperative management. Our impression is that it is as though the already-implanted patient feels responsible for the newer one.

Postoperative management is provided by the rehabilitation team which is already familiar with the patient before the operation. Therefore, first fitting and successive adjustments, as well as training, are carried out by the same therapist.

First Setting and Adjustments

The patient will have been counselled, and accepted, that '[s]he will hear everything but will understand nothing'. She will have been advised that sounds through the cochlear implant are different from those previously heard. Further, the patient will be able to understand the auditory information transmitted through the cochlear implant only after having worn the device regularly and having attended training. In spite of this, and although patients are cautioned that in no case will the auditory sensations sound normal, some of them are disappointed during the first setting.

Our team carries out the first fitting of the cochlear implant on the tenth day following surgery: a quick procedure to check the amplitude of current necessary for obtaining responses and to verify that all electrodes are operating. The patient feels reassured because she hears sounds, because setting thresholds for the dynamic range are non-invasive and because she feels no pain. Fitting sessions are repeated daily until we obtain the first satisfactory programme that is to be used for starting the rehabilitative training. This usually requires three or four fitting sessions.

Further adjustments take place to compensate for difficulties in perception encountered during training and to better adjust the comfort and quality of sound according to each patient's needs. Without going into details about the setting of different devices, either all electrodes are activated from the beginning of training or some basal electrodes are provisionally inactivated for the time required by patients to adapt to high-pitched frequencies.

Information and Psychological Support

Even if the patient has already seen the external device he/she will have to wear, it is necessary to explain repeatedly the mode of operation of the speech processor, the batteries and their recharging characteristics, the number of hours of recommended use (from one hour during the first few days to constant daytime use) and the various modes of use relative to the listening situations.

We explain to the patient the value of personal involvement separate from the rehabilitation and, together, we define the type of exercises to be carried out. We ask patients to show curiosity, to be on the alert for all patterns of sound information and to listen to environmental sounds, whether domestic or street noises. We ask them to watch television, not to withdraw into isolation, to talk with their family and to make note of their impressions of whatever sounds they hear in the form of a diary.

The patient is requested to wear the device as frequently and as long as possible. It is often necessary to reassure both patients and their family because, in spite of the numerous preoperative conversations and explanations, some anxiety still persists when patients are due to leave the hospital with the device. In particular, they may have a fear of not handling it properly.

Training Protocols

Patients leave hospital soon after the first setting. They return to daily training after of about two months from the day they leave hospital. The training for these patients has changed considerably in 20 years, less with regards to the various types of exercises than to the speed at which the patients progress from simple to more complex exercises. For example, we have become more demanding in terms of speech understanding without resorting to lipreading as compared with developing skills for environmental sounds discrimination. Environmental sound rehabilitation appeared rather extraordinary to us 20 years ago but it seems to be ridiculously limited today when we are tempted to speak of failure whenever a postlingual patient is unable to hold a conversation without using lipreading or faces some difficulties in using the telephone.

Our aims have changed and our requirements greatly increased with the technical progress in cochlear implants. The first phase of the current postoperative training lasts from 2 weeks to 2 months, depending on the difficulties faced by the patient. Table 20.1 lists the steps involved in the training protocol which progresses from environmental noise discrimination, discrimination of male from female voices, pitch discrimination, intonation and other prosodic discriminations including musical instruments, to the understanding of speech. We also include some training for voice control. When leaving our team, a postlingually deafened patient should be able to understand sentences spoken at random without lipreading and be able to use the device throughout the day.

Training is continued at a less intensive pace, i.e. twice a week, and for as long as is required for satisfactory rehabilitation. The ongoing training is either with our team, if the patient lives in our geographic area, or with a local speech therapist. We maintain close relations with the local speech therapist who takes over the treatment. Together, we define the type of training, the type of exercises to be carried out and the time sequence of the rehabilitation protocol. We always see the patients at 3, 6, 9, 12, 18, 24 and 36 months after implantation.

Evaluation Protocols

Although evaluation protocols are indispensable, it would be detrimental to place patients in a permanent testing situation. We developed an evaluation for French-speaking individuals in cooperation with Professor Frachet's team at Avicenne's Hospital in Bobigny. It is called the French Cochlear Implant Assessment Procedure (Vormes et al., 1990; Monneron et al., 1995). We always test our patients under the same conditions, using different randomisations of the test materials. This makes it possible to perform periodic assessments without the possibility for the patient to become accustomed to the test items. If such evaluations take place on a regular basis, it enables the progress achieved by the patient to be closely monitored.

Table 20.1: Training protocol for postlingually deafened individuals

Skill	Tasks
Environmental sounds discrimination	The patients work alone with familiar sounds that occur in their own environment as well as with sounds recorded on tape. The patients listen to different sounds that have specific, but different characteristics, such as: long/short, repeated, dull, metallic or resonating, scrapings, clickings. Many of these sounds are recorded on tape
Discrimination of female and male voices	Personal observations. Listening to recorded voices
Pitch discrimination	This is an essential part of our training. We use tasks for differentiating low and high tones, ascending and descending scales, melodies and progressive classification of tones ranging from the lowest to the highest pitch. We use a tape recorder and a synthesiser for these exercises
Intonation and prosody discrimination	Recorded words and sentences with different stress and rhythm such as questions, exclamations or statements
Musical discriminations	Listening to recorded melodies performed with different musical instruments
Voice control	Control of their own singing voice to differentiate loud from soft voice and high- from low-pitched voices. We ask patients first to sing a single note, then to vary between two notes and then three. Finally, we introduce more complex melodies
Phonetic and speech discrimination. (These represent the most important part of our training because the results obtained clearly objectify the possibilities for speech understanding.) The training progresses hierarchically from easy to difficult. Lipreading is never used during this type of training	(1) Closed lists of heterosyllabic words, homosyllabic words, short heterosyllabic sentences, short homosyllabic sentences, keyword recognition in a sentence (word in initial, medial or final position), review of a text read aloud by the speech therapist; (2) cued open-set lists of words with theme (countries, professions, vegetables, fruits), sentences with the help of a known word or a known context, incomplete sentences, missing words in a text; (3) lists of open-set; short then long sentences; sentences spoken at slow then fast speed; open-set words in quiet and then in noise; understanding of a read text first slowly then at normal speed; (4) conversation training without lipreading; (5) telephone-use training

Our assessment method allows for a maximum score of 1000 points. The points are assigned according to results of specific tests. A 1000-point score represents the performance of a so-called star patient. Results are calculated on a semi-logarithmic scale, graduated from 0 for communication limited to lipreading to 1000 for normal, interactive communication. The scores on the tests are accumulated to derive a single score. Because scores are cumulative, results are given as a 1 to 3 digit number. Table 20.2 shows the scoring system.

Table 20.2: Scoring criteria used with the evaluation protocol for postlingual adults

Skill	Point	Total
The unit (single digits) 0–10		
Alarm function: 5 unknown noises identified during a conversation must be noticed by the patient	1	
Discrimination of voices from noises: 10 voices and noises with identical rhythms	1	
Male/female voice discrimination	1	
Familiar noises: 10 noises from current life	2	
Voice improvement	2	
Lipreading skills	2	
Hours of use per day	1	10
The tens (double digits): 0–90		
Pitch discrimination: 10 questions/statements	10	
Closed-set words: 10 words in a closed set without lipreading	10	
Consonant/vowel discrimination: 20 word pairs differing only in either a vowel or a consonant (without lipreading)	20	
Cued open set (with a theme): 10 words with topic known by the patient (without lipreading)	20	
Open-set list of sentences: 10 sentences without lipreading	30	90
The hundreds (three digits): 0–900		
Open-set words: 10	100	
Open-set sentences: 10	100	
Open-set words from JC Lafon Test (Lafon, 1958)	200	
Telephone use with context	100	
Telephone use: free, interactive use	400	900
Grand total		1000

We have observed that the cumulative score, achieved by tested patients according to this method, always corresponds to the subjective impression made by the rehabilitation team concerning the patient's communication potential. For adults, this number is not meant to quantify either the patient's level of satisfaction or the psychological implications of implantation. The patient's satisfaction and the psychological repercussions are often greater than could be expected from the score obtained. The cumulative score is derived from objective performance measures.

This protocol is carried out at 3 and 6 months, and then at six-month intervals until the two-year interval and finally, at year three.

Management of children suffering from prelingual deafness

The protocol for this group applies to children between $2\frac{1}{2}$ and 12 years of age. Postoperative management is developed during the presurgical consultations. It is made possible in most cases through preoperative cooperation with deaf children's institutions.

The presurgical evaluation protocol helps us to decide on the value of using a cochlear implant for a particular patient. It also serves as a reference to calculate the results obtained after placing a cochlear implant and it guides us in selecting postoperative management options.

The interviews during the evaluation periods help us to estimate the quality of the family environment; and particularly the behaviour of parents, their availability for rehabilitation and their motivation for wanting their child to receive a cochlear implant. Further, interviews and presurgical evaluations help to establish an understanding of the true level of the child's perception, comprehension, expression capabilities and behavioural characteristics. Each child is subjected to a series of examinations before the decision to implant in order to assess the potential for postoperative clinical results.

In practice, we use one evaluation procedure for parents to assess clearly the familial environment, the sociocultural level and the parents' motivation, and another procedure for children to estimate their performance levels, particularly in relation to speech production and spoken language. We are also concerned with the type of communication used and the child's interest in communicating.

Prior to surgery, it is essential to specify the guidelines for postoperative management, the time sequence of the various steps in the adjustment of the device and the practical application of the long-term training. When full cooperation with the teaching team of the institution responsible for the child exists, this time sequence is defined jointly. At the end of the preoperative counselling, we must be certain that parents have realistic expectations relative to the cochlear implant and that they are aware of both its potential and limitations. Postoperative management differs according to the child's maturational age and language level. In practice, two groups are defined: children aged $2\frac{1}{2}$ to 5 years and children between 6 and 12 years of age.

First Fitting and Adjustments

The first fitting takes place at a later stage than for adults, e.g. about 3 weeks after surgery. The child requires a different team for rehabilitation than the one that performed the surgery in order to reduce her fears and worries.

The first fitting is always carried out in the presence of the parents and with extreme care to avoid any attitudes leading to the rejection of the speech processor. The child handles the device, becomes accustomed to it and to the antenna-microphone before any setting takes place. The first fitting, as well as the subsequent adjustments, are always performed by the child's rehabilitationists. This is a person, or persons, that the child met prior to surgery. The familiarity creates a climate of confidence that is very important, particularly when adjustments are based solely on the child's responses. In our team, thresholds are set according to the child's response. This accounts for the importance we place on creating an excellent climate of confidence between the child, the parents and ourselves.

In all cases, we check the functioning of the electrodes after about 3 weeks, keeping the fitting process short and using low intensities for the first stimulation. The fitting process is carried out during short sessions, several times a day, if necessary. Adjustment sessions are far more frequent for children than for adults and totally integrated into the rehabilitation programme during the 2–3 months after surgery.

Speech processor adjustments and postoperative training are always interdependent. In order for successive adjustments to be relevant for improving the child's successful use of the device, it is necessary to be familiar with both the progress and the difficulties the child faces during the rehabilitation sessions. This close cooperation is essential to achieve effective adjustments that are adapted to the real capabilities of the child and of the cochlear implant.

Parental Guidance

Parents receive precise answers to the many questions they ask about cochlear implants before the operation. They are fully informed about appropriate expectations, and particularly about language acquisition. Even with such counselling, their enthusiasm often must be tempered. We ask them to help their child discover its sound environment through games. This should be done without the tasks becoming work or exercises. We ask the parents to develop the child's curiosity as regards environmental sounds, even the most unusual ones. We ask them to be even more attentive to their child, to speak to her as often as possible, using a lively and attractive voice, varying the melody of the voice, exaggerating intonations. They are also asked not to put the child in a permanent test situation. We insist on the importance of the child feeling that the parents are available for her, on the need to provide the child with numerous explanations and to answer any questions without expecting the child to return systematic responses too quickly.

Parents must help the child to handle the external device, teach her to modify the volume according to listening situations and the sound environment, and to quickly gain greater autonomy. The child does not always accept the constraint of wearing a traditional hearing aid and may also have the same attitude towards the cochlear implant which is only a 'rather special' hearing aid. We insist, therefore, that the child use it incrementally, first at times which are comfortable, then during periods when enjoyable listening is also the focus. There should be a differentiation between these periods and the training work so that hearing becomes a pleasant experience throughout the day. Parents are encouraged to help their child discover the world of sound, and they must also participate in the rehabilitaion to facilitate the hearing education of their child. They will always have to temper their impatience and must avoid placing their child in a situation of constant failure.

Relationships with Educational Institutions

In the interests of these children, it is desirable that relationships between centres for the education of deaf children, families and the hospital unit that placed the cochlear implant be in close communication. They should also share a sense of confidence in each other. At present, these relationships serve functions as minimal as simply providing information about the cochlear implant to the ideal circumstance of making joint decisions regarding the type and extent of training needed for each child.

Good relations are essential because they allow the child to benefit from the best training conditions. They provide the therapist in charge of adjusting the cochlear implant with as much information as possible relative to real and potential difficulties met during rehabilitation. They also reassure families and create psychological conditions that are very favourable for the child.

Training Protocols

The training begins about 3 or 4 weeks after the operation. A child undergoes an intensive rehabilitation programme every day for 2 months in our department. This is followed by stays of one week every 3 months during the first postoperative year and then one week every 6 months during the following years. In the meantime, the child continues his/her rehabilitation with a speech therapist close to home or in the educational facility. The younger the child, the greater is the similarity to rehabilitation practices for prelingual, non-implanted children wearing traditional hearing aids. Younger children require several months before they take responsibility for not losing their external equipment. The oldest children become totally self-sufficient in maintaining the external parts of the implant system soon after being fitted.

Preoperative counselling provides the foundations for postoperative training. In cooperation with the families, decisions are already made about the timing of training periods. Parents are advised about when and where the child should use the device and about how long the child should be exposed to auditory stimulation. The training is always different according to the age and the language level of the child but the same areas for training are included. These areas are: auditory training, prosodic imitation and identification, speech perception training, and speech and language development.

Auditory training

Auditory training uses tape-recorded materials, live-voice training and a synthesiser. Work begins on developing an alerting function by assisting the child in distinguishing between widely differing signals such as noise and silence, voiced and unvoiced sounds; by encouraging spontaneous reactions to environmental sounds and drawing attention to the location and origin of sounds. Other activities include responding to familiar sounds (voices, doorbells and telephones ringing, dogs barking, etc.).

Prosody and pitch perception

Prosody is practised by providing the child with opportunities to reproduce simple and complex rhythms and to distinguish between fast and slow rhythms. The perception of simple intensity differences is practised with widely differing loud and soft sounds and changes from ascending to descending intensities. Pitch perception exercises help to teach differences between low- and high-pitched signals.

Speech perception

Speech perception training uses closed-set lists supported by pictures, first with the help of lipreading and progressively without it, depending on the results obtained. The most basic skill is to expand the prosody training to include voice affectation associated with exclamations/ commands, anger, sadness, singing and other distinctions. Word identification progresses from common words in closed sets, to cued open-set words with a theme and, finally, open-set words. Sentence identification begins with simple sentences containing a subject and a verb in a closed-set, cued open-set and open-set format. More complex sentences are formed with a subject, verb and one or more complements. A final set of exercises is centred around identifying simple commands.

Speech and language

Spoken and receptive language acquisition exercises start with training in voice control focusing on intensity and pitch control. This may be augmented with visual support provided by an IBM computer: the so-called Speechviewer II – version 1.01 – from IBM. Children are asked to imitate prosodic changes that occur in simple stories and then to reproduce words and sentences spoken by the therapist. Further exercises use counting and learning nursery rhymes and poems. At the same time, vocabulary acquisition, syntax understanding, articulation and lipreading are taught with classical techniques developed for deaf children (Aimard & Morgon, 1983).

Assessment Protocols

Evaluation protocols are essential for the device adjustments and to adapt the training from the observed results. They are also valuable in providing information about the effectiveness of the rehabilitation by comparing postoperative findings with preoperative data. We summarise the results through the use of two test protocols. In these assessment procedures, four fields of interest are included: comprehension, auditory perception, expressive abilities and behaviour. One protocol assesses children under the age of 5 years old who either lack or have poor linguistic skills and another protocol is for children between 6 and 12 years of age.

Evaluation protocol for children under 6 years

This assessment allows us to compare scores obtained at the preoperative level with subsequent training results and, more importantly, with scores obtained by normal-hearing children of the same age (Lenenberg, 1967; Busquet & Mottier, 1978). Several different measures are obtained for comprehension, general auditory perception, expressive abilities and behaviour.

Comprehension is evaluated with the help of lipreading and includes the following tests: knowledge of body parts (hair, hands, feet, mouth, etc.), colour recognition, space notion (where?), quantity notion (how much?), property notion (whom?), tactile notion (soft, rough), word identification using objects and pictures, recognition of simple commands (from pictures), simple sentence identification (from pictures) and complex sentence recognition (using pictures as clues) (Borel-Maisonny, 1967; Lege & Dague, 1978).

Auditory perception is evaluated without the help of lipreading. The test materials are different from those used during rehabilitation training. The tests include alerting function, i.e. reaction to sound, localisation, noise/no noise, voice/no voice and familiar sounds (rings, voice, engine, etc.); intensity differentiation (tape-recorded familiar sounds and synthesiser-produced sounds); prosodic identification (live voice and synthesiser produced); pitch reproduction (live-voice); intonation differentiation (live-voice and tape-recorded materials); and phonetic differentiation using simple and complex sentences, vowels and consonants.

Expressive abilities are estimated by comparing the cochlear implant child with similar-aged children with normal hearing. The score ranges from early linguistic abilities between the ages of 1 and 5 months to complete language usage by age 4 years (Chouard & McLeod, 1973; Lafon, 1985).

Behaviour and interpersonal relationships are considered important in the overall rehabilitation of children because they show the quality of the cochlear implant efficiency. They are evaluated by questionnaire, interview or subjective impressions provided by the rehabilitation team at the hospital, parents and teachers. Characteristics considered are: communication attitude (pleasure or disinterest in communication), type of communication (oral, sign, mixed) and parent–child interaction. The quality of the communication is also considered during the training and the evaluation protocol period.

Evaluation protocol for children from 6 to 12 years old

For these children, we summarise progess using the assessment procedures contained in an adapted version of the so-called French Cochlear Implant Protocol. The procedure is similar to that used for adults. The scoring criteria are found in Table 20.3. For some teenagers who have an adequate language level, understanding of speech and some auditory abilities, we use the French evaluation procedure designed for adults with postlingual deafness.

Conclusion

The postlingually deaf patient rehabilitation is usually short, a few weeks to some months post-device fitting. This is particularly true if deafness was of short duration, if the patient had a high sociocultural level and if good preoperative motivation was present. The results for these subjects can be obtained quite rapidly and are easy to compare with preoperative data.

The prelingually deaf children require a longer training period. It is slightly similar to the training for a child wearing a traditional hearing aid but with a very important emphasis on auditory training for high frequencies. It is necessary to have a thorough knowledge of deaf children and to master a deep understanding of the device that was chosen for implantation to obtain the best results with a cochlear implant.

Further, it is necessary to maintain close follow-up contact in order to monitor the patients' reactions and evaluate their performance at regular intervals.

Table 20.3: Scoring criteria used in the evaluation protocol for children between 6 and 12 years of age

Skill	Point	Total
The unit (single digits): 0–10		
Initial reaction	1	
Alarm function: 5 unexpected, unknown sounds identified during a rehabilitation session must be noticed by the child	1	
Rhythm discrimination: simple/complex: long/short	1	
Rhythm identification: rhythm in a word	1	
Intensity discrimination: loud/soft	2	
Pitch discrimination: different frequencies (male/female)	1	
Intonation discrimination	1	
Familiar sounds: environmental sounds of current life spontaneously recognised	1	
Familiar sounds: closed-set list of 10 sounds	1	10
The tens (double digits): 0–90		
Vowel discrimination	5	
• two vowels (phoneme only)	5	
• vowels opposed by pairs	5	
Consonant discrimination		
• voiced/unvoiced	7.5	
• plosive/sibilant	7.5	
Word identification: closed set of 10 words or pictured words (without lipreading)	15	
Sentence identification: closed set of 10 familiar sentences (without lipreading)	15	
Cued open-set list of words with context (known theme) – with and without lipreading	15 + 15	90
The hundreds (three digits): 0–900		
Number of use hours per day	150	
Lipreading improvement	100	
Voice control	100	
Spontaneous speech capability	150	
Language improvement ability	150	
Behavioural improvement	150	
Family appreciation	100	900
Grand total		1000

If we can say that adults require re-education, then children require basic education. Our rehabilitation programme is designed to reduce the required time for language acquisition in children. A cochlear implant provides the basis for children to learn language through audition and to reach near-normal conditions for language learning.

The management of postlingually deaf adults and prelingually deaf children is obviously different because of the history of deafness (onset, duration) and the progress of the training (duration, timing). However, it is similar in its aim: to provide speech communication that is as close as possible to the communication of normal-hearing individuals.

References

Aimard P, Morgon A (1983) Approche méthodologique des troubles du langage chez l'enfant. Paris: Masson.

Borel-Maisonny S (1967) Langage oral et écrit. Tests de langage, Vol. 2. Neuchatel: Delachaux et Niestlé.

Busquet D, Mottier C (1978) L'enfant sourd. Développement psychologique et rééducation. Paris: Baillère.

Chouard CH, McLeod P (1973) La réhabilitation des surdités totales: essai de l'implantation cochleaire d'électrodes multiples. Presse Médicine 49: 12–58.

Chouard CH, McLeod P (1976) Implantation of multiple intra-cochlear electrodes for rehabilitation of total deafness. Laryngoscope 86: 1143-48.

Chouard CH, Fugain C, Meyer B, Lacombe H (1983) Long term results of the multichannel cochlear implant. Annals of the New York Academy of Sciences 405: 387–411.

Lafon JC (1958) Test phonétique. Paris: Compagnie Française d'Audiophonologie.

Lafon JC (1985) Les enfants déficients auditifs. Paris: SIMEP.

Lege Y, Dague P (1978) Test de vocabulaire en images. Paris: Centre de psychologie appliquée.

Lenenberg EH (1967) Biological Foundations of Language. New York: Wiley.

Monneron L, Toffin C, Guegan F, Fugain C, Meyer B, Chouard Cl-H (1995) Protocole d'évaluation de l'implant cochléaire chez l'enfant de moins de 5 ans. Ann Otolaryngol. Chirurgie Cervicofacial 112: 28–35.

Pialoux P, Chouard CH, McLeod P (1976) Physiological and clinical aspects of the rehabilitation of the total deafness by implantation of multiple intra cochlear electrodes. Acta Otolaryngologica 81: 236–47.

Vormes A, Fugain C, Frachet B, et al. (1990) Présentation d'un protocole francophone d'évaluation de l'amélioration de la communication chez les sourds implantés. Annals of Otolaryngology 107: 466–68.

Index